SEXUALITY,
SOCIAL EXCLUSION
& HUMAN RIGHTS

Sexuality, Social Exclusion & Human Rights

Vulnerability in the Caribbean Context of HIV

EDITED BY

CHRISTINE BARROW, MARJAN DE BRUIN, ROBERT CARR

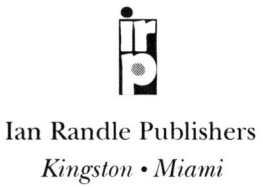

Ian Randle Publishers

Kingston • Miami

First published in Jamaica, 2009 by
Ian Randle Publishers
11 Cunningham Avenue
Box 686
Kingston 6
www.ianrandlepublishers.com

ISBN 978-976-637-395-5 (pbk)

National Library of Jamaica Cataloguing-in-Publication Data

Sexuality, social exclusion & human rights: vulnerability in the Caribbean
        context of HIV / edited by Christine Barrow, Marjan de Bruin, Robert Carr

        p. ; cm.

        ISBN 978-976-637-395-5 (pbk)

1. HIV infections – Caribbean Area – Prevention 2. Human rights – Caribbean Area 3. Gender identity – Social aspects – Caribbean aspects 4. Sex role – Caribbean Area 5. Youth – Sexual behaviour – Caribbean Area
I.. Barrow, Christine II. De Bruin, Marjan III. Carr, Robert

362.196972 dc 22

Cover and Book Design by Ian Randle Publishers
Printed and Bound in the United States of America

TABLE OF CONTENTS

LIST OF TABLES... viii

LIST OF FIGURES... ix

FOREWORD xi
Brendan Bain

PREFACE xiii
Sir George Alleyne

INTRODUCTION xvii
Christine Barrow, Marjan de Bruin, Robert Carr

ACRONYMS... xxxiii

HUMAN RIGHTS, CITIZENSHIP AND SOCIAL EXCLUSION

Chapter 1   Authorized Sex: Same-Sex Sexuality and Law
in the Caribbean 3
Tracy Robinson

Chapter 2   Drugs Obscure the Human Rights Issues for Drug Users:
Are Demons and Jumbies Rights Holders? 23
Marcus Day

Chapter 3   Charting a Legal Response to HIV and AIDS and Work
from the Perspective of Vulnerability 38
Rose-Marie Antoine

Chapter 4   Social Exclusion, Citizenship and Rights:
Grappling with Vulnerability in the
Epidemic of HIV 71
Robert Carr

Rethinking Communication

Chapter 5   Speaking Sexuality:
The Heteronationalism of MSM **95**
Andil Gosine

Chapter 6   Positively Limited:
Gender, Sexuality and HIV and AIDS Discourses in
Barbados **116**
David Murray

Chapter 7   Communication and HIV:
Multi-Dimensional Frustration **130**
Marjan de Bruin

Chapter 8   Tackling the Social Complexities of HIV and AIDS:
Understanding the Social Roots of the Epidemic and
Learning from Developments in HIV Communication.. **153**
Robin Vincent

Reconceptualizing Sex

Chapter 9   Centering Praxis in Policies and Studies of Caribbean
Sexuality **179**
Kamala Kempadoo

Chapter 10   Afro-Surinamese Women's Sexual Culture and the
Long Shadows of the Past **192**
Gloria Wekker

Chapter 11   Contradictory Sexualities: From Vulnerability to
Empowerment for Adolescent Girls in Barbados **215**
Christine Barrow

Chapter 12   How Risk and Vulnerability Become 'socially
embedded': Insights into the Resilient Gap between
Awareness and Safety in HIV **239**
David Plummer

POLICY AND MACRO-PERSPECTIVES

Chapter 13 Risking Education:
           Placing Young MSM in the HIV Prevention Equation.. **259**
           R. Anthony Lewis

Chapter 14 HIV and AIDS, Vulnerability and the Governance
           Agenda: A Critical Perspective on Barbados **277**
           Philip Nanton

Chapter 15 HIV and AIDS in the Caribbean:
           An Assessment of the Risk Environment **295**
           Roger McLean, Karl Theodore,
           Caroline Allen, Martin Franklin and Christine Laptiste

CONTRIBUTORS.. **314**

INDEX.. **318**

LIST OF TABLES

Table 12.1
Key indicators for HIV-related awareness, knowledge and practice
among 15-24 years olds in 6 eastern Caribbean countries............... 241

Table 14.1
Population by Religion: 1960, 1970, 1980, 1990
and 2000 Censuses: Barbados 286

Table 15.1
Employment status by sex of respondent.. 302

Table 15.2
Income level of family by sex of respondent................................... 303

Table 15.3
Quality of life by sex of respondent... 304

Table 15.4
Satisfied with health by sex of respondent..................................... 305

Table 15.5
Feelings about living with HIV disease... 306

Table 15.6
Used condom at last sex by sex of respondent................................ 307

Table 15.7
Used condom at last sex by highest level of education..................... 308

Table 15.8
Use of condom at last sex by income level of family........................ 309

Table 15.9
Used condom at last sex by knowledge of
current partner's HIV status.. 310

LIST OF FIGURES

Figure 12.1
The gap between HIV-related awareness and practice
among 15-24 years olds in 6 eastern Caribbean countries.............. 242

Foreword

Brendan Bain
Regional Coordinator, The University of the West Indies
HIV/AIDS Response Programme (UWI HARP)

This publication was made possible through the collaboration of a team from the University of the West Indies HIV/AIDS Response Programme (UWI HARP). UWI HARP was launched in 2001 based on the premise that HIV and AIDS are much more than medical problems. From its inception, campus-based teams in Barbados, Jamaica and Trinidad and Tobago framed HIV and AIDS as a multifaceted societal problem requiring a multidisciplinary response. The recent colloquium 'From Risk to Vulnerability: Power, Culture and Gender in the Spread of HIV and AIDS in the Caribbean' which took place at the Mona campus of the University of the West Indies, Kingston, Jamaica in September 2007, and this book, which is its sequel, are the result of a deliberate attempt to view the epidemic from many angles.

In addition to linking staff and students from this University around a common theme, one of the stated aims of UWI HARP is to partner with Government and non-Governmental organizations in the response to HIV. For this reason, we welcome the contributions of colleagues from other institutions and agencies to the colloquium and to the book. We are especially pleased about the input from NGO-based researchers, from persons in the multilingual and multicultural Caribbean and from writers based in North America, the UK and The Netherlands who are familiar with the Caribbean diaspora.

Recently, UWI HARP's approach has shifted from a traditional compartmentalized or segregated multidisciplinary way of working to an interdisciplinary approach in which genuine dialogue is being attempted between and among scholars belonging to a variety of disciplines. In fact, the newly revised UWI HARP mission statement commits us to 'positively impacting the health and wellness of the University population and the wider Caribbean society through interdisciplinary research, education and training; sharing information; and advocacy.' The interdisciplinary approach is evident as one reads this volume.

Exchanges of ideas across disciplines will help us to decipher and unravel the complex social and environmental context in which individuals must make choices and in which the epidemic has been unfolding. A wider array of players must also be brought into our national teams if we are to make the necessary inroads in understanding and responding to the epidemic. Greater insight gained from this interaction would then lead to a more strategic approach to tackling the several interactive causes of HIV and to addressing the ramifications of the epidemic.

From one perspective, the epidemic is about a new microbial invader surreptitiously entering the human social environment and causing disruption in the lives of individuals, sub-groups and entire communities. The challenge is both to recognize its presence and come to grips with the circumstances in which it is transmitted and to arrest its spread. There is the simultaneous responsibility to support persons and families already infected and affected by the invading agent, to respect their right to dignity and survival, and to counteract the fear and reject the stigma with which the infection has become associated. We need to understand risk and vulnerability. We must also understand how to practice compassion without self-righteousness or patronage. At the same time, we must strive to learn lessons from those who are not capitulating to the threat of HIV and to share those lessons widely.

This book offers thought-provoking contributions to the dialogue about HIV and AIDS. The writers do not hesitate to raise controversial issues that have hardly begun to be confronted in the Caribbean context. This creates a healthy opportunity for constructive debate, which may allow policy makers and community leaders to clarify their perspectives and take action based on research evidence, clearer reasoning and larger development objectives of well-functioning societies. Although it is written from a Caribbean perspective, readership should not be limited to persons from this part of the world. Many of the themes will resonate with persons from other societies and, indeed, are being debated worldwide.

JUNE 2008

Preface

Sir George Alleyne
Chancellor of the University of the West Indies (UWI),
UN Secretary-General's Special Envoy for AIDS in Latin
America and the Caribbean

It is a pleasure and a challenge to write a preface for this book. The pleasure derives from several sources. First it is gratifying to see the breadth and depth of Caribbean thinking that addresses one of the fundamental problems of our time. Second the complexity of the issue and the closeness of some of the arguments make for intellectual titillation if not stimulation. Third, I am pleased to see a serious attempt made to explore and explode issues that our societies and cultures have made sensitive although they may not be inherently so.

The challenge lies in the fact that many of the assertions confront some of my own beliefs which as a biologist I think I can justify with data. It is always a challenge for a biological scientist to enter the lists with social scientists, but I always take heart by reflecting on the quotation which I have used so often and comes from one of history's greatest social reformers — Virchow — 'Medicine is a social science. And politics is nothing but medicine on a grand scale.'

The problem appeared to be fairly straightforward to some people at the outset as there was no debate about the agent, the host or the mode of transmission, thus the approach consisted essentially of attacking the agent or interrupting the mode of transmission. Of course that approach has been shown to be extremely simplistic and this book describes in detail the vacuousness of that simplicity. It is pleasing to see acceptance of the view that it is critically important to change the enabling environment in addition to addressing the behavior of the agent or the host.

The book makes it clear that there can be no aspect of the life of a being that is not impacted upon or impacts the expression of sexuality.

The term being is used as the same assertion holds for many species besides ours. The study of human sexuality has a recent but a respected tradition, but on reading this book it becomes crystal clear why the juxtaposition of Eros and Thanatos has shaken the world.

The book touches on the most difficult social issues surrounding sexuality. One of the most dominant themes throughout the various parts of the book relates to the construct of gender and the extent to which this impacts on HIV transmission. But what is delightfully clear is that there is no universality of this construct. It was refreshing or rather depressing to read that in spite of the tomes written about it there was a paucity of evidence that there were interventions that had or had potential to change the power relationship that is at the root of the female vulnerability. Given the rate of increase of prevalence in girls, this is sad news indeed and perhaps it might have been useful to see reference to means by which women could not so much change the power relationships in society, but have power over their own selfhood and the mechanisms to ensure that they could or could not express their sexuality freely without fear of infection. I was intrigued that there was considerable attention to sexuality and less to the fact that sexuality and sex are not coterminous.

Stigma and discrimination receive considerable attention and some of the writing which advocates for social justice almost in Rawlsian terms is very moving. The fact that hierarchical division among all creatures is a universal finding makes it challenging to posit that it is the selection of the criteria by which these divisions are determined that has to be a matter of concern for all citizens who wish to live in a just society. The constant reference to the need to understand society as a complex open system was well put. If the communication strategies are to be effective, then this dimension has to be appreciated. There was considerable attention paid to the fact that provision of information was not enough. There was less attention paid to what has to be a source of concern to those who propose communication as an intervention strategy. In all human endeavor, the action that follows on internalization of information to create knowledge depends on the willingness to pay the cost of that action. It would have been good to see some debate about the cost to the individual of internalizing and acting on the information and why most of the interventions are not such as to convince the individual to pay the cost of the action that would result in what is presumed to be healthy or appropriate behaviour. The perception of society as an open system and its relevance to the problem of reducing HIV transmission is well set out in several places. I always urge that we remember that open systems are deceptive and induce us to make inputs into those places that are least likely to have an impact.

I would recommend this book highly. It is extremely well written and the several chapters very well referenced. There is logic to its sequencing and it explores the critical issues without cant and in language that is easily followed. Its full import and possible impact can not be gained through a single reading. I hope that it is widely read by persons involved in trying to confront the HIV epidemic as well as scientists interested in human behaviour with respect to one of our most basic urges. I also hope that some of its basic tenets are set out and disseminated in a form that the general public, especially school children can appreciate. This will probably cause disquiet and discomfort in some quarters, but such is the way to progress.

June 2008

Introduction

Sexualities, Social Exclusion and Human Rights: Vulnerabilities in the Caribbean Context of HIV

Christine Barrow, Marjan de Bruin and Robert Carr

This book looks at risk, sexuality, rights, power, culture and vulnerability in the context of the epidemic of HIV in the Caribbean. It examines how power, gender, sexuality and other cultural determinants promote risk taking in sexual behaviour, sustain vulnerabilities and undermine resilience in dealing with the pandemic. The discussion is also set within questions of citizenship and human rights.

As such, this volume represents an attempt at a different kind of conversation about HIV, meant to take our understanding of the epidemic substantively further. It brings together a diverse group of academics and activist scholars — lawyers, anthropologists, economists, communication specialists, frontline service providers, specialists in education — who were asked to analyse the Caribbean response to the epidemics of HIV and AIDS and to delve, from their discipline and perspective, into what 'vulnerability' means and what constructs it.

This volume explores the dynamics of marginalisation and the realities of the excluded, peeling back layers of silences to see what we might learn about how vulnerabilities are constructed. The book, thus, examines some of the most virulently outcast yet impacted groups facing infection rates several times higher than the general population around them — drug users, sex workers, gay men and other men who have sex with men — and those whose exclusion is more obscured, complex and normalised, particularly women, especially young women, and girls.

For some time, discussions of 'risk' in relation to HIV have been the frame through which responses to HIV have been developed. 'Risk' here has come to be equated with individual behavioural risks, such as inconsistent condom use or multiple partners. The physical act of unprotected sex initially became the major focus for intervention aimed at behaviour modification. HIV prevention was seen, predominantly, as a (public) health issue, focusing on an individualised view of sexuality. The assumption was that 'high-risk' sexual behaviour could be changed into safer sexual behaviour by encouraging desired behaviours through the provision of knowledge. This approach, based on the medical model with its epistemological certainties, turned to psychology for insights into effective prevention strategies and focused on individual behaviour change, understood as rational and volitional responses to risk, amenable to change through information and education. Models of programmes for prevention have been based on the assumption of a rational subject, motivated by self-protection and enjoying the freedom to choose exactly when, how and with whom to engage in sex. This often does not hold up under scrutiny however, as desire proves deeply irrational.

At the national and regional planning levels, while situational analyses have incorporated some recognition of vulnerability as a result of complex economic, social and cultural drivers of the epidemic, the national strategic plans themselves have been limited in their response by presenting a similarly narrow understanding of risk and, therefore, of risk reduction. For instance, in examining gender, while many national strategic plans state that power inequities between men and women play a substantial role in increasing women's risk, there is little or no programming designed to address this in the national response. Most focus on promoting condom use, faithfulness or partner reduction, or else abstinence. But this is exactly where the link between risk reduction and vulnerability reduction needs to be made: the imperative to consider what it actually means for women to abstain, be faithful or use a condom. None of these options takes place in a vacuum; each of them exists and is lived in specific socio-cultural, economic and political contexts which predispose, enable and/or reinforce behaviour and constrain free choice. In many instances, the open — and underground — gendered cultural norms of power and sexuality will make it difficult, or impossible, for women to act on these behavioural suggestions as viable options. In such situations, vulnerabilities and risks become complementary concepts in which individualised calls for behaviour change and the mere provision of knowledge become irrelevant. Cultural norms of power, unequal gender relations, social expectations, desire and unequal access to economic and cultural resources render knowledge alone inadequate, especially among poor women. As such, vulnerability speaks to larger scale inequities and structural determinants of choices and behaviours in which risky practices occur that, once addressed, can reduce social exclusion and risk more broadly, as well as strengthen social inclusion, for example, in health and justice systems. Those dynamics have not been recognized in the past. In the words of Paul Farmer (2001, 51): 'The means by which confluent social forces — here, gender inequality and poverty — come to be embodied as risk for infection with this emerging pathogen have been neglected in the biomedical, epidemiologic, and even social science literature on AIDS.'

A CARIBBEAN GENEALOGY OF RISK AND VULNERABILITY

Traditionally, the Caribbean responses to HIV prevention were based on studies with a heavy emphasis on quantitative approaches, large-scale surveys describing individual behaviour, especially focussing on knowledge, attitudes and practices (KAP). Often the many studies done steered clear of the structural relationships that set the context for behaviour.

In this approach certain priorities of what constituted viable knowledge — especially statistics — dominated the design and evaluation of interventions and programmes: the number of AIDS cases by gender and age; the reported modes of infection; the percentage of the public able to correctly identify modes of transmission; the percentage of the population reporting condom use at last sex; beliefs in myths, and so on. What was not recognized in these modes of mapping and interpreting HIV transmission was the complexity of sexual relationships; the fact that they are embedded in and are products of negotiated relationships to power, economic dependencies and social inequality that contextualise and influence, if not determine, sexual behaviour. Quantitative data provided an important part of the picture but, by definition, left out the underlying layer(s) of motives and drivers of behaviour. The need for a deeper understanding, as signalled during the 1990s by various authors on adolescents' sexual behaviour (Chevannes 1994, 1996; Jackson et al. 1998; Senderowitz et al.1998) eventually paved the way for more qualitative in-depth studies. These new approaches provided breakthrough insights as to the role of economics, gender inequity, peer pressure, power and other variables that compound prevention programming. Nevertheless, these insights had little or no impact on programming itself.

The primacy of positivist, quantitative biomedical research approaches in the Caribbean stemmed from health-based responses to the epidemic, seeing HIV as a sexually transmitted infection and AIDS as a medical condition requiring medical treatment. As a result, much emphasis has been placed on capacity building for the health sector, including training of doctors, nurses and other health care workers; on reducing stigma and discrimination in health care settings, as well as the greater involvement of people living with HIV, their families and communities in care and support. The focus on epidemiology reflected the belief that understanding the numbers would lead to understanding the epidemic. This was tied to a concern to identify who exactly was HIV-positive and to understand their demographics and behaviours. In Cuba, they were quarantined; in other countries, including the United States, politicians debated legislating a compulsory tattoo to mark all those known to be living with HIV, eventually settling for making it illegal for HIV-positive people to enter the United States.

As has been pointed out by many analysts of the response to HIV, the emergence of the epidemic on the global stage through the activism of professional, white, gay men in the US and Europe and the conceptual lens of the US Centre for Disease Control (CDC) fed into the idea of identifying 'high-risk' groups, such as 'men who have sex with men,' 'sex workers' and 'promiscuous young people'. It led to calls for dedicated programming aimed at what became discrete sub-populations seen through an epidemiological lens — reinforcing the misperception that only they were at risk and 'the rest of us' were largely immune once we stayed away from 'them' as 'vectors of infection'. The persistent association of HIV with socially excluded groups — men who have sex with men, sex workers, and other 'dirty people' (Carr 2002; White and Carr 2005) — also meant that many government ministries which were slated to launch programming were resistant, yielding little progress on broadening the response in most countries.

The main message, repeated around the world, was 'AIDS kills'. The reality had not yet been grasped that we are all interconnected, especially in an environment that drives risk behaviours underground. It was only under what is called the 'second generation' of communication programmes that the 'ABC' approach was introduced (Bertrand et al. 2006). With the arrival of this approach, a détente was reached where those who believed HIV was the result of immoral attitudes towards sex promoted abstinence, those who believed marriage was a panacea stressed faithfulness within marriage as the solution, and for those sexual dissidents who insisted on having sex otherwise, condoms could be an answer, under certain circumstances. The instruments for the dissemination of these options were 'IEC' campaigns, providing information, education and communication in a variety of settings: schools (HFLE), workplaces, church congregations, other agencies and through the print and electronic media as well as peer educator models.

All of these programmatic responses were based on the assumption that addressing certain key constructs that could be quantitatively operationalised as variables, such as self-efficacy, attitudes towards condom use, knowledge of transmission modes would lead to behaviour changes thus reducing risk and achieving greater compliance with the ABC approach. What remained unaddressed was how power and inequality contributed to the spread of HIV; leaving out of focus the role that gender plays in normalizing — and thus accepting — unequal power relations; ignoring the realities that undermine the ability of men and women, boys and girls, to make informed and empowered sexual and relational decisions. It forced us to think about the need for changes in perspective and framework: if sexual expressions and cultures, relationship dynamics, gender identities, inequalities, and hetero-normativity are so influential in sexual decision making, what does this mean for conceptualizing changes in sexual behaviour?

Analysing and demystifying power and gender can mean examining violence against women and youth but also against men, for example where gang violence is driven by the construction of masculinity and power in Caribbean social spaces. It can also mean examining forced sex, dominant ideologies and invested narratives of the 'normal' and 'subaltern' and expressions of masculinities and femininities, gender equity/justice, pleasure/violence in relationships, and so on.

The risk-focused strategies yielded critical successes in creating greater access to treatment; raising knowledge levels on HIV-related matters; increasing condom availability and use — up to a certain point; reaching more people who were willing to be tested for HIV. On the other hand, knowledge levels may be high but myths are hard to eradicate and knowledge does not always lead to behaviour change; condom use is not always consistent; stigma and discrimination are still reported as strong at the community level and numbers of people living with HIV are still coming for treatment only at very late stages of the disease.

The biomedical approach has turned out to be necessary but has also proven to be insufficient to adequately address the complex and layered challenges presented by the invisible spread of HIV. The number of new infections continues to rise, pointing again to the challenge of treating a medical condition — stemming AIDS — and at the same time changing the way and conditions under which people have sex — stemming HIV.

UNAIDS (2005), in its policy position paper on HIV prevention, argues, repeatedly, that effective prevention programmes must address 'deep seated causes of vulnerability.' In the global debate, there is agreement on principles: developing a broad-based, multi-method approach, including enabling environments, taking into account sociocultural contexts, emphasizing knowing your epidemic; encouraging evidenced-based programming; messaging by target groups, and integrating prevention, support and care.

The papers in this volume reflect an attempt to examine in greater depth the component of the response that has received the least concrete analysis in the Caribbean and from a Caribbean perspective: vulnerability and its reduction. Addressing and grounding the analysis of vulnerability in the Caribbean context means crossing the borders from the certainties and comfort of a rational world with rational beings on which the bio-medical and early psychological approach have been premised. It means learning from anthropologists, sociologists, social workers, feminists and gender analysts, human rights activists and lawyers, social geographers and historians. It means centering the work of communication specialists who appreciate that change communication is not a product but a community-driven process, and including a new kind of development economist as exemplified in the approaches of Amartya Sen, Stephen Leavitt and Jeffrey Sachs. This opens the door to qualitative researchers and community activists for a seat at the table and for important targetted knowledge that provides us with deeper insights into the contexts for human behaviour, including and especially human sexual behaviour to help us understand the dynamics behind — and limitations of — the emphasis on numbers.

The new contributions to understanding vulnerability and the persistence of risk behaviours made by these disciplines are at their most useful when they open up the complexities of everyday life in which the spread of HIV, like human desire, is embedded, even as the sharp boundaries between oversimplified categories of individuals by neatly constructed modes of infection break down. The lessons to be learned from the voices of those who have been silenced, marginalised and socially excluded by the discourse of 'risk groups' and 'vectors' of illness can then begin to be heard. There is now no way around the reality that sex workers have husbands and lovers, and that husbands also have intimate sexual relationships with men. With a growing appreciation of the role of gender and power, the extent to which the artifice of the 'good woman' and the 'real man' puts wives at particular risk has also become a central problematic. Similarly, the diversity and subtlety of relationships between desire, emotions, trust, lust, intimacy, erotics and fidelity in the context of economic drivers in sexual decision-making and power differentials in relationships are emerging as central to stymieing IEC messaging on 100 per cent condom use.

Increasingly, government responses and NGOs are interested in vulnerability as a model for understanding HIV and AIDS. For example, some among the leadership of people living with HIV have challenged the limitations of living testimony, pointing out that the real challenge is in policy reform, gender inequalities, and a widespread lack of political will. Among coalitions of civil society groups working with sex workers, youth and men who have sex with men there is a similar recognition that effective programming needs to address issues of entrenched social injustice and inequities, also speaking to the politics of social inclusion and exclusion embedded in institutional behaviour.

This volume provides the opportunity to bring together some of the best minds in the Caribbean and beyond to work on the issue of understanding the epidemic through that lens and from different disciplinary perspectives. It explores some of the key drivers of HIV and AIDS by examining vulnerability, power, culture and gender in the Caribbean. It means grappling with processes of social inclusion, social exclusion and building resilience, including macro-socioeconomic factors such as education and employment opportunities, governance, information/knowledge, religion/media/popular culture, mobility and migration, fear/social outcasting/discrimination, social unrest/crime/ societal violence, survival/transactional sex, poverty and other key issues.

HUMAN RIGHTS, CITIZENSHIP AND SOCIAL EXCLUSION

The first section of the book focuses on one of the most intractable challenges in national and regional programming in the Caribbean, the issues of stigma and discrimination, or, more precisely, the issues of citizenship, human rights, legislation and state-sanctioned social exclusion. While national strategic plans as well as the Regional Strategic Framework have recognised the strategic importance of addressing this issue, most countries — The Bahamas is an important exception — have made little or no progress on anti-discrimination legislation to protect the rights of the vulnerable, including people living with HIV and affected groups.

This section of the book opens with a gender and human rights analysis by Tracy Robinson, who examines the trends across the region in legislative reform purporting to address family law and violence against women that also became the means by which, in some countries, Caribbean Parliaments decided to legislate desire and used the power of the law to sharpen 'the notion of and danger of the homosexual Other'. She argues that an analysis of the wave of legislative reform of the 1980s 'demonstrate[s] how impoverished notions of gender equality have become a modern mechanism for "redrafting morality" ' (p. 5). '"New-old" laws', she argues, 'also represent contemporary ways of thinking about national progress and citizenship' where the spectres of the sex worker and the homosexual are invented in contemporary Caribbean law as antithetical to the nation (p. 5).

Marcus Day picks up on the issue of legislating humanity and humanity's outcasts in his chapter on policy and legislative approaches to people who use drugs in the region, especially homeless crack users. The adoption of US-sponsored policy frameworks on drugs in the Caribbean has led in part to the invisibility of the epidemic among crack users but also, as elsewhere, to the entrenchment of destructive policies that both stymies an effective response to HIV among crack users and makes the situation more severe for the people on the other side of those branded criminal. In this context, created by the state, he asks the pointed question of whether 'demons and jumbies' can be 'rights-holders'. Vulnerability, he argues, becomes a creation of the legislative imperative of the state.

Rose-Marie Antoine then examines in depth the issue of rights for people living with HIV, looking at how the structure of Caribbean law both hinders and facilitates meaningful legislative action on protection from discrimination. She argues strongly that the law 'cannot merely depend on a consensus in a society to shape itself…[especially] where it has to embrace normative and highly controversial ideas.' Thus the legislative solution to discrimination, she argues, must be focused on 'a legislative strategy centred on general equality concerns [that can] more effectively embrace issues of risk in relation to HIV' (p. 38).

Closing this section on challenges in rights policies and legislation, Robert Carr examines rights debates in the Caribbean context through the lens of subalternity. He introduces the reader to the perspective of fundamental principles, examining the conflict at the heart of Caribbean debates over rights legislation between Enlightenment principles that propose progress to mean tolerance, and the pressure to found legislation on fundamentalist interpretations of the Bible, and the legislation of morality. To illustrate his point he analyses a debate over licensing sex workers in two of the most respected newspapers in the region, Barbados's *Nation* and Jamaica's *Daily Gleaner*. Both cases illustrate, he argues, 'a central irony of our history…that we have adopted political structures such as parliamentary democracies, yet cling to the [colonial] history of social exclusion embedded in…our assumptions about the value of the human lives around us' (p. 88).

Rethinking communication

The second section of the book concentrates on 'Communication'. This discipline, or rather, interdisciplinary field of inquiry, in HIV discussions has for far too long been conceptualised very narrowly. Since the onset of the epidemic more than a quarter of a century ago, until even nowadays 'communication' in HIV prevention has been seen merely as the transmission of messages — as nothing more than the provision of information by senders who would target audiences using media as conduits. A more sophisticated view has developed more recently which underlines the need to differentiate audiences, to tailor messages which should be 'culturally relevant' and, if possible, to include target groups from the early stages of message design. Although this approach is more refined and closer to the complexities of reality, it still limits communication to the exchange of messages.

However, communication encompasses much more; it should be seen as a — smaller or larger — network of interactive processes in which people exchange information the meaning of which, however, will depend on how those involved frame the debate and what sense they make of it.

These processes, which form the context of our daily lives, take place at many different levels, include many different actors, use a range of modes, are interwoven with culture and influenced by many variables — gender, class, age, location, race, among others. They outline for us what we take for granted, provide for us a way of seeing, and make us familiar with norms and standards. Often this happens in such a way that it is difficult to step back and critically analyse the ways of seeing we have been taught and which have become our points of departure in understanding the world.

The four chapters in this section address different aspects of communication. The first two try to show us the many layers of what appears to be simple and straightforward communication. Andil Gosine focuses on what, at first sight, just seems to be one of these abbreviations that slipped into the contemporary discourses of the response to HIV: the epidemiological category of 'men who have sex with men' (MSM). He dissects the discourse in several Caribbean countries and contends that the figure of the MSM 'works to facilitate, rather than challenge, the heteronationalist intent of anti-sodomy laws and other measures used to strip homosexual actors of citizenship and human rights in many Anglo-Caribbean states' (p. 97). His motive for demonstrating the hidden power of language is not to denounce it or to demonstrate the 'right' language for discussing HIV and AIDS in the Caribbean. Instead, he warns how an 'unproblematic epidemiological category' may have serious implications for the rights and welfare of Caribbean people (p. 113).

David Murray's chapter explains how prevention education is used to convey 'moral agendas in which certain bodies are privileged as model citizens of the nation state while others are labelled dangerous through their association with improper gendered and sexual behaviour which renders them diseased and deadly.' (p. 141). The Government, through its statements and publications, actually produces gendered and sexual citizenship which perpetuates heteronormativity in policy and planning in the HIV arena. The dangerous implication of this is that 'same-sex sexual minorities are, for the most part, unmentioned or unmentionable, and that when they are visible their visibility tends to be only in association with HIV as 'risk' groups whose sexuality ends up being represented as a problem or threat.' Fundamental issues of justice and human rights have become framed as part and parcel of treating AIDS, thereby clouding the question or 'transparent universality as to what rights mean' (p. 149).

This section closes with two chapters in search of new conceptual frameworks and theoretical approaches. Marjan de Bruin points to some of the puzzling data in Caribbean research on sexual behaviour: especially in findings from the Knowledge, Attitude, Practice and Behaviour (KAPB) surveys which seem to demonstrate the need to revise some of the traditional concepts and assumptions in this area: individual behaviour change communication intervention are insufficient to achieve change in structural conditions. She summarizes the international debates over the last decade which focused on similar issues. De Bruin analyses a selection of national and regional policy frameworks in the Caribbean which make it clear that the role ascribed to communication is narrow and limited, not recognizing its potential for use in interventions for change at various levels.

The need to develop new approaches to address social challenges underpinning vulnerability to HIV is the main theme of Robin Vincent's closing chapter in this section. Vincent makes the case for looking 'beyond narrow, short-term interventions focused on individual behaviours, [to] understand some of the social and structural underpinnings of an effective public health response to HIV and AIDS' (p. 153). His chapter draws on developments in participatory communication for social change, the dynamics of HIV social movements, and attempts to apply the theory of complex systems to understand social change. Vincent shows the need to strengthen key social foundations, such as universal provision of basic health and education. 'Equally, political will is needed to address the inequity and poverty that drive the epidemic and to work for legal and institutional policy frameworks that will address the social and structural barriers to the response' (p. 172).

Reconceptualizing sex

The third section of the book addresses sexualities and sexual expressions. Kamala Kempadoo begins with a conceptual overview in which she agrees that gender and gender mainstreaming are critical, but argues that unless attention is turned to the overlapping though distinct terrain of sexuality, little headway will be made in stemming HIV. Examining sexuality and the relations of power and ideologies that shape it, within a framework of Caribbean sexual cultures enables a more complete understanding of sexual praxis. By opening the discourse of sex to the analysis of race, economics and transactional sex, sexual commodification and exploitation locally and globally, and sexual inequality and discrimination in law, centering sexuality could engender a reformulation of the response to HIV prevention.

Gloria Wekker's chapter draws on longitudinal, in-depth research on sexual subjectivity among African-Surinamese working-class women. Historical circumstances in Suriname, she argues, enabled women to counter the heteronormative contract, and to freely explore sex as pleasure with each other and with men. For women, *mati work* is a historically and culturally embedded source of sexual empowerment, agency and autonomy. The claim articulated in her chapter is that a more informed, socio-historical understanding of sexual configurations is necessary in order to successfully respond to HIV.

Taking the high rates of HIV infection among adolescent girls in Barbados as a starting point, Christine Barrow explores how their sexuality is configured by culture, gender and generation against the backdrop of a heteronormative femininity that values abstinence, virginity and respectability, and the counter-construct of *bashment* that promotes an early, active and assertive sexual practice. Girls' vulnerability to HIV, abuse and violence is revealed as their sexual and life choices navigate between these contradictory scripts, both of which, Barrow argues, are *unsafe* sexual identities. To be effective, HIV prevention strategies must centre issues of vulnerability and resilience within a public discourse on gender equality and the empowerment of women and girls, human rights and social justice.

In the final chapter of this section David Plummer challenges researchers to interrogate the gap between sexual awareness and safe practise in HIV — the KAP gap. Research on Caribbean masculinities reveals that despite high levels of knowledge and awareness, risk and vulnerability are entrenched in peer group pressure, gender roles, social taboos and stigma, economic factors and religion. Explanations on the *social embeddedness* of risk and vulnerability can lead to improved HIV interventions, aiming for broader social change and behavioural outcomes including 'refashioning dominant masculinities so that sexual prowess and risk taking are replaced with more positive qualities' (p. 255).

POLICY AND MACRO-PERSPECTIVES

This closing section of the book focuses on issues at policy levels. External pressures from the World Bank and other major donors for a 'multisectoral' response pushed 'expanded' national responses that attempted to include other ministries, departments and units, with the intention of integrating an understanding of HIV, in particular, as the responsibility of many different sectors in society. R. Anthony Lewis's opening chapter zooms in on the education sector. Lewis tackles the controversial intersection of Health and Family Life Education (HFLE) in a context where young gay and bisexual men are seeking information and find themselves pathologised or erased altogether by society's gatekeepers in the media and the school system. Given the epidemiological reality of concentrated epidemics — often found among MSM, including young MSM — Lewis asks us to consider the implications of the young men at the crux of debates about what it means to drive sex education underground in a context in which schools play a central role in providing young people with the information they need to manage risk. Exacerbating the vulnerability of young MSM is the heated expulsion of gay and bisexual sexuality from the body of knowledge that makes up the HFLE curriculum, even to the point of the bowdlerizing the definition of what constitutes sex itself. The effects of such policies, he argues, show up in AIDS statistics a decade later.

Approaching the response to HIV from the position of governance, Philip Nanton argues that the concept of vulnerability may serve both as 'an instrument of hegemony' and a 'trigger to resistance and resilience' (p. 277). Nanton's chapter examines how the response is negotiated in Barbados, highlighting the tension between the state's concern to regulate risky sexual practice and promote morality, and the need to encourage harm reduction by grappling with a variety of sexual expressions and desires, from conventional to transgressive, in this context of entrenched conservative attitudes towards sexuality.

The interplay between perceived vulnerability and risk behaviour, as it relates to HIV, is extremely complicated — at the analytical and theoretical level as well as at policy and intervention level. Roger McLean, Karl Theodore, Caroline Allen, Martin Franklin and Christine Laptiste search for some of the causal factors that make certain groups more vulnerable than others to HIV. Central to this discussion is the issue of the risk environment and those factors that influence this environment. They signal the fact that HIV and AIDS have spawned changes on families, communities and entire societies 'that have reconfigured long-standing social and economic structures and now threatens the very social fabric of some countries' (p. 295). Their chapter uses the results of a survey among persons living with HIV in Trinidad and Tobago, looking specifically at their risk environment in an effort to identify the factors that are key in determining the link between vulnerability and risk behaviour in this community.

Finally, the editors would like to thank all the contributors to this volume for sharing their work and tackling admittedly complex issues. We would also like to thank the Pan Caribbean Partnership Against HIV/AIDS (PANCAP) and the European Union, as well as the United Nations Educational, Cultural and Scientific Organisation (UNESCO) for their generous support in the production of this volume, and the holding of an international colloquium where the authors could share ideas and learn from each other which strengthened their contributions and the book as a whole.

REFERENCES

Bertrand, Jane, Kevin O'Reilly, Julie Denison, Rebecca Anhang and Michael Sweat. 2006. 'Systematic review of the effectiveness of mass communication programs to change HIV/AIDS-related behaviors in developing countries'. *Health Education Research, Theory and Practice* 21, no.4: 567–97.

Carr, Robert. 2002. Stigma, Coping and Gender: A Study of HIV+ Jamaicans. *Race, Gender and Class. Special Issue on The Intersection of Race, Gender & Class in Social Services and Social Welfare* 9, no. 1:122–44.

Chevannes, Barry. 1994. 'Sexual Decision-Making Among Jamaicans 1990–1994'. UCLA Report. Submitted to FHI /UCLA/ISER. Final report, Part I, II, III (unpublished manuscript).

———. 1996. *The Women's Centre Foundation of Jamaica: An Evaluation.* Commissioned by UNICER/UNFPA.

Farmer, Paul. 2001. *Infections and Inequalities – The Modern Plagues.* Berkeley, CA: University of California Press.

Jackson, Jean, Joan Leitch, Amy Lee, Elizabeth Eggleston et al. 1998. *The Jamaica Adolescent Study Final Report.* International, Research Triangle Park, NC, USA: Family Health.

Joint United Nations Programme on HIV/AIDS. 2005. *Intensifying HIV Prevention: UNAIDS Policy Position Paper.* Geneva: UNAIDS.

Senderowitz, Judith, Elsie Le Franc and James Sitrick Jr. 1998. *A Program to Address Adolescent Reproductive Health in Jamaica.* Prepared for USAID/Jamaica.

White, Ruth C. and Robert Carr. 2005. 'Homosexuality and HIV/AIDS Stigma in Jamaica'. *Culture, Health and Sexuality* 7: 347–59.

Acronyms

AAA	American Anthropological Association
BCC	Behaviour Change Communication
BMSM	Black men who have sex with men
BSS	Behavioural Surveillance Surveys
CARE	Comfort Assist Reach out Educate
CAREC	Caribbean Epidemiology Centre
CARICOM	Caribbean Community
CBOs	Community-based organizations
CCB	Child Care Board
CDC	Center for Disease Control
CFCS	Communication for Social Change
CHRC	Caribbean Health Research Council
CSWs	Commercial Sex Workers
CVC	Caribbean Vulnerable Communities Coalition
DFID	Department for International Development
EMCDDA	European Monitoring Centre for Drugs and Drug Addiction
FHI	Family Health International
FRESH	Focusing Resources on Effective School Health
GFI	Goodness-of-fit index
GRID	Gay Related Immune Deficiency
GLBT	Gay, lesbian, bisexual and transgender
HAART	Highly active antiretroviral therapy
HCV	Hepatitis
HDI	Human Development Index
HFLE	Health and Family Life Education
HPS	Health Promoting School

IAMCR	International Association of Media and Communication Researchers.
ICCPR	International Covenant on Civil and Political Rights
ICRW	International Centre for Research on Women
IDU	Injecting Drug Use
IEC	Information, Education and Communication
ILO	International Labour Organization
JASL	Jamaica AIDS Support for Life
KAPB	Knowledge, Attitude, Practice and Behaviour
MARP	Most At Risk Populations
MSM	Men who have sex with men
MSMNPA	Men who have sex with men–No Political Agenda
MTCT	Mother-to-child transmission
NACC	National AIDS Coordinating Committee
NHAC	National HIV/AIDS Commission
NSP	National Strategic Plan
OECS	Organisation of Eastern Caribbean States
PAHO	Pan American Health Organization
PANCAP	Pan-Caribbean Partnership Against HIV/AIDS
PEPFAR	President's Emergency Plan for AIDS Relief
PLWHA	People Living with HIV and AIDS
PLWHIV	People Living with HIV
RSF	Regional Strategic Framework
SASOD	Society Against Sexual Orientation Discrimination
TB	Tuberculosis
UN	United Nations
UNFPA	United Nations Population Fund
UNIFEM	United Nations Development Fund for Women
USAID	US Agency for International Development
UWIHARP	University of the West Indies HIV/AIDS Response Programme
WAND	Women and Development Unit
WCC	World Cup Cricket
WHO	World Health Organization

HUMAN RIGHTS, CITIZENSHIP AND SOCIAL EXCLUSION

Chapter 1
Authorized Sex
Same-Sex Sexuality and Law in the Caribbean

Tracy Robinson

We should be free to define our own identity and concept of life and self — including our sexuality — without the compulsion of the state.[1] When the state insists, through law or otherwise, that we must be sexed in a specific way — be it heterosexual, monogamous, nuclear family-oriented, married, or mother — it strikes at the heart of our dignity as human beings, and treats us as unworthy as persons *and* as citizens (Cornell 1995, 10). 'Erotic autonomy', as Jacqui Alexander describes it, is, therefore, a crucial benchmark of our citizenship (Alexander 1997). Autonomy here is not simply 'the right to occupy an envelope of space in which a socially detached individual can act freely from interference by the state' because, as Albie Sachs J points out, '... people live in their bodies, their communities, their cultures, their places and their times'.[2] Alexander's notion of erotic autonomy strongly suggests that individuals are entitled to choose lives of intimacy, closeness and community with others.

Alexander's (1991, 1994, 1997) seminal critiques of the Trinidad and Tobago Sexual Offences Act 1986 and The Bahamas Sexual Offences and Domestic Violence Act 1991 — prominent legislative responses to local and global violence against women campaigns — demonstrate that this state initiated woman-protection was fundamentally entangled with and compromised by the use of the state power to re-authorize heteropatriarchy, retrench sexual freedom, and outlaw sexual dissidence. Yasmin Tambiah's (2002) very fine study of the 1986 Trinidad and Tobago law reads much more closely the processes of reform that led to the 1986 Act — the progress of debates in and outside Parliament, the shades of opinion and the alterations in the draft legislation —as social discourse nuanced by place and time and hierarchies and relations of race, gender and sexuality. While Alexander's analysis underscores the force of law as overwhelming and coercive state power, Tambiah plainly shows that law is deeply embedded in, and connected to, the everyday and social processes as well. In this way law also influences and shapes sexual decision-making, expressions, cultures and identities in the Caribbean.)

Both Alexander (1991, 1994) and Tambiah (2002) reveal the instability of law and legal understandings, confirming that contemporary lawmaking in the Caribbean provides critical insights into Caribbean sexualities. Tambiah's appraisal of the making of the Trinidad and Tobago Sexual Offence Act shows how national and idiosyncratic the lawmaking process is. Notwithstanding that, some lawmaking projects in the Caribbean can be understood in regional terms as well. The Trinidad and Tobago Act was the first modern sexual offences law in the Caribbean in 1986.[3] In 1991, The Bahamas enacted new legislation and so did Barbados in 1992.[4] Antigua and Barbuda enacted new sexual offences legislation in 1995, Dominica in 1998, Belize amended the provisions of its criminal code in 1999, and Saint Lucia enacted a new criminal code in 2004.[5] Each of these statutes represents a lawmaking process that is dense and distinctive and, undeniably, offers its own story. A regional angle provides another view of the relationship between law and sexuality in the Caribbean.

This essay turns our attention to how the region-wide overhauling of laws dealing with violence against women and the family over the last 25 years revised the focus and boundaries of authorized sex and sharpened the notion and danger of the homosexual *other*. Historically, the criminal law proscribed unnatural non-procreative sexual behaviour and who was doing it and with whom was generally irrelevant. The spectre of 'the homosexual' is, legally speaking, a relatively modern one. I look not only at the modern sexual offences laws but a wave of family law reforms since 1980 that are giving growing recognition to 'common law unions' and even 'visiting relationships'. This specialized vocabulary of Caribbean conjugality, valorizing heterosexual reproductive intimacy, becomes a signifier of Caribbean authenticity. One consequence of this is that the homosexual is now more discernible as the counterpoint to the reproducing heterosexual citizen. These law-reform initiatives in criminal and family law professed to have the improvement of the status of women as their focus. They, unfortunately, demonstrate how impoverished notions of gender equality have become a modern mechanism for 'redrafting morality' and retrenching erotic autonomy.

Many conversations on Caribbean sexuality hold law as a constant, the antithesis of a vibrant and shifting social environment. As a consequence, law looms large as a giant fossil or contemptible relic, outdated and disengaged from life. Or, alternatively, in interrogating Caribbean sexualities, law generates indifference and escapes close analysis. The broad contour of most criminal laws dealing with sexual offences in the Caribbean is at least a hundred years old, some bearing strong similarities to the UK Offences Against the Person Act 1861. But the law has not stood still. Even the most ancient criminal codes in the Caribbean have been refined over the years. Ironically, we may learn as much about the formulation of the homosexual as a dangerous outlaw from contemporary lawmaking, including family law, as we would from the antecedents of the current laws.

In our analyses of HIV and law, it is imperative to appreciate that laws delineating allowable and impermissible sex are in flux. There is a strong tendency to identify outdated laws dealing with unnatural sex and sex work as seriously hampering a meaningful response to the epidemics. Though not entirely misguided, that perspective is, to some, extent misinformed because most of the countries in the independent English-speaking Caribbean have recently reformed sexual offences laws. The re-enactment of old laws in new statutes, as is more common with the legal regime for sex work, is more than the continuity of the legal status quo. 'New-old' laws also represent contemporary ways of thinking about national progress and citizenship. Moreover, it would be a grave error to ignore Alexander's (1997, 96, 97) and Tambiah's (2002, 39–40) claim that anxiety about HIV and AIDS has already been instrumental in the construction of authorized sex in contemporary lawmaking and that danger has been already reified in the homosexual body and sex worker.

UNPRODUCTIVE SEX

The early- to mid-twentieth century Caribbean criminal codes did not target homosexuality per se, the focus was unnatural, non-procreative sex. Same-sex sexuality was included, but it was not a singular object of laws prohibiting unnatural crimes. Buggery, for instance, was simply sexual intercourse *per anum* by a man's or boy's penis. The offence was committed if the anus penetrated was that of 'humankind', male or female, including a wife, or 'any other living creature', thus including animals. Consent was irrelevant to its commission and it was the same offence when committed between adults and with a child.

The penalties imposed by nineteenth-century Caribbean criminal codes for buggery were extremely harsh. In Guyana's 1893 Indictable Offences Ordinance, buggery was punishable by 'penal servitude for life'.[6] Antigua and Barbuda's 1840 Offences Against the Person Act made the 'abominable crime of buggery' a capital crime, punishable by death.[7] By the early- to mid-twentieth century, consistent with changing attitudes about penal justice, sentences were significantly reduced. In Antigua, for example, the maximum sentence was reduced to 10 years by 1863.[8]

In addition to buggery, some Caribbean criminal codes criminalised non-penetrative sexual acts under the rubric of indecency. Relative to buggery, indecency was a minor offence. In Guyana it was, and still is, an offence to commit an indecent act in a public place or in any other place with the intention to insult or offend others.[9] This is a misdemeanour punishable by a maximum imprisonment of two years. This crime can be committed in any configuration of persons: by two men, two women or a male and a female.

Gross indecency was generally the only named offence in twentieth-century Caribbean criminal statutes that was defined as one committed only by a male in relation to another male. It could be committed in public or private and consent was irrelevant. It included sexual activities short of anal penetration and could even be committed without physical contact, for example where a man exposed his penis to another. Like committing an indecent act, conviction could give rise to imprisonment of up to two years in Guyana.[10]

REPRODUCING THE NATION

Heterosexual reproduction was a preoccupation of the nation project in the Caribbean. While colonial criminal laws in the early- to mid-twentieth century Caribbean deemed non-procreative sex, even between heterosexuals and married persons, a crime against the nation and an assault to the public interest, the reproductive sex of unmarried black men and women was being treated as deviant and destructive to the possibilities of nationhood and social and economic development. In the period of incipient nationalism of the early- to mid- 1900s, weak father/child ties, marginal men, hyper-visible mothers and un-manned households, though communicated as social deficits, were, plainly, also considered a political predicament (Robinson 2006, 24). High rates of illegitimacy were continually attributed to rampant black concubinage, and signaled both immorality and underdevelopment.

But reproduction could also be a site of redemption for working-class Blacks in the Caribbean. A central idea of Caribbean nationalism was that men and women could be *made* into worthy citizens through marriage, social uplift, awakening their ambition, reproducing responsibly in marriage and living proper lives for the betterment of their children, the future citizens, as expressed in an article entitled 'Women's Liberal Club Aim at Mass Wedding' published in the *Daily Gleaner* of September 6, 1939. It was thought that converting concubines into spouses could stem illegitimacy and, conversely, affiliate bastard children with putative fathers, obliging them to pay child support, and, thus, might discourage concubinage (Robinson 2006, 11).

In the post-slavery period, legal marriage was so determinedly being urged on Caribbean working-class blacks and Indians that to be achievable it had to become more accessible. In the late nineteenth and early twentieth century, Caribbean laws governing marriage were under constant revision, broadening the circumstances under which men of faith could marry beyond the established church and, ultimately, beyond Christianity, providing for the registration of non-Christian religious marriages, and regularising Blacks in 'de facto marriages' immediately after slavery and,

7

retrospectively, legitimizing their children. Schemes like the mass marriage movement in Jamaica in the late 1930s to early 1950s targeted persons engaging in practices on the edge of marriage, like concubinage, and encouraged them to translate their proximate relationships into *de jure* marriage for the sake of the nation.

These efforts were less accommodation and more regulation, but they put certain forms of extra-legal heterosexual reproductive conjugality conceptually in closer proximity to marriage (Robinson 2006, 10). As criminal laws reinforced the idea that non-reproductive sexual practices were unnatural and perverse, the categories of recognisable conjugality were being broadened to ensure that men and women in heterosexual reproductive unions could be counted. In 1943, the earliest modern census in the Caribbean, 'common law husbands' and 'common law wives' were included as a category of conjugal condition in the Jamaica Census, to be followed in the rest of the British West Indies in the 1946 censuses. 'Visiting relationships' were added as a category of conjugality in small sample surveys in the late 1950s and in Caribbean censuses from 1970 to capture the excess of reproductive 'single' women who were not in common law unions.

CALIBRATED CITIZENSHIP

The region-wide overhauling of laws dealing with violence against women is a prominent symbol of feminist mobilization in the 1980s and '90s. The passage of domestic violence laws and new sexual offences provisions were a direct response to the violence against women campaign and the global movement pressing for greater recognition of women's rights. There is no single issue on which there has been greater feminist engagement with the state in the English-speaking Caribbean region in the last two decades than violence against women. In the early 1990s, CARICOM, through its Women's Desk, drafted a series of model laws on areas relating to gender equality, including domestic violence and sexual offences. About one half of the region has significantly reformed sexual offences laws.[11] New laws on domestic violence have been enacted throughout the entire Commonwealth Caribbean allowing victims of violence to apply for protection orders and relief ancillary to protection orders. They are now the most important legislative initiative to advance the rights of women in the 1990s as well as the most significant family law reform effort in the region in that period.[12]

The reformed provisions on sexual offences tried to ameliorate the victimisation complainants experienced in the justice system by providing for in-camera hearings in certain sexual offences, limited use of the past sexual history of victims and the protection of the privacy of victims by restricting reports on their identity. Some also abolished the requirement of corroboration for rape and the recent complaint rule. The new laws were not an indisputable victory for feminists. There was a strong current of formal equality in the new laws: that men and women should be treated exactly the same. Gender neutral rape laws emerged. Rape is now defined in the Dominica Sexual Offences Act 1998 as having taken place when a 'person' has sexual intercourse with 'another' without their consent. The gender neutral rape laws were awkward, failing to make it clear in what circumstances a woman could commit the crime; and by presenting men and women as de-gendered bodies, people with different body parts, neutrality threatened to obscure the gendered reality of sexual violence — that it is more often than not the exercise of masculine power against women, other men and children.

Much more devastating for feminist advocates, lawmakers sought to affirm the inviolability of patriarchal marriage in the new sexual offences statutes with narrow definitions of marital rape. The women's movement in Trinidad and Tobago mobilized to fight for a broadened definition of marital rape with limited success (see Mohammed 1991). The 1986 Act created an offence of sexual assault, and not rape, for which the maximum sentence was 15 years in contrast with life imprisonment for rape.[13] Furthermore, no proceedings could be brought without the authorization of the director of public prosecutions. By 1992, in a decision that is likely to be viewed as good law in the Commonwealth Caribbean, the English House of Lords ruled that men and women were to be considered equals in a marriage and the marital rape exemption was anachronistic.[14] Non-consensual sex between husband and wife was in all circumstances to be considered rape at common law. Notwithstanding this ruling, Antigua and Barbuda, Dominica and Saint Lucia all enacted legislation after the decision adopting a much more conservative position, that rape only occurred in limited circumstances, for example if there was a separation agreement, decree nisi of divorce or a protection order.

The primacy of heterosexual marriage and conjugal unions that resembled heterosexual marriage was vigorously expressed in the family laws of the same period, from the 1980s into the new millennium. The earliest and most striking recognition of an expanded notion of heterosexual conjugality was the Barbados Family Law Act 1981.[15] The legal definition of family dramatically expanded, so that persons in 'unions other than marriage', a term of art coined by the Act, and their children now fell under the Family Law Act.[16] In almost all respects — maintenance, property adjustment, child support and custody and protection against domestic violence — these long-term heterosexual unions had all the same rights and duties as persons married. A 'union other than marriage' was defined as a man and a woman living together continuously for a period of at least five years. The goal of the new Act was to 'give the widest possible protection and assistance to the family as the natural and fundamental group unit of society, particularly while it is responsible for the care and education of dependant children',[17] but it also emphasized 'the need to preserve and protect the institution of marriage as the union of a man and a woman to the exclusion of all others voluntarily entered into for life'.[18]

To slightly different degrees, Trinidad and Tobago, Jamaica, Guyana and Belize have all recognized legal duties and rights relating to property and financial provision from these long-term cohabiting heterosexual relationships.[19] Trinidad and Tobago in 1998 enacted a Cohabitational Relationships Act which gave those in 'cohabitational relationships' rights to make claims to property and financial provision at the end of the relationship. Similar to the Barbados 'union other than marriage' a cohabitant is a man or a woman living with someone of the opposite sex on a bona fide basis as husband and wife.[20] Highlighting the centrality of reproduction to the legal definition of conjugality, persons in relatively short cohabiting relationships could qualify for relief under the Act if they had children together.[21] 'Cohabitant' is a new term of art that has been mainstreamed in other statutes. The 2000 amendments to the Trinidad and Tobago Sexual Offences Act now include it, affirming that the offence of rape and grievous sexual assault can be committed by parties to a marriage or cohabitational relationship.[22]

The most dramatic expansion in the definition of conjugality in family law came in the 1990s with the passage of domestic violence statutes. Virtually every Commonwealth Caribbean country has enacted, since 1991, legislation that provides protection against domestic violence for a man and a woman who are living or once lived together. Marriage has been somewhat subverted by this development, but, at the same time, heterosexual marriage has gained currency as the paradigmatic anchor for national development and progress by the growing recognition of marriage-like relationships.

In 1999, a new Domestic Violence Act was passed in Trinidad and Tobago repealing its previous law made in 1991.[23] The 1999 Act, which has become the new model for regional reform in the area, now provides relief for a wider range of relationships — not just cohabitational relationships but persons in visiting relationships, persons with a biological child in common and members of the household. 'Members of a household' must be persons related by blood to each other, thus excluding same-sex partners.[24] Trinidad and Tobago preferred the term 'visiting relationships' to that of 'close personal relationships' which had been proposed by the Ad Hoc Committee set up to reform the 1991 Domestic Violence Act (Trinidad and Tobago 1997, 16). The indicators for close personal relationships tended to be functional — the nature, intensity and duration of the relationship.[25] The Trinidad and Tobago lawmakers preferred 'visiting relationships', a culturally and sociologically resonant marker of heterosexual reproductive intimacies, which was curiously defined as a non-cohabitational union between a man and a woman that is otherwise similar to the relationship between husband and wife. To qualify to make an application under the Act the visiting relationship must have subsisted for at least 12 months.[26]

The categories gained ascendancy in demography where they served as heuristic devices that revealed valuable data on fertility (Robinson 2006, 50). Questions of conjugality by the mid-twentieth country were being regionally understood as ones about how women of child bearing age organized their reproductive lives with men, making non-reproducing bodies uncountable and same-sex relationships statistically impossible (Robinson 2006, 51). The couching of expanded notions of conjugality in anthropologically and culturally significant language like 'common law' and 'visiting' unions in lawmaking further anchors the normality of patriarchal heterosexual reproduction. 'Common law' and 'visiting' were in law made contingent on similarity to marriage. As analogues for marriage they signified a sexual division of labour, male control and female domesticity and dependency. Same-sex intimacies in these processes of family law making gained more clarity as an alterity, the *other* consolidating and shoring up the legitimacy of legal categories of heterosexual conjugality. A homosexual relationship, as compared with persons engaging in unnatural acts, sharpens conceptually to represent the unthinkable, the legally impossible and what family *is not*.

THE SEXUAL OUTLAWS

In the early twentieth century the sex you *did* and its contribution to reproducing the nation helped to define your worth as a citizen. By the 1990s *whom* you had sex with was being increasingly affirmed as a yardstick for belonging in criminal and family laws. The 1986 Trinidad and Tobago Sexual Offences Act was the first major post-independence reform to sexual offences law in the region. The wave of sexual offences reforms beginning in 1986 was not uniform but on the whole the new legislation significantly refined the definition of buggery or the unnatural crime and increased the severity of the punishment. Some important changes occurred before 1985. In Belize, for example, the offence of 'unnatural crime' covered only non-consensual anal sex with a person, but a 1944 amendment repealed the requirement of lack of consent or force and made consent irrelevant to the commission of the crime.[27]

Before 1986, buggery in Trinidad and Tobago was an amorphous crime covering a miscellany of conduct. It included anal sex between men and men, women, children, and animals, and consent was no defence to the crime. Those convicted were liable to a maximum of five years imprisonment. In the 1986 Act, buggery and bestiality as offences were separated.[28] A gradated crime for buggery was introduced that depended on whether a minor was involved. The maximum sentence for buggery between consenting and non-consenting adults increased to ten years imprisonment.[29]

Although in Barbados the sentence for buggery under the new sexual offences statute did not increase, it was already very onerous and, by contrast, sentences for bestiality were reduced. Prior to 1992, the 'abominable crime of buggery' was committed either with mankind or animals and gave rise to a maximum sentence of imprisonment for life.[30] The 1992 Sexual Offences Act created two separate offences and introduced a maximum term of imprisonment for bestiality of ten years.[31] Buggery, on the other hand, maintained a maximum sentence of imprisonment for life. In Antigua and Barbuda, prior to 1998 there was one category for the crime of buggery and it gave rise to a maximum term of imprisonment of ten years.[32] The 1998 Sexual Offences Act distinguished buggery and bestiality and the penalty for the latter remained ten years imprisonment, and that for consensual and non-consensual buggery between adults rose to 15 years.[33]

The Bahamas is the only territory where there has been some decriminalization of unnatural crimes. Under the Sexual Offences and Domestic Violence Act 1991 an 'unnatural crime' is committed by an adult male who has sexual intercourse with a minor of the same sex, or an adult female who has sexual intercourse with a minor of the same sex.[34] Sexual intercourse between two adult males or females amounts to an unnatural crime only if it takes place in public.[35] In essence, the Act decriminalized consensual anal sex between two men in private, but it also expanded the definition of sexual intercourse to cover anal sex and oral and manual stimulation of the genitals. This allowed sexual activities between two women, which hitherto did not amount to an unnatural crime, to be criminalized for the first time. The consent of the attorney general is required to pursue a prosecution under this new provision.[36]

From the very opaque previous law that described prohibited unnatural behaviours, The Bahamas now clearly identifies men who have sex with men and women who have sex with women as the nub of unnatural crimes. Enlarging the definition of 'sex' was essential to this move. It was not enough to speak of unnatural connections between women or men. It was crucial to create proximity to the essence of heterosexual intimacy by separating bestiality from buggery and also by describing a wide range of sexual contact as sexual intercourse. Through this proximity to heterosexual conjugality, homosexual sex could be more precisely defined and proscribed. The Bahamas had, and still has, in its Penal Code the offence of gross indecency.[37] It includes almost all of the behaviour covered by the unnatural crime under the Sexual Offences and Domestic Violence Act, except it could include heterosexual sexual behaviour in public. But gross indecency is a misdemeanour punishable by a fine while the unnatural crime carries a term of imprisonment of up to 25 years. Given the existence of the lesser offence of gross indecency, the inclusion of the unnatural crime sends a clear message that public displays of homosexual sex, in contrast to indecent behaviour, amount to a very serious offence.

While The Bahamas narrowed the unnatural crime to homosexual sex engaged in by men or women, the 2004 Criminal Code in Saint Lucia limited it to male homosexual sexual intercourse.[38] Prior to 2004, the Code criminalized unnatural connections generally, and this included anal sex between a man and a woman. The 2004 Criminal Code now defines buggery as sexual intercourse per anus by a male person with another male person. Gender neutral rape laws further distilled the objects of the new buggery and unnatural offences as a male homosexual. Rape at common law was defined as non-consensual penetration by a male of a female's vagina. The 1992 Sexual Offence Act of Barbados made rape gender neutral and it now included non-consensual anal sex by a male with another male or male with a female.[39] This meant that there was no need for a buggery provision that covered non-consensual anal sex. The unique sphere of application of the buggery law was in effect the prohibition of consensual anal sex.

Almost identically, Caribbean territories reformed the offence of gross indecency and replaced it with one of serious indecency. Prior to 1986 in Trinidad and Tobago, the offence of gross indecency by a male with another male had a maximum sentence of two years.[40] After 1986 it was replaced by the crime of serious indecency defined as an act other than sexual intercourse by a person involving the use of the genital organs to arouse or gratify sexual desire.[41] Again this was a gradated crime based on age of parties. This new offence was not restricted to activities between men, but for the first time included sexual activities between women. The new law explicitly excluded acts of serious indecency between husbands and wives and men and women over age 16 engaged in sexual activities from its purview.[42] The punishment for serious indecency for consenting adults was increased to five years.[43]

Like Trinidad and Tobago, the 1992 Barbados Act replaced the misdemeanour of gross indecency, which was committed by a male in relation to another male and gave rise to imprisonment of up to two years, with the new one of serious indecency.[44] Serious indecency was also gender neutral. The penalty substantially increased from two years to imprisonment to up to ten years if the offence was committed between persons over age 16, and 15 years if a minor under age 16 was involved. Serious indecency was the use of genital organs for sexual desire, but unlike Trinidad and Tobago, no exception was made for heterosexual sexual activities. Saint Lucia, Dominica and Antigua and Barbuda all adopted statutes similar to Trinidad and Tobago on gross/serious indecency excepting consensual heterosexual sexual relations in private.[45]

Yasmin Tambiah (2002) suggests that there were differences in the thinking behind the criminalization of male versus female homosexual sex in Trinidad and Tobago. The scripting of HIV and AIDS as gay diseases, fears about the risks homosexual anal sex posed to the well being of the nation and the sanctity of heterosexual marriage loomed large in the debates in that country (Tambiah 2002, 39–40). A legacy of a number of modern sexual offences statutes is the criminalization of the transmission of HIV.

The Bahamas Sexual Offences and Domestic Violence Act now provides that a person who knows they are infected with HIV and has consensual sex without disclosing this to the other party commits an offence and is liable to be detained for up to five years.[46] It is now an aggravated assault in Saint Lucia to intentionally or recklessly infect another with the HIV virus and it is no defence to prove that the other person consented to the sexual encounter.[47] Tambiah (2002, 41, 53) ascribes the nascent criminality of lesbianism to an obsession with gender equality and resentment that men were being stereotyped as sexual predators and perpetrators, notwithstanding the demand for women's equality. Gender equality meant that both men and women were to be culpable in the same way for sexual offences. Erotic autonomy for both men and women was not seen as a dimension of gender equality.

A second stage of sexual offences law reform occurred in Trinidad and Tobago in 2000. While the 1986 Sexual Offences Act excited considerable interest and advocacy from the women's movement in Trinidad and Tobago, the dramatic reforms in 2000 went largely under the radar. It takes a stronger stance on sex crime, broadening the range of existing crimes, creating new ones and substantially increasing the penalties. While the provisions are ostensibly to better protect victims of sexual violence, consensual same-sex sexual activities are caught within this new evangelism and have become more criminalized than ever. In 2000, new offences, like grievous sexual assault, were created in Trinidad and Tobago.[48] Rape now fully includes violations within marriage and it is also now defined in gender neutral terms.[49] Non-consensual anal sex now falls under rape where the penalty can be as high as imprisonment for your natural life.[50] Given the expansion of rape, one might have expected the old buggery law to be repealed or given less prominence. On the contrary, the punishment for buggery between two adults, which given the broadened definition of rape especially targets consensual anal sexual relations, has increased from ten to 25 years.[51]

In 2000, a new provision was introduced in Trinidad and Tobago requiring judges at sentencing to impose notification requirements on certain sex offenders, and this includes persons convicted of buggery and possibly serious indecency.[52] The new law now also requires a judge to order a medical examination of a person convicted of certain sex crimes, which includes buggery.[53] Where that person is living with HIV or any other communicable disease, the other party will be notified.[54] And, where the complainant has contracted a disease from the defendant, he or she can be ordered to pay compensation.[55]

The reforms to the Belize Criminal Code since 1999 follow a similar pattern, increasing the penalties for sexual offences and creating new sexual offences. In 2001, the Code was amended to create the offence of deliberate or reckless spreading of HIV.[56] The Code now provides that certain habitual sex offenders, and this includes those convicted of buggery, must undergo counselling and medical and psychiatric treatment, and the offender has an obligation to notify, among others, the commissioner of police if he or she intends to change his or her place of residence.[57]

Under the guise of protection of the vulnerable, more of the sex we choose and agree to is being regulated and surveyed. Where there are no individual complainants, the state is positioning itself, and the nation, as the victimized and violated.

THE LIMITS OF SEX

In 2000, the Trinidad and Tobago Equal Opportunities Act was enacted.[58] 'Sex' is described as a prohibited ground of discrimination but the law explicitly states that 'sex' does not include 'sexual orientation'.[59] There are proposals of the same order for constitutional reform in Jamaica (see Butler 2006), but no Caribbean statute is quite as forthright in severing sexual expression from gender equality. The same ideology has less overtly guided reforms in criminal and family laws over the last 25 years in the Commonwealth Caribbean which have used the context of purportedly improving the status of women as a tool for controlling sexuality and to justify heightened surveillance of sexual expression.

I see these law reforms as a worrying dimension to post-feminist mobilizations of gender. 'Gender' has taken hold of bureaucratic imagination in at least two unfortunate ways. First is the neutralizing of gender's analytical gravitas — its focus on relations of power, including sexualized power, and the uneven burdens of sex stereotyping — with the equation 'gender = men + women'. This has promoted an expanded recognition of women's sexual agency in extremely negative ways, understood only as danger; which means that women can now legally be rapists and 'sodomites', just like men. Secondly, it has compromised the legitimacy of woman-centred work, the repeated charge being that the latter is one-sided and unbalanced. The spaces in which women are being recognized as legal subjects are narrowing. 'Gender' is being bureaucratically mined to present a flattened idea of woman determined by suffering, entirely a victim. Women have become a paradigm of the vulnerable, those in need of protection, and the state assumes the role of a benevolent progressive patriarch (Alexander 1997). By pathologizing womanness in this way, vulnerability is feminized. But the imagery can also be turned on its head so that women stand proxy for the nation, which is presented as victim and sufferer, at serious risk from disease, foreign values and depravity. It is never enough to point out that contemporary laws are making sex between certain consenting adults more criminal because the essence of the complaint is that the nation is the victim and that the national body has been violated.

Gender equality is also being burdened with nationalist conceptions of women as citizens having a special responsibility as guardians of the moral code and as producers and reproducers of the nation (Robinson 2003). Contemporary sexual offences laws are embodied moral codes and 'women become the terrain upon which ideas about sexuality, gendered behaviour, construction of family, and consequently a citizen's worth are contested and negotiated' (Tambiah 2002, 27). The history of feminist advocacy and the women's movement in the Caribbean has been one of resistance to these constrained notions of womanhood (Alexander 1997; Mohammed 1991; Tambiah 2002). However feminist actors are less and less driving the invocation of what I call 'gender somethings', goals related to gender that have gained wide bureaucratic currency because they are signifiers of progress and development and provide opportunities for political rectitude.

'Gender' is not politically spent. On the contrary, the developments described suggest that we urgently need to re-politicize the concept. Sexed and eroticized bodies are gender's subjects, and the idea and burdens of womanhood serve as rudiments for modern conceptions of sexuality in the Caribbean. Our agendas for social justice will be ethically weak and politically fractured if we do not vigorously resist the circling of 'gender' and 'sexuality' as discrete concerns.

Law in the Caribbean appreciably mediates notions of what is permissible or acceptable sex. The legal framework that has been refined in the late-twentieth century in relation to crimes and the family is progressively more punitive towards those who step outside the boundaries of what is deemed acceptable sex, and affirming of those who meet heteronormative standards of family. The much heralded expansion of definitions of family in family property laws and domestic violence laws 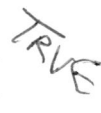 to include men and women in long-term relationships re-inscribe heterosexual reproduction as the lynchpin of suitable family life. Many of the initiatives in contemporary Caribbean sexual offences laws to tackle sexual violence are valuable. However, by so determinedly overreaching into the sex adults choose — constructing the state as the victim of a refined crime of buggery and an expanded crime of serious indecency — the reformed sexual offences laws undermined their valuable initiatives to protect victims of sexual violence and ensure perpetrators were punished.

The fact that what is seen as progressive lawmaking has, at the level of formal law, left many less free to live lives of their choice, is a reminder that lawmaking in democratic societies is intrinsically a process involving compromises and concessions. It can adversely affect constituencies and communities who are unaware that their bodies, lives and possibilities are under ruthless review. A reappraisal of what we mean by gender justice and giving serious consideration to the place of erotic autonomy in what it means to be a citizen are crucial to changing the terms of engagement of lawmakers and others on the question of same-sex sexuality.

Notes

1. *Planned Parenthood v Casey* (505 US 833) (1992) (Supreme Court, USA).
2. *National Coalition for Gay and Lesbian Equality and Another v Minister of Justice and Others* 1998 (12) BCLR 1517 [117] (Constitutional Court, Republic of South Africa).
3. Trinidad and Tobago Sexual Offences Act 1986–27.
4. The Bahamas Sexual Offences and Domestic Violence Act 1991, 2000 Revised Laws of The Bahamas, cap. 99; Barbados Sexual Offences Act 1992, 1971 Rev. (with cumulative supplements to 2002), cap. 154.
5. Antigua and Barbuda Sexual Offences Act 1995-9; Dominica Sexual Offences Act 1998–91; Belize Criminal Code (Amendment) Act 1999-36; Saint Lucia Criminal Code 2004, 2005 Rev., cap. 3:01.
6. Indictable Offences Ordinance 1893-18, 1891–1894, Laws of British Guiana, vol. IV, s. 359.
7. Antigua Offences Against the Person Act 1840-884, 1846 Rev., vol. IV, s. xiii.
8. Antigua Offences Against the Person Act 1863-190, s. 57.
9. Guyana Criminal Law (Offences) Act 1894, 1973 Rev., cap. 8:01, s. 360.
10. Ibid., s. 353.
11. See notes 3–5 above.
12. Antigua and Barbuda Domestic Violence (Summary Proceedings) Act 1999-3; The Bahamas Domestic Violence (Protection Orders) Act 2007-24 (this Act has not yet come into force), Sexual Offences and Domestic Violence Act 1991; Barbados Domestic Violence (Protection Orders) Act 1992, 1971 Rev. (with cumulative supplement to 2002), cap 130A; Belize Domestic Violence Act 1992, 2000 Rev, cap. 178; Bermuda Domestic Violence Act 1997-1; British Virgin Islands Domestic Violence Summary Proceedings Act 1996-2; Cayman Islands Summary Jurisdiction (Domestic Violence) Law 1992-20; Dominica Protection Against Domestic Violence Act 2001-22; Grenada Domestic Violence Act 2001-15; Guyana Domestic Violence Act 1996-18; Jamaica Domestic Violence Act, 1995-15; St Christopher-Nevis Domestic Violence Act 2000-3; Saint Lucia Domestic Violence (Summary Proceedings) Act 1995, 2005 Rev., cap. 4:04; St. Vincent and the Grenadines Domestic Violence and Matrimonial Proceedings Act 1984, 1990 Rev, cap. 165, Domestic Violence (Summary Proceedings) Act 1995-13; Trinidad and Tobago Domestic Violence Act 1999-27.
13. Trinidad and Tobago Sexual Offences Act 1986, s. 5.
14. *R v R* [1991] 1 All ER 747; [1992] 1 AC 599 (House of Lords, England).
15. Barbados Family Law Act 1981, 1971 Rev. (with cumulative supplements to 2002), cap. 214.
16. Ibid., s. 39.
17. Ibid., s. 22(b).
18. Ibid., s. 22(a).

19. Belize Supreme Court of Judicature (Amendment) Act, No. 8 of 2001-8; Guyana Married Persons (Property)(Amendment) Act 1990-20; Jamaica Property (Rights of Spouses) Act 2004-4, Maintenance Act, 2005-30; Trinidad and Tobago Cohabitational Relationships Act 1998-30.
20. Trinidad and Tobago Cohabitational Relationships Act 1998, s. 2.
21. Ibid., s. 7(b).
22. Trinidad and Tobago Sexual Offences (Amendment) Act 2000-31.
23. Trinidad and Tobago Domestic Violence Act 1999-27.
24. Ibid., s. 3
25. See e.g. Bermuda Domestic Violence Act 1997-1, s. 4(4).
26. Trinidad and Tobago Domestic Violence Act 1999, ss. 3 & 4(2)(g).
27. Belize Criminal Code Amendment Ordinance 1944-14.
28. Trinidad and Tobago Sexual Offences Act 1986, ss. 13 & 14.
29. Ibid., s. 13.
30. Barbados Offences Against the Person Act 1868, 1971 Rev., cap. 141, s. 64.
31. Barbados Sexual Offences Act, 1971 Rev (with cumulative supplements to 2002), cap. 154, ss. 9 & 10.
32. Antigua and Barbuda Offences Against the Persons Act 1873, 1992 Rev., cap. 300, s. 59.
33. Antigua and Barbuda Sexual Offences Act 1995, ss. 12 & 13.
34. The Bahamas Sexual Offences and Domestic Violence Act, s. 16.
35. Ibid.
36. Ibid.
37. The Bahamas Penal Code, 2000 Rev., cap 85, s. 490.
38. Saint Lucia Criminal Code, s. 133(3).
39. Barbados Sexual Offences Act 1992, s. 3.
40. Trinidad and Tobago Offences Against the Person Act, 1980 Rev. (updated to 1986), chap. 11:08, s. 61.
41. Trinidad and Tobago Sexual Offences Act 1986, s. 13.
42. Ibid.
43. Ibid.
44. Barbados Sexual Offences Act 1992, s. 12.
45. Saint Lucia Criminal Code, s. 132; Dominica Sexual Offences Act, s. 14; Antigua and Barbuda Sexual Offences Act, s. 15.
46. The Bahamas Sexual Offences and Domestic Violence Act, s. 8(2).
47. Saint Lucia Criminal Code 2004, article 140.
48. Trinidad and Tobago Sexual Offences (Amendment) Act 2000, s. 3.
49. Ibid., s. 4.
50. Ibid.
51. Ibid., s. 13.
52. Ibid., s. 20.
53. Ibid., s. 20 which introduces the new Sexual Offences Act, s. 34E.

54. Ibid.
55. Ibid.
56. Belize Criminal Code (Amendment) Act 2001-42.
57. Belize Criminal Code (Amendment) Act 1999-36.
58. Trinidad and Tobago Equal Opportunities Act 2000-69.
59. The Privy Council has recently upheld the constitutionality of the law, including this provision, in *Suratt and others v Attorney General of Trinidad and Tobago* [2007] UKPC 55.

REFERENCES

Alexander, M. J. 1991. 'Redrafting Morality: The Postcolonial State and the Sexual Offences Bill of Trinidad and Tobago'. In *Third World Women and the Politics of Feminism*, eds. Chandra Talpade Mohanty, Ann Russo and Lourdes Torres, 133–52. Bloomington and Indianapolis: Indiana University Press.

———. 1994. 'Not Just (Any) *Body* can be a Citizen: The Politics of Law, Sexuality and Postcoloniality in Trinidad and Tobago and The Bahamas'. *Feminist Review* 48: 5–23.

———. 1997. 'Erotic Autonomy as Politics of Decolonization: An Anatomy of Feminist and State Practice in The Bahamas Tourist Economy'. In *Feminist Genealogies, Colonial Legacies, Democratic Futures*, eds. M. Jacqui Alexander and Chandra Talpade Mohanty, 63–100. New York and London: Routledge.

Butler, De-Andra. 2006. 'The Charter of Rights and the Right to Privacy Polemic'. LLB. Thesis, University of the West Indies.

Cornell, Drucilla. 1995. *The Imaginary Domain: Abortion, Pornography & Sexual Harassment*. New York and London: Routledge.

Daily Gleaner. 1939. 'Women's Liberal Club Aim at Mass Wedding' September 6 , 16–17.

Mohammed, Patricia. 1991. 'Reflection on the Women's Movement in Trinidad: Calypsos, Changes and Sexual Violence'. *Feminist Review* 38: 22–39.

Robinson, Tracy. 2006. 'Taxonomies of Conjugality'. Hauser Global Law Working Paper 11/06.

Tambiah, Yasmin. 2002. 'Redefining the Female Body Politic: Women, Sexuality and the State'. SEPHIS Postdoctoral Project.

Trinidad and Tobago. 1997. 'Report of the Ad Hoc Committee for the Reform of the Domestic Violence Act 1991, and related legislation'. Port of Spain: Ministry of Legal Affairs.

CHAPTER 2

DRUGS OBSCURE THE HUMAN RIGHTS ISSUES FOR DRUG USERS

Are Demons and Jumbies Rights Holders?

MARCUS DAY

D rug users as a population can be viewed as vulnerable as a result of their illegal, and therefore criminal, drug use and resultant lifestyle. The view that drug users are entitled to the same human rights as the general population is a relatively new concept that has grown out of and around the development of harm reduction interventions that address the needs of drug users from a non-judgemental perspective that focuses on reducing drug-related harms and not the legality of drug use.

This chapter addresses the question of whether drug users in the Caribbean, and by extension all drug users, are rights holders. To accomplish this we will explore the current status of drug users in the Caribbean, their vulnerability to HIV and how the international conventions and laws prohibiting drug use dramatically increase the vulnerability of drug users to HIV and social exclusion.

We will start a short discourse on vulnerability and how prohibitionist legislation creates a greater vulnerability than the behaviour it prohibits, a discussion of drug use (primarily non-injecting crack cocaine use) and HIV risk in the context of the Commonwealth Caribbean, and an outline of the international drug conventions and how the Caribbean's wholesale acceptance of these conventions place drug users at increased risk.

Vulnerability is viewed as a result of complex economic, social and cultural drivers of the epidemic. The author contends that the *state* needs to be added to that list as the creator of legislation that tramples, rather than protects, human rights.

Examples of laws that are guilty of creating or increasing vulnerability include:

- laws that restrict minors from accessing sexual and reproductive health services without parental consent;
- buggery laws that seek to legislate conduct in one's bedroom; and
- prostitution laws that criminalize a financial transaction between a willing buyer and a willing seller. Even the transmission of HIV is now being criminalized.

What is less considered is how drug prohibition, the state's attempt to penalize a private act of substance use, creates an environment that places people more at risk than the harm caused by the very substances those laws seek to protect us from.

DRUGS IN THE CARIBBEAN REGION

The nations and the territories of the Caribbean are located between the producers of cocaine and heroin in South America and the main consumers of the drug in North America and Europe. In the past three decades the Caribbean has been increasingly used for the transhipment of cocaine.

Research has shown that the misuse of alcohol and crack cocaine represents serious threats to social cohesion. Drug misuse causes harm to both individuals and society. It is associated with physical and mental health problems, greater risks of HIV infection and developing AIDS through unprotected and risky sex and, due to its prohibited status, leads to criminal behaviours and possibly to incarceration, as drug users may commit crimes to obtain money for drugs. The high profits associated with the distribution and sale of drugs in communities may also lead to social dislocation due to the emergence, in some communities, of gangsters and a violent culture based on fear of reprisal and gang membership. As we will show later, some of these harms are associated with the substance itself, while others are created and aggravated by the prohibitionist laws forced upon the Caribbean by the drug war mentality embedded in the three international drug conventions currently enforced.

While the use of crack presents the main challenge in the Caribbean region, use of other substances — marijuana, alcohol and over-the-counter and prescription drugs — also present serious problems. In addition, inhalants such as thinners, glue, and gasolene are commonly used by street children in the larger and more populated countries of Jamaica, the Dominican Republic and Haiti. The author has also come into contact with evidence of heroin use and of injecting drug use (IDU) in Trinidad and Tobago, and Guyana and both countries have reported HCV in the blood supply, a clear marker for IDU.

Extent of drug-use in the region

After more than 10 years of the Barbados Plan of Action (1996) it is still not possible to ascertain the number of drug users in the region. Research in the region has focused on school populations and on admissions to treatment centres. Other than a number of rapid assessments undertaken in selected communities in the late nineties, there is little information about the 'hidden population' of users, the diversion of pharmaceuticals, little information about the extent and nature of crack cocaine use, less information on the HIV overlap and almost no information on heroin use and what appears to be a growing incidence of injecting behaviours.

Our research has determined a pattern to crack/cocaine initiation in the Caribbean. While 50 per cent of female users are enticed by males into using crack, almost 20 per cent of males are enticed by females. Twenty per cent of crack users start out selling crack and, due to the exposure opportunity, are lulled into experimentation. That crack use starts as a result of economic activity among the poorer sectors of society is a measure of the inadequacy of legitimate outlets for young entrepreneurial-minded males, in particular. The mixture of crack cocaine with marijuana contributes to the addiction of another 20 per cent of the using population. This is an indictment on an abstinence-based drug education programme that attributes similar harms to all drug use regardless of substance and neglects substance-specific messages.

Local individuals, who are involved in the transhipment of cocaine, receive cocaine as an in-kind payment for their facilitation. In order to convert this product into cash, cocaine is sold on the local market at a price well below that of the countries of final destination. Thus, cocaine is easily affordable to the local population and has found its way into most urban centres and rural areas alike.

Thus, cocaine trafficking in the Caribbean has, in recent years, led to its increasing local use. In studies conducted either on the streets or in secondary schools, half of the sampled population said that they knew of a crack user and knew where to buy crack. It should also be noted that the association between crack cocaine as an economic activity and crack use complicates the treatment and rehabilitation process. Many clients who have undergone treatment and have been successfully discharged have been known to resort to selling crack again in order to survive economically. Existing skills-based rehabilitation services are limited in their capacity to address this situation.

In all Caribbean countries and territories, with the exception of the smallest (for example Montserrat and Saba) crack/cocaine is easily available. Other drugs of use include inhalant use, especially among the young homeless population in some countries.

Reports have also been received of isolated incidences of Colombian heroin coming on to the black market in Trinidad and Tobago and Guyana where interdictions of this substance points to its availability. Currently, North American heroin markets are satisfied by supplies transiting Central America while the European heroin market receives their drugs from Afghanistan. As long as this remains unchanged the Caribbean is unlikely to see major movements of heroin through its waters. If Europe seeks its heroin elsewhere it could present a problem for the Caribbean that has no experience with harm-reduction interventions and views drug abstinence as the only drug policy. Thus, once again, the Caribbean may be used as a transhipment point of the European market. If the 'model' of paying in kind for transhipment services is replicated, it is likely that heroin will become readily available at an affordable price to the general population.

Most local experts hold the view that there is a general aversion to injection among the Caribbean population and, therefore, injection drug use is unlikely to become popular. However, there are already reports of an increase in injection use in the region and no reason to suppose that it will not spread further, should it become an economic necessity for drug users.

In some Caribbean countries, access to drugs has also been linked to those involved in service industries. For example, many states are associated with 'drug-tourism' and also linked to sex industries. In many cases the sex industry is linked to the drug industry if for no other reason than both activities are illegal and, therefore, are controlled by the same 'criminals'.

THE EXTENT OF HIV IN THE CARIBBEAN

After Africa, the Caribbean has the second highest burden of HIV infection in the world, with a regional prevalence of 1.6 per cent (UNAIDS Report 2006). The highest prevalence rates in the region are reported to be in Haiti (3.8 per cent) and The Bahamas (3.3 per cent). The epidemic appears to be levelling off in some countries, such as Haiti and Jamaica, but is of increasing concern in other countries such as Guyana. The epidemic is being fuelled by sexual transmission, migration, and both intravenous drug use (Inciardi, Syvertsen, Surratt 2005), and non-intravenous drug use. While there have been attempts to create a regional response to the epidemic, the diversity of language, culture and socio-economic standing among the Caribbean islands make a regional response difficult to implement. Even if a coordinated, regional response were possible, it would first require strengthening of each nation's capacity to deal with the epidemic within its own territory. A report on the quality of HIV surveillance concluded that in the Caribbean region, only the Dominican Republic and Jamaica had 'fully implemented systems' able to accurately track the epidemic (Walker, Garcia-Calleja, Heaton et al.). As a result, quality information on the HIV epidemic is lacking (Inciardi, Syvertsen, Surratt 2005; Calleja, Walker, Cuchi, et al. 2002; Hacker, Malta, Enriquez, et al. 2005).

While intravenous drug use is rare in the Caribbean — exceptions include Puerto Rico (Inciardi, Syvertsen, Surratt 2005), the use of crack cocaine is extensive as cocaine transits the region on its way to North America and Europe. In 2005, this knowledge gap of the role of crack cocaine in the Caribbean HIV and AIDS problem was identified as a priority area of the Caribbean Regional Strategic Framework for HIV and AIDS, stated as follows: 'To strengthen understanding of the role of substance use and drug use in [the] regional epidemiology of HIV, and to use [the] information in appropriate prevention and care strategies' (Caribbean Regional Strategic Framework).

DRUG USE AND ITS ROLE IN THE HIV EPIDEMIC IN THE CARIBBEAN REGION

A comprehensive review of the literature on the relationship between drug use and HIV and AIDS in the South American and Caribbean regions was published recently (Hacker, Malta, Enriquez, et al. 2005). There is an extensive literature for South America indicating a role for both injection and non-injection drug use in the HIV epidemic there, especially in Argentina and Brazil (Calleja, Walker, Cuchi 2002; Hacker, Malta, Enriquez, 2005; Montano, Sanchez, Laguna-Torres, et al. 2005). The limited available literature from the Caribbean indicates that, in general, intravenous drug use is uncommon. Puerto Rico, Bermuda, and The Bahamas are among the exceptions. The major drug of use is cocaine. What is striking in this report and others (Calleja, Walker, Cuchi 2002) is the lack of information from the Caribbean region with which to evaluate the importance of non-injection drug use in the HIV epidemic. There are isolated reports from The Bahamas (Gomez, Kimball, Orlander, et al. 2002), and Trinidad and Tobago (Cleghorn, Jack, Murphy, et al. 1995), but a comprehensive evaluation of the problem in the Caribbean is not possible due to lack of data. Thus, the extent of non-injection cocaine use and its importance in the HIV epidemic at this time is not known. In 2005 this knowledge gap was identified as a priority research area of the *Caribbean Regional Strategic Framework for HIV/AIDS* (Caribbean Regional Strategic Framework 2005).

The problem of crack cocaine in the Caribbean

The Caribbean islands are recognized as a transit point for drugs (CIA Fact Book for Saint Lucia). Cocaine arrives by sea and is offloaded to smaller local vessels along the coasts for onward shipment to Europe and North America. It is increasingly common that with each shipment some percentage of goods stays behind as a payment in kind. As most facilitators are not users, the cocaine is 'dumped' on the local market. High grade powder cocaine is converted into crack cocaine with a 'crack rock' costing from US$1 in Trinidad and Tobago to US$5 in Saint Thomas.

Association of Crack Cocaine and HIV infection in the Caribbean

Prior to conducting our research in Saint Lucia the author found little data on the association between crack cocaine and HIV infection in the English-speaking Caribbean. There are reports of an association between the use of crack cocaine and HIV infection in The Bahamas (Gomez, Kimball, Orlander et al. 2002) and Trinidad and Tobago (Cleghorn, Jack, Murphy et al. 1995).

In the Trinidadian study of STD clinic attendees cited above (Cleghorn, Jack, Murphy et al. 1995), crack cocaine use was a significant independent predictor of HIV infection among men, but not among women in whom risk factors were age — 14 years at first sex — commercial sex work, and having a history of non-gonococcal cervicitis. The men were asked about paying for sex, but commercial sex work or being paid for sex with money or drugs was not evaluated in the men. A second study conducted in Trinidad and Tobago among crack cocaine users in rehabilitation found that exchange of sex for money among men who do not identify themselves as homosexual does indeed occur in the crack cocaine using population of that island (Djumalieva, Imamshah, Wagner et al. 2002).

In The Bahamas, a concordance was observed between the new cases of treatment for smoked cocaine use, and new cases of gonorrhoea or genital ulcer diseases during the period 1984–87 (Gomez, Kimball,

Orlander et al. 2002). Using a case-control study design among attendees of a public STD clinic, the authors found an odds ratio of 10.2 (95 per cent CI: 4.5–23.4) in men and 5.7 (95 per cent CI: 2.2–14.9) in women for the association of crack cocaine use with HIV infection. These odds ratios were derived in clinic attendees with no other concurrent STD diagnoses, and were adjusted ratios for age and year of HIV diagnosis. Other known risk factors for HIV, including number of sex partners or commercial sex work, were not evaluated in that study. Another Bahamian study among women attending an antenatal health clinic also found an association between crack cocaine use and HIV (Gomez, Bain, Major et al. 1996). As with the previous study, no account was made for number of sex partners or commercial sex work.

It is debatable whether sex work is a potential confounder of the association between cocaine and HIV infection or whether it is an intermediate that lies in the mechanistic pathway between cocaine use and HIV infection. If cocaine use leads to exchanging sex for money or drugs to support an addiction, then sex work could be thought of as an intermediate in the pathway between cocaine and HIV infection.

A behavioural and seroprevalence study of crack cocaine users undertaken in Saint Lucia (referred to above) in 2007 found that 75 per cent of the females and 50 per cent of the males engaged in transactional sex or sex for drugs exchanges with only 11 per cent of the females and 23 per cent of the males reporting that they used condoms consistently every time they had sex. The interesting fact is that none of these women were involved in sex for drugs transactions prior to smoking crack and that the average price for penetrative vaginal or anal sex was between US$2 and US$4 — basically equal to the cost of one or two crack 'rocks'.

Now that we have an overview of the drug and HIV situation in Caribbean let's examine the relative harms associated with drug use. Basically these harms fall into two categories:

- Medical or physical harms
- Legal harms or harms created by legislation

The physical or medical harms of drug simply stated are:

- Any smoking, whether from marijuana or crack cocaine, causes tar to build up in your lungs, decreasing the lungs ability to absorb oxygen;
- Persons with a pre-disposition to mental illness may experience psychotic episodes from marijuana or crack use that are sometimes irreversible;
- Crack smoke has a detrimental effect on your teeth;
- Crack smoking effects the dopamine receptor in the brain and leads to an inability to feel pleasure except when smoking and;
- Crack smoking (or cocaine use in general) when done in combination with alcohol drinking has been attributed to a high level of heart attacks.

Granted, none of this is good but, basically, these are self-inflicted inflicted harms with little societal impact.

In terms of harms created by legislation

- Imprisonment — and all the physical and mental harms that are associated with it. In the Caribbean a person is still imprisoned for simple possession of marijuana let alone crack cocaine.
- Because it is illegal, crack, in particular, is so expensive that people are willing to do all manner of things to get more:
  - stealing anything for the next rock,
  - selling sex for the cost of a rock,
  - selling everything you own until you are homeless.
- Violence — due to its high cost and the potential for earning extraordinary amounts of money there is a culture of violence associated with crack.
- Corruption of the institutions of government and law enforcement due to the inordinate amounts of cash involved in the drug trade.

Each of the harms created by legislation would disappear if drugs were no longer illegal. There would be no inordinate profits, no terms of imprisonment, no gang warfare, no drug induced crime and, surely, no

Legalize e Drogas.

drugs for sex exchanges with its incumbent HIV-risk if cocaine users could receive their drugs as prescription medicine. If the legislative harms create more harm than good, why do we have these laws that prohibit drug use and create the environment of illegality, violence and corruption? Basically, the countries of the Caribbean — as the rest of the world — are bound by three international drug conventions:

- 1961 Single Convention on Narcotic Drugs, as amended by the 1972 Protocol;
- 1971 Convention on Psychotropic Substances; and
- 1988 Convention against Illicit Traffic in Narcotic Drugs and Psychotropic Substances.

As of the end of 2007, 183 nations are party to the first and second of the three conventions and 182 nations to the third convention. At face value, one might consider these conventions to be good and wholesome and created to save the world's people from the perniciousness of illegal drug use.

However, international drug control conventions hamper or prohibit measures that have proven effective in reducing the spread of HIV. The prohibitionist paradigm engenders policies and practices that inhibit access to care, treatment, and support. The perfect example of this is depriving injecting drug users access to clean syringes.

LACK OF HUMAN RIGHTS IN THE WAR ON DRUGS

There is no mention of human rights in any of these drug control conventions, with the exception of 1988 Convention that mentions human rights in relation to growers.

As with all international conventions, the UN Charter takes precedence. This is clearly stated in article 103. In relation to human rights, Articles 55–56 protect human rights.

Human rights abuses, perpetrated in the name of law enforcement, supply reduction or treatment programmes, include:

- mass incarceration,
- extra-judicial killings,

- coercive drug treatment, and
- death penalty for drug offences.

CREATING CRIMINALS

The conventions signed and ratified since 1961 and the laws that nation states have followed have succeeded in criminalizing two generations of persons who use drugs and are now in the process of criminalizing and incarcerating the third generation.

Do these drug laws actually work?

European experience

According to the EMCDDA the five-year trend in Europe shows a decline in the street price for cannabis, heroin, amphetamine, ecstasy and cocaine.

In fact, data from some of the high-prevalence countries suggests that cocaine and ecstasy were considerably more expensive in the late 1980s and early 1990s than they are today. 'Drug use in Europe is cheaper than ever before' the EMCDDA concludes.

US EXPERIENCE

According to the US National Drug Threat Assessment 'Despite the highest recorded level of cocaine interdiction and seizure in 2005 — the fifth consecutive record-setting increase — there have been no sustained cocaine shortages or indications of stretched supplies in domestic drug markets. These seemingly inconsistent trends suggest greater source country supply than was previously estimated.'[1]

THE CARIBBEAN

In the Caribbean we have no data as to the effectiveness of drug prohibition but the fact that one can walk in any Caribbean city, town or village and buy marijuana, crack and, now in some Caribbean states, heroin speaks to the success (or actually lack thereof) of enforcement efforts to reduce supplies of drugs.

Prevention messages that contribute to the problem

As drugs are against the law, the state, through its various enforcement organs, seems obligated not only to incarcerate drug users but to discourage all people, mostly young people, from initiating drug use. A common and popular methodology is using scare tactics to keep people from drugs. Blanket statements such as 'drugs will kill you', 'drugs will make you crazy' and 'drugs will make you drug "addicts"' are evil and demonize drug users in an effort to scare our children into not using. In the Caribbean drug addicts are given derogatory names such as 'Jumbie' and 'Zombie' two names that refer to demons or the walking dead but not humans. In an effort to keep people from using drugs we have characterized drug users as less then human. Unfortunately, this type of anti-drug message begs the question: If drug users are not human are they entitled to human rights? Are demons seen as rights holders?

Human rights and the global system of drug control

Many aspects of the global drug control system potentially contradict the human rights and judicial standards promoted in other parts of the UN system. For example, while the International Covenant on Civil and Political Rights (ICCPR) does not require the abolition of the death penalty it clearly states that the death sentence may be imposed only for the most serious crimes in accordance with the law in force at the time of the commission of the crime.[2] Nonetheless, more than 30 member states still retain the death penalty for drug law offences, clearly outside the domain of 'the most serious crimes'. It is common for police and military action that is, purportedly, aimed at tackling drug markets to involve gun battles and accounts of extra-judicial killings, and torture and detention without charge or trial are not rare. The most recent, blatant example of this was in February 2003, when, in Thailand, a violent state-sponsored 'war on drugs' resulted in the unexplained killing of more than 2,000 persons.[3] In addition, law enforcement efforts to identify, arrest and punish drug users can lead to the breach of rights to privacy, of normal standards of criminal justice process, and of proportionality in sentencing.

Campaigns to eradicate marijuana crops in the Caribbean have resulted in the aerial spraying of harmful chemicals not only on the marijuana crops but on agricultural crops. In addition, in a recent eradication exercise in St Vincent by the Regional Security System not only were the marijuana crops destroyed but the troops also knocked down 120 'shacks'. It is hard to argue against the eradication of illegal crops, but what right do the authorities have to deprive persons of their residence. Clearly, this was a violation of the human rights of those farmers and their families.

In the Caribbean the Rastafarians claim the right to use marijuana in their religious ceremonies. While every country of the Caribbean has constitutional protections in place for religious freedom, the right of the Rastafarians to worship as they please is easily abridged because they are seen as 'drug users' and, therefore, not entitled to the right to cultural self-determination.

Unintended consequences of criminal penalties

In the conventions and in most of our countries, marijuana and cocaine are considered schedule one substances. Consequently, both substances carry the same penalties. So, since crack is more profitable and easier to transport than marijuana, people are encouraged to deal in the more harmful substance. Because both substances are illegal the markets for both converge and it creates the opportunity for people purchasing marijuana to be exposed to the much more dangerous substance — cocaine.

In closing, it is important for states to develop a drug policy that is evidenced based and views each substance separately and educates the public about each substance and their relative harms. In their drug prevention messages marijuana and cocaine are lumped together as drugs and the state claim 'drugs kill' ascribes the same harms to all substances

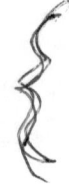

regardless of the actual harm they cause.

Drug policy should shift in focus from reducing the scale of the drug market to reducing the negative consequences of drug use. Supply reduction should not focus on punishment of growers and demand reduction should not focus on punishment of users.

NOTES

1. National Drug Intelligence Centre, US Dept. of Justice. National Drug Threat Assessment 2007: 3.
2. UN General Assembly Resolution 2200 A (XXI) of 16 December 1966. Entered into force on 23 March 1976).
3. http://www.hrw.org/campaigns/aids/2004/thai.htm

REFERENCES

Anonymous. 2005. 'Caribbean Regional Strategic Framework (CRSF) – priority areas and strategic objectives'. *PANCAP Perspective* 1 no. 1.

Calleja, J. M., N. Walker, P. Cuchi et al. 2002. 'Status of the HIV/AIDS epidemic and methods to monitor it in the Latin American and Caribbean region'. *AIDS* 16: S3-S12.

CIA Fact Book for Saint Lucia http://www.cia.gov/cia/publications/factbook/print/st.html

Cleghorn F. R., N. Jack, J. R. Murphy et al. 1995. 'HIV-1 prevalence and risk factors among sexually transmitted disease clinic attenders in Trinidad'. *AIDS* 9: 389–94.

Djumalieva D, W. Imamshah, U. Wagner et al. 2002. 'Drug use and HIV risk in Trinidad and Tobago: qualitative study'. *International Journal of STD and AIDS* 13: 633–39.

Gomez P. M., R.M. Bain, C. Major et al. 1996. 'Characteristics of HIV-infected women in The Bahamas'. *Journal of Acquired Immune Deficiency Syndrome and Human Retrovirology* 12: 400–405.

Gomez M. P., A. Kimball, H. Orlander et al. 2002. 'Epidemic crack cocaine use linked with epidemics of genital ulcer disease and heterosexual HIV infection in The Bahamas'. *Sexually Transmitted Diseases* 29: 259–264.

Hacker M.A., M. Malta, M Enriquez et al. 2005. 'Human immunodeficiency virus, AIDS, and drug consumption in South America and the Caribbean: epidemiological evidence and initiatives to curb the epidemic'. *Panamerican Journal of Public Health* 18: 3003–313.

Inciardi J.A., J. L. Syvertsen and H.L. Surratt. 2005. 'HIV/AIDS in the Caribbean Basin'. *AIDS Care* 17 (Supplement 1): S9–S25.

Montano S. M., J.L. Sanchez, Laguna-Torres et al. 2005. 'Prevalences, genotypes, and risk factors for HIV transmission in South America'. *J Aquir Immune Defic Syndr* 40: 57–64.

Walker N., J. M.Garcia-Calleja, L Heaton. et al. (n.d) *Epidemiological analysis of the quality of HIV sero-surveillance in the world: how well do we track the epidemic?*

UNAIDS Report for 2006 Fact Sheet Caribbean (Available online at: http://data.unaids.org/pub/GlobalReport/2006/200605-FS_Caribbean_en.pdf)

Chapter 3

Charting a Legal Response to HIV and AIDS and Work From the Perspective of Vulnerability

Rose-Marie Antoine

The Context of Risk and Vulnerability

The issues of HIV remain complex ones, firmly grounded in obstinate and wide-ranging problems related to social organization. Of these social problems, perhaps none is more relevant or damaging than that of enduring inequities in society, particularly gender inequities and issues of sexuality. Such inequities create groupings which are more vulnerable to HIV. Within this paradigm it is difficult for the law to regulate, or even locate and define, HIV in the legal spectrum. Nonetheless, we must construct an appropriate legal framework for HIV.

This legal programme should also re-evaluate our mindsets and prejudicial practices in more general areas. The law needs first to identify the vulnerabilities in the society which present risks in terms of HIV. Law is not merely a passive response to social problems but must embrace a proactive and participatory approach. The law cannot merely depend on a consensus in a society to shape itself. This is particularly important where it has to embrace normative and highly controversial ideas. Indeed, the law must help to shape the very society from which it springs. There is, thus, a need for a legislative strategy centred on general equality concerns. Such a strategy will more effectively embrace issues of risk in relation to HIV.

This chapter takes a two-pronged approach. First, some important conceptual questions and even philosophical questions need to be addressed. These will help to define the direction that the law must take. The more pragmatic legal concerns relating to HIV and the law in the region are then addressed.

WHY FOCUS ON HIV AT THE WORKPLACE?

This chapter focuses on HIV in the work sphere. However, the issues that arise are mirrored in the wider society, as indeed, the workplace is a microcosm of that society. The world of work occupies much of the space of our lives. In addressing access to work, treatment at work and termination of employment, we encounter many of the societal assumptions and inequities that challenge the society and create vulnerabilities to HIV. For example, issues which involve sexual orientation, gender, race and class are confronted at the workplace. The law relating to work, the labour law, is itself broad, encompassing sex work, immigration, social welfare, even constitutional and human rights.

It is instructive, too, that even legal concepts utlized in labour law, which we believe to be objective, such as the concept of reasonableness, are, in fact, based on social values. Thus, if a person is dismissed because of his or her HIV status or sexual orientation, or fails to be dismissed when he or she sexually harasses another, the question of whether that dismissal is reasonable very much depends on the values current in that society, not some neutral, extremely rational universal truth. One sees this very clearly in the BICO case[1] from Barbados, where a female magistrate referred to a male worker's actions in making remarks about his female co-workers private parts, peeping at them when they changed, etc., as merely 'ungentlemanly conduct'. That magistrate believed that such a worker should not be dismissed for such conduct.

More pragmatic concerns prioritize the choice of examining HIV at the workplace. HIV and AIDS are impacting on the most productive parts of our societies, that is, our young people and our female population. Acknowledging this leaves us with no choice but to take steps to harness the potential of our young people and women, indeed anyone, affected by AIDS. They will be given the opportunity to contribute to the society so that the society, as a whole, can benefit from their potential productivity.

Workers who do not receive treatment for HIV, or consideration in the workplace, are less likely to be able to perform at work, either because they are more ill than needs be, or because of psychological factors, thereby having hugely negative impacts on productivity. For example, more sick days, will be lost, thus directly impacting on the workplace. They are also less likely to remain at the workplace either because of direct discrimination such as with dismissal, or 'voluntary' separation. Certainly, too, they are less likely to be hired, thus depriving the workforce of potential productive elements.

Thus, the law has an active role to play in the endeavour to encourage and compel those intimately involved in the employment sphere and, indeed, the wider society, to ensure that people living with HIV form an integral and useful part of the work environment. It is in the workplace that we are likely to see the greatest impact of HIV and AIDS and that is where we must turn if we are to minimize the disastrous effects on our economies and societies.

QUESTIONING THE HUMAN RIGHTS PARADIGM IN RELATION TO HIV

The 'rights' approach to HIV has been made fashionable by the International Labour Organization (ILO) and other United Nations (UN) organizations. Thus, we typically speak of ensuring 'rights' for persons with HIV as being a part of some form of definable basket of rights. While I understand the philosophy of the human rights approach to HIV, I am somewhat cautious about the context of this approach and even whether it is the most pragmatic route. The problem is not with rights, generally. I suggest that while the rights approach is necessary, it is not sufficient in addressing HIV and AIDS and is certainly not a panacea for all ills. The rights approach should be carefully scrutinized and its limitations noted.

If we accept the premise stated above, that vulnerability to HIV is a consequence of deeper, wider vulnerabilities and inequities in the society, the question would then be: should the focus be on HIV or on broader grounds of discrimination and inequity, such as gender and race? If persons are susceptible to the disease because of certain social constructs, based on gender, etc. shouldn't the law be first addressing these social constructs? The so-called rights approach in its rudimentary form singles out the symptom and not the cause for protection. Thus, if we accept the 'rights' paradigm, it is perhaps more important to advocate 'rights' in relation to gender equality and the like and not specifically for persons with HIV.

Further, it is somewhat incongruous to be speaking of 'special interests' or rights based on HIV when most of the laws in the region do not even acknowledge such rights for other persons. Some of the human rights we are advocating for persons living with HIV are not generally available to others in the society. These include, for example, the right to employment (unfair dismissal), privacy, gender equality and sexual orientation rights. Are we, therefore, putting the cart before the horse?

Thus, the risk and vulnerability to HIV that continued stereotypical gender roles and other unequal relationships impose are not ameliorated by taking an insular, stop-gap, 'handout of rights' approach to HIV and AIDS.

Special rights – Us versus them

As HIV becomes more and more a special interests argument in the rights analysis, we should also be concerned that in our quest for these special interests, we are not underscoring difference, utilizing an 'us and them' approach. In the context of HIV, there is really only one human right that we are fighting for –– the right to equality, or to non-discrimination. We want persons living with HIV to be treated equally to other persons in society, not for the promulgation of some special human right. There is some intellectual difficulty in using these terms loosely and we need to be careful that in our language we are not making a case for difference in our quest not to be treated differently, that is, to find equality.

LOBBYING FOR RIGHTS IN THE COLLECTIVE

By arguing that a particular person with HIV has a right to A or B, such as a right to work or housing, we are, in effect, adopting an extremely narrow focus. It emphasizes a very individualistic notion of rights and ignores broader social concerns which can only really be resolved in the collective. It should be reiterated that the argument is not that HIV-positive persons should not have rights; it is that they have rights *despite* their illness and not *because of* their illness.

The danger is that we might seek to secure rights only for a minority when the disempowered majority, based on more general criteria, is left out in the cold. If we do embrace a rights approach we should consider as a strategy the impact of focusing on collective rights which accrue to the community at large rather than individualistic rights of persons living with HIV. For example, arguments are often made for the rights of persons living with HIV to health and to a healthy environment. This involves public expenditure. In this vein should we be speaking about rights to health care because of HIV, or general rights to healthcare? Given what I said before about not arguing for a special basket of rights, or if we want to address vulnerability at its source, a better strategy to emphasize the right of the public to a safe and healthy environment. Public expenditure is more likely to be utilized for conditions that benefit persons living with HIV with the understanding that if we manage to prevent HIV or AIDS then the entire community benefits. The members of a society which is deprived of adequate health and a healthy environment are more likely to be at risk of contracting HIV.

Indeed, such an individualistic conception of rights allows us to escape some of the deep social challenges that exist. For example, we need not focus too much on issues of sexual orientation if we can look instead at an individual's HIV status. Already the law is focusing on such narrow questions, asking only whether the individual worker who is HIV-positive can perform the job.[2]

In immigration questions, discussed further below, cracks in this rights-based approach are already apparent. A number of persons have approached the courts in the UK and other countries for political asylum, claiming that it is cruel and inhuman and, therefore, constitutionally untenable to deport them because they will be persecuted on account of their homosexuality. Instead of the courts viewing these cases as issues involving discrimination against a group on the ground of sexual orientation, they have produced a narrow test which gives skewed and even absurd results. This involves inquiring into and attempting to measure the 'degree' of suffering of the individual applicant, a rather different approach to emphasizing positive rights of the persons of that group.[3]

Rights secured only against the state

The rights approach is also limited in that rights are secured only against the state. This does not help if it is a private employer or a co-worker who is trampling upon a person's rights. If we are focusing on rights in the constitutional sense, we need to be careful that we are not stymied by existing constitutional limitations, discussed below. Constitutional reform may be too difficult or inaccessible, suggesting that we need to put our energies into ordinary legislation.

We need also to determine what we really mean by human rights? Rights conjure up the idea of constitutional protection. However, it may well be that the so-called rights about which we speak are located well outside of the boundaries of the Constitution. As we shall see, much of what we want to secure cannot be identified or located adequately in our constitutions. We may need to rely, more specifically, on ordinary legislation which targets issues important to the HIV phenomenon in a more pragmatic, direct way.

In many cases, what have been committed are simply legal wrongs for which the law already prescribes remedies. For example, there is no legal basis upon which a child can be denied her inheritance merely because she has been orphaned as a result of AIDS. Not only are these issues about 'rights' in the constitutional sense, but further, they relate to legal matters which often are not even contentious. In such cases, the answer is more advocacy and not more law.

Moral, ethical and religious norms underlying rights

The assumption that rights are inherently neutral, or even universal and, consequently, if one focuses on rights, one moves away from the limitations of morality and religion which often fuel gender and other inequities, is also fundamentally flawed. Rights are based on underlying moral precepts, value-laden norms which often encompass foreign notions of morality which are not necessarily grounded in our own social environments. They are, for example, usually Anglo-Saxon norms of morality.[4] Indeed, I have argued elsewhere that increasingly, the notion of rights embodied in our apparently 'home-grown' constitutions is becoming hijacked by concepts adopted wholesale from international conventions which may bear little relation to our cultural and social realities and beliefs.[5]

Curiously, in the context of gender equality and sexuality, these more 'universal', liberal ideas have failed to penetrate our constitutional interpretations and the legal psyche. This helps to explain damaging decisions such as *Girard and the St. Lucia Teachers Union v. A.G.,*[6] a case from Saint Lucia, where the courts failed to locate a right to non-discrimination on the basis of sex when unmarried school teachers were dismissed upon becoming pregnant. One of the grounds used to successfully abort any such constitutional protection was public morality. Further, the court saw the category of sex mentioned in the introduction or preamble of the Constitution as merely declaratory and not enforceable.[7]

Thus, in *Girard,* the real issue (as to whether dismissal in the particular circumstances of pregnancy could amount to discrimination), was, in effect, avoided. While the 'correctness' of the decision in terms of strict constitutional interpretation of the rule on the presumption of constitutionality could be defended, a huge question mark remains. What is the threshold for rebutting that presumption where women's rights are concerned? This was a seemingly easy case of discrimination. However, the legal response to the attempt to secure what is viewed as a fundamental right for women, supported by international norms and for which there is support in Caribbean society, was woefully inadequate.

Morality, as encapsulated in our understanding of rights, also fails to address and explain the fear which underlines the rationales presented for discrimination against persons living with HIV and against those affected by HIV.

These few examples demonstrate that the law and its agents can find ways of denying basic equality even within an apparently liberal conception of rights. This is particularly so where issues of gender and sexuality are involved, issues which speak to well-entrenched prejudices in the society.

Our notion of rights in the equality domain thus remain fairly static and cannot, without significant reorientation, address issues of HIV which depend upon more fluid concepts of rights and equality.

The insular rights approach fails, further, to acknowledge the preventative aspect of the HIV response, so that we are expected to 'give rights' only to persons who are already living with HIV.

Equality of treatment or equality of outcomes

Another concern about a simplistic rights route involves the philosophical approach to equality and non-discrimination. Rather than an expectation that everyone is to be treated in identical fashion, the 'equality of treatment' approach, it is more desirable that the justification for equality be based on an outcomes approach. This approach recognizes that persons start off from unequal stances and, therefore, differences must be treated differently. In many cases, the law actually requires that persons living with HIV be treated differently, but then demands further that there be some comparator to determine the extent of accommodation.

For example, utilizing the equality of treatment approach, the earlier cases, for example, *Chalk v USDC*[8] suggest that in dismissal cases we treat people living with HIV at the workplace exactly as we would treat other terminally ill patients, such as cancer patients. This, however, ignores the social reality of stigma and the presumptions of inequality which attach to HIV. Often, people living with HIV, as with women and girls and other minorities, may need to be treated differently in the first instance, if equality and rights are to be achieved. This is different from saying, simply, that people living with HIV should have special interests and rights. It is in this context that the 'accommodation principle' in anti-discrimination law is useful. This principle demands that the employer accommodates employees' differences which are based on some ground of discrimination, whether that difference is in relation to race, gender or sex, HIV status, etc. This is provided that such accommodation does not impose 'undue hardship' on the enterprise. The question of 'undue hardship' is of course, a question of law.

BALANCING RIGHTS IN THE HIV CONTEXT

A rights approach assumes that competing rights will be balanced. However, in a very narrow, individualistic construct of rights, when rights conflict, often the result is that we are led right back to our narrow, prejudicial assumptions. It is difficult for the rights of persons with HIV to survive the clash of value-laden rights.

Several conflicts exist in relation to rights and HIV. The right of a person with HIV to privacy conflicts with the right of the public/state/ employer to know. This right to information is often predicated on the need to prevent harm, protect public health, ensure social order, and even morality. These are broad-based rationales for abrogating rights which are even enshrined in our constitutions based on concepts of reasonableness, that is, the proviso that rights can be limited if 'reasonably required' in the wider interest of the society.

The assumption that laws, particularly rights, are neutral and can easily provide a sanctuary for people living with HIV is, therefore, suspect. The task is to put forward a broad equality and rights agenda which liberates, rather than cements, the underlying prejudices and inequities in the society.

Culture of silence

Laws which seek to prohibit discrimination or disadvantage meted out to employees with HIV must also speak to the culture of silence surrounding the disease. Thus, the law cannot merely seek to protect persons diagnosed with HIV. Such a law will fail to recognize that many potentially infected persons will refuse testing. In circumstances where confidentiality is not secured, this means that they expose themselves to the very discrimination that the law attempts to ban. Assessing vulnerabilities must also take this phenomenon into account. To counter such negative consequences, wording often used in recent laws concerned with HIV includes: that a worker 'is perceived to be' or is living with HIV.

On the other hand, the law has an important role to play in diminishing the dangerous silence which surrounds HIV. To this end, we can question the liberal precept that confidentiality as a legal principle in HIV cases is necessarily a desirable objective. Entrapping HIV with such an all-encompassing confidentiality ethic, one that goes well beyond the usual norms which attach to other medical illnesses, can indeed underscore the 'hush hush', 'unspeakable' nature of the disease leading to further prejudice and inequity.

POVERTY, CLASS, GENDER AND VULNERABILITY

While law, including non-discrimination law, does not comfortably address issues such as class, it is apparent that this is also an important aspect of our discussion on inequity and its implications for risk of contracting HIV. This is particularly important in our region where class discrimination is often linked to race and, of course, class stratification raises issues of poverty. Poverty has been demonstrated to be a factor which raises the vulnerability ranking of groups at risk of HIV.[9] Interestingly, studies have also noted the link between gender inequity and poverty,[10] making the problem of poverty an all-pervasive one which is decidedly not neutral and which cannot be ignored in constructing a legal framework for HIV. How does the law locate such persons if trapped in certain presumptions about race, class, and so on.

It is also true that the developing world is particularly vulnerable to HIV because of poverty and other financially driven problems. Thus, the issue is one that transcends individual risks and takes on broader dimensions speaking to global inequity.

On the other hand, we must be wary about certain stereotypical assumptions about vulnerable groups which are made to fit our legal and social constructs. In one telling ILO study which looked at child labour in a number of Caribbean countries, including The Bahamas and

Barbados, it was found that child prostitution was often not the result of poverty, but about young persons wanting to cultivate 'brand name lifestyles'. A sizeable proportion of middle-class children were involved.[11]

Having laid out the conceptual framework for a legal policy which can adequately address HIV and AIDS, we can turn now to examine some individual aspects of that legal programme in more detail.

CURRENT LEGAL INFRASTRUCTURE

Currently, the legal infrastructure in the region is not adequate to meet the challenges posed by what has become known as the HIV pandemic. The meagre initiatives have tended to be negative. By that, I mean that we have focussed on what may be viewed as penalizing persons with HIV or AIDS. For example, the region has been quite eager to enact legislation to authorise provisions which require notification of the disease. Several countries, including Saint Lucia, Grenada, Jamaica and Guyana[12] have notification requirements in place for public health reasons.

We have also embarked on a vigorous, and somewhat sensational, discussion to ensure that persons who deliberately infect others with HIV incur criminal liability. Our emphasis here is on punishment. For example, section 140 of the new Criminal Code of Saint Lucia makes it an offence for anyone to intentionally or recklessly infect someone else with HIV. This is, no doubt, important and just. However, such a legislative direction will do little to curb the HIV pandemic and will most likely alienate persons living with HIV. Moreover, it is improbable that there is a large percentage of persons going around searching for persons to infect. It is far more likely that there is a larger group of persons who, because they are fearful of discrimination and stigma, will fail to get tested, never know that they have the disease and infect others in that way.

Such laws and practices marginalize persons with HIV and imply an 'us and them' approach. Significantly, they are ineffective at curbing the disease or addressing its causes. It is, therefore, imperative that a large parcel of laws and policies on HIV should centre on broad issues of non-discrimination which treat with vulnerability and aim at integrating persons living with HIV into the society.

Several areas of law may be viewed as being relevant to the discussion of HIV and AIDS. They include anti-discrimination laws, unfair dismissal law, the Constitution, ordinary contract law, especially the contract of employment and implied terms therein, health and safety laws, immigration law, sick leave and benefits, unemployment/social security benefits, child labour, movement of labour legislation, disability law and practice, insurance law and judicial review.

The face of the law today with respect to HIV and employment is, however, bleak. The Bahamas is the only country, thus far, which has enacted specific legislative provisions on HIV in employment. This is in the form of a brief clause under section 6 of the Employment Act 2001 that includes HIV as one of the prohibited grounds of discrimination. The proposed Labour Code of Saint Lucia, passed in 2006, but still to be implemented, also contains a clause prohibiting discrimination on the ground of HIV. Barbados does not have specific HIV legislation, but its Industrial Relations Code of Practice, which is a non-binding but persuasive document, prohibits discrimination on the ground of HIV. Elsewhere in the region, legislative reform is still at the discussion stage.

In addition, the laws and legal practices which could compensate for this gap in HIV-specific legislation are generally lacking in the region. Innovative routes may be put forward to approach the problem. In the main, this requires creative ways of utilizing already existing laws and legal norms in order to address the relatively recent phenomenon that is HIV. For example, one may derive a right not to be discriminated against on account of one's HIV status from a broader right against discrimination. Such solutions presented to overcome the paucity of the legal framework with respect to HIV and AIDS should in no way undermine the need for new legislative policy specific to HIV and AIDS.

However, even more alarming, given the thrust of this chapter that HIV should be viewed as one component of broader social problems of inequity, is the paucity of laws on equality and non-discrimination in the region. This is particularly the case in relation to gender equality and sexual orientation. Further, because notions of equality are not well entrenched in the social consciousness, it is less likely that broad, elastic labour law legal principles, which depend on that social conscience, such as requirements for fairness in dismissals or implying fundamental terms into the contract of employment, can be easily or adequately employed to address HIV at the workplace.

In sum, with few exceptions, the region lacks (1) specific laws on HIV in employment; (2) general laws on non-discrimination; and (3) a developed jurisprudence and case law which can be read into general employment law precepts.

Discrimination as an umbrella issue in the legal programme

While many areas of law impact upon and are impacted by the issues of HIV and AIDS, one of the broadest problems that we need to address is the discrimination practised against persons because of their HIV status. Such discrimination is evident in public institutions and services, private relationships, whether in housing, rentals, or in the health services.

There are a number of reasons why anti-discrimination policies in respect of HIV are important. First: discriminatory practices because of HIV have a counter-productive effect on health and safety measures as people living with HIV are less likely to come forward to be tested and to access available treatment and other benefits. This, in turn, increases the risk of spreading the disease as it can cause infected persons to inadvertently infect others. Consequently, in the long run, more persons will be impacted. Further, as noted previously, it undermines productivity and drives away persons from the workplace.

Discrimination against people living with HIV is wide and varied and practised by both private employers and the state. Such discrimination affects not merely how one is treated at the job, but goes to the heart of job security and access to employment (hiring and firing questions). Discriminatory attitudes may also prevent employers and policy makers from introducing and implementing more sensitive and practical policies to deal with HIV at the workplace, whether these are privacy policies or practical policies of job restructuring. Discrimination thus becomes a broad umbrella term under which we can address many of the legal issues of HIV and AIDS at the workplace.

Unfortunately, there is still much ignorance and stigmatisation associated with HIV in all of the countries in the region. In Guyana, for example, it was reported that some employees refused to share sanitary facilities with infected workers and there was little respect for their privacy.[13] This suggests an underlying need for public education to change the culture surrounding HIV. The law cannot stand alone. On the one hand, the law can compel attitudinal changes. On the other, the law can reflect the realities and changes in society.

GENERAL ANTI-DISCRIMINATION PROVISIONS AS A SHIELD AGAINST HIV DISCRIMINATION

It is to be expected that where general provisions against discrimination in employment exist, that workers with HIV can look to these provisions for some assistance. However, an initial obstacle to be met is that very few countries in the region, Saint Lucia, Trinidad and Tobago and Guyana being laudable exceptions, have enacted such general anti-discrimination laws or policies.[14] In Guyana, the Prevention of Discrimination Act 1997 lays down general criteria prohibiting discrimination in employment and elsewhere. In Saint Lucia, the Equality of Opportunity and Treatment in Employment and Occupation Act 2000 prohibits discrimination and inequality in employment in broad terms.[15]

Even where such general anti-discrimination provisions exist, they do not mention HIV as a ground of discrimination. As anti-discrimination law generally depends on the grounds of discrimination being enumerated, HIV cannot be inferred easily from any of the stated grounds of discrimination unless it can be demonstrated that the protection is reasonably incidental to another stated ground. However, some grounds of discrimination which speak directly to groups most vulnerable to HIV are addressed, in particular, sex, gender and race, which is an important first step.

Where disability is put forward as a ground of discrimination as is the case in the Guyana and Saint Lucia legislation, HIV protection may be inferred if the courts adopt the approach found in many jurisdictions around the world, where discrimination on the grounds of HIV has been treated as an aspect of disability.[16] However, this route to protection would be on firmer ground if the definition of disability were to specifically include HIV.

Fear and prejudice — Medical myths and health and safety

In the case of socially excluded groups which are particularly vulnerable to HIV, the law must deal not only with the prejudices and xenophobia surrounding the group or class, but also the fear and myths surrounding the disease. Often, it is such fear that fuels the discriminatory action of an employer or co-worker toward an HIV infected employee. The employer or co-worker may be afraid that he or she, or other persons under his or her care will 'catch' the disease or that customers may believe that they will become infected because of the presence of an infected employee, thereby resulting in a loss to his business. Consequently, the legal response must take into account the medical aspect of HIV since the fear engendered by HIV stems mainly from the ignorance and myths which still surrounds the disease.

Significantly, in emphasizing the medical aspects of the issue, the courts have begun to address directly the myths and prejudices associated with HIV. This leads to questions of law such as whether the employer has the right to dismiss on grounds of safety and health where he merely suspects danger and whether an employee has a right to privacy in such a situation. The courts have insisted that it is the medical realities of HIV and not uninformed fears that will ground the legal issues.

As a first principle, courts will ascertain whether the fear of HIV is based on ignorance or prejudice or real danger and risk. Under the law, only the latter will suffice to legitimize a dismissal, a refusal to employ, or other discriminatory action taken with regard to HIV infected persons. Certain occupations are clearly riskier than others and discrimination law recognizes this. However, these are very well defined and are the exceptions rather than the rule. Case law demonstrates that health-care workers provide the most common and acceptable examples. Their employment is considered potentially risky both if they have the disease and if they are working with others who have the disease. However, even in these occupations, and particularly as knowledge of the disease increases, prohibiting someone from working because of HIV requires a high legal threshold to cross.[17] Yet, the courts have often found other ways to exploit what is essentially an health and safety argument.

For persons in employment outside of these special risky occupations, the courts have shown very little tolerance toward those who discriminate against or penalize workers with AIDS, based on fear and ignorance. In fact, these courts have argued that the law has a duty to stamp out the stigma of prejudice based on ignorance and lack of scientific data, highlighted in the case of *Hoffman v SA Airways*.[18] It is, therefore, insufficient that the employer or his customers merely believe or are fearful that they can get the disease from an employee who is HIV-positive.

Further, the law differentiates depending on the stage of the disease in order to pose effective legal solutions. Different variables, whether risk related or capacity to perform on the job, are at play. The law assumes that an employee whose immune system is severely compromised should not be treated in the same way as someone whose immune system is still healthy. Such a person in the work environment may also be at a greater health risk. The latter may also provide legal grounds from excluding persons from work or particular kinds of work.

The principle of accommodation

The principle of accommodation is a key aspect of general anti-discrimination law. The principle mandates that the employer must do all in his or her power to facilitate the particular employee in relation to that employee's 'differences' which are relevant to the ground of discrimination. So, for example, persons living with HIV should be allowed to work at home if presence at the workplace is difficult or if they prefer the privacy of home, away from inquisitive stares, questions and humiliation. The employer will also need to consider more flexible work arrangements such as job restructuring, modifying work schedules/plans and even the reassignment of duties. Similarly, the employer may need to be more lenient with regard to sick leave absences. The principle of accommodation, is, however, buttressed by an undue hardship limitation, since the employer's duty is only to reasonably accommodate.

In considering how to accommodate persons living with HIV, another principle of anti-discrimination law comes into focus. This is the comparator principle. To avoid a claim of discrimination, therefore, the employer is only required to treat the employer with HIV in similar vein to how he would treat anyone else in a similar position such as another employee with some other terminal disease.

This is not to suggest that the unique aspects of HIV, such as stigma, would be ignored. Rather, these are factored into the equation. There may be a higher burden to accommodate someone living with HIV at home, for example, because of the stigma attached.

HIV discrimination and women's vulnerabilities

Statistics demonstrate that women in the region, like elsewhere in the world, are especially vulnerable to contracting the disease.[19] This pattern means that in real terms many women are suffering from the disease or will contract the disease in the future. Women's susceptibility to HIV is due to physiological as well as to social and cultural factors.

As intimated earlier, the question of HIV and women's vulnerability to the disease is a subject intimately connected to the right of women to be free from discrimination. Special note must be taken of the way in which HIV affects women in the workplace and in the society at large.

The social and cultural factors which make women more vulnerable to HIV must be considered against the backdrop of women's general unequal status in society and, in a specific context, in employment.

Rationales for this vulnerability in the employment sphere include their unequal earning status and employment opportunities, which make them more economically dependent on men. The ILO contends that the greater the gender discrimination in societies and the lower the position of women, the more negatively they are affected by HIV.[20]

Thus, women are impacted more negatively due to both social and economic factors although we see that economic vulnerability is largely a function of the social factors. In terms of economic factors, for example, several may be noted:

(i)   Women are still less readily employed than men, despite relatively higher qualifications;

(ii) When employed, women still earn less than men for equal work: This is true both in developed and developing countries;

(iii) Women are still more unlikely to be unemployed or underemployed and found more often in forms of work which attract less pay and benefits, e.g. casual work, informal work (services whether domestic, tourism etc.), part-time employment.[21]

All of this means that women are still economically fragile and often need to rely on men for financial support. It is therefore hardly surprising that they are unable to negotiate safe sex or no sex, even when HIV is a risk.

These discriminatory phenomena are as a result of women's inferior status in society and must be confronted. In terms of law, it means that non-discrimination law should include, as a first premise, non-discriminatory pay, in the form of equal remuneration for work of equal value. Such inequity involves addressing the phenomenon of the 'feminization of casual labour' whereby women more typically fall into the lowest paying jobs, which in turn, are those in the informal sector. The agenda for non-discrimination and gender equality is therefore broad.[21]

Relationship paradigms and sexual stigmas

Women's general unequal place in society is also manifested in their relationship paradigms: whether with casual sex, commercial sex or sex in formal, ostensibly 'protected' relationships such as in marriage. Men are viewed as being in control of the sexual relationship, leading to a tendency of women to relinquish control over their bodies and sexual relations. Certain cultural stereotypes emphasize this unequal relationship: Promiscuous men are 'studs' but such women are 'loose'. To add to this, there is a high percentage of single mothers, many of whom are unemployed or underemployed [22] and a high degree of incest, mainly involving girls.

These paradigms also lead to women being more susceptible to sex work, hence making them a high risk group for HIV. Indeed, women's sexuality is seen as a commercial and / or bargaining commodity.

Women may also fall victim to more discernible patterns of discrimination when they have already contracted HIV.[23] This may be explained by cultural notions of what is appropriate sexual behaviour for women and the consequent stereotyping when women contract a sex-related disease. The UWI study showed women living with HIV suffered more discrimination in hospitals and even by female nurses. This is double jeopardy, in that there is generally more discrimination against women and, therefore, an increased likelihood for HIV, and when women are living with HIV, they suffer more discrimination.

The UWI study even found discrimination among women living with HIV. There are, for example, distinctions between the way they contracted the virus, and the way 'those women' contracted it. In reality, these are the same issues of gender inequities, stereotyping and vulnerabilities.

It is to be expected that this more pronounced discrimination for women with HIV is also played out at the workplace.

In sum, the reactions to HIV exacerbate the already detrimental paradigm in which women are exposed to various forms of discrimination and unequal treatment in society and at the workplace. We can see, therefore, that the goals of gender equality and gender empowerment have concrete implications for responding to HIV as gender inequality actually leads to women being more vulnerable to HIV.

Girl children and HIV and AIDS

Such gender inequities also spill over to problems of child labour where we find that girl children are particularly vulnerable to HIV. One reason is the higher incidence of child labour in relation to girl children, such labour often amounting to sexual exploitation and statutory rape.

Sexual orientation

HIV has long been associated with homosexuality because of the fact that when the disease first emerged as an issue in the mass media, it was identified with homosexual men. Although HIV is now a disease that affects everyone, the myth that only homosexuals are susceptible to HIV presents its own form of discrimination and vulnerability. This can lead to double discrimination on the ground of a person's sexual orientation. Persons of homosexual orientation or those perceived to be homosexual are more likely to be denied employment, fired, or otherwise discriminated against.

Sexual orientation as a ground of discrimination is also excluded both in the various constitutions and in the existing anti-discrimination legislation. Indeed, this is a controversial issue in the region. Consequently, while some persons still erroneously link HIV with homosexuality, if a person is discriminated against because of such a link, there is no specific protection which can be granted on that ground. Employers are seemingly free to dismiss or otherwise penalize persons because of their sexual orientation. It is only if such a reason can be brought under another heading of law, such as, for example, if the reason is found to be unjust under unfair dismissal law, that redress can be sought successfully. As yet, few judicial norms exist which would include sexual orientation within the more generally accepted ground of sex discrimination and the *Surrat* case, discussed below, suggests that it is not likely to be forthcoming soon. [25]

The case law in this area is particularly under-developed in the region. In Trinidad and Tobago, an initial attempt to introduce general equality legislation specifically excluded the ground of sexual orientation. When the law was not implemented by a later government, in a legal challenge, the High Court accepted that sex did not include sexual orientation and that homosexuality was against the law. This was the case of *Surrat v AG of Trinidad and Tobago*[26] where the government argued successfully against implementing the state's own law (passed by the previous party in government) which sought to introduce equality and non-discrimination, including non-discrimination on the ground of sexual orientation. On the issue of sexual orientation the court held in favour of the status quo and was clear that 'homosexuality is illegal' and could not therefore be read as part of the constitutional protection against discrimination on grounds of sex. An important element of this reasoning was that the 'unconstitutional' law banning homosexuality was regarded as preserved. This 'chicken and egg' argument failed to inquire seriously into whether such discrimination violated fundamental norms of the laws and ignored the fact that the Constitution is supposed to measure the legality of other laws and more importantly, is meant to be a dynamic instrument.[27]

THE INADEQUACY OF THE CONSTITUTION IN PROTECTING AGAINST HIV-RELATED DISCRIMINATION

A popular assumption is that our constitutions will be able to address issues relevant to HIV and AIDS. In particular, it is expected that problems such as discrimination and privacy violations may be addressed. However, for a number of reasons, our constitutions will not be particularly useful tools to address these problems. First, under the state action doctrine, our constitutions typically address only human rights violations by the state vis-à-vis the citizen. Hence, perceived encroachments of freedoms by private employers cannot be challenged successfully in the courts. This excludes a great majority of workers and people living with HIV.

Secondly, perhaps unsurprisingly, nowhere in our constitutions are the terms HIV or AIDS addressed. This means that we will have to turn to more general constitutional provisions, such as those on privacy and discrimination for assistance. Here too, we may run into difficulty. The various constitutions, of course, specifically mention both discrimination and privacy. However, neither the anti-discrimination nor the privacy provisions enshrined in these constitutions are particularly strong provisions, either in their scope or in their interpretation.

Perhaps more surprisingly, given our initial discussion of the broader social problems still evident in the society, the Constitution fails to protect adequately against discrimination on the ground of gender, sex or sexual orientation. This is partly because such grounds of discrimination are not specifically mentioned in the Constitution, or because they are mentioned only in the preamble or introductory clause to the Constitution and not in its body. The latter is the case, for example, in relation to discrimination on the ground of sex. As the decision of *Girard*[28] demonstrates, the courts have found that in such a scenario the ground of discrimination is not protected as it is not justiciable? Indeed, there is little legal authority for asserting protection against discrimination on the ground of sex. A case from Belize, *Wade v Roches*,[29] is a rare exception.

Other constitutional protections pertinent to HIV are similarly disenfranchised. Privacy, for example, is not a well established ground of constitutional redress in the Commonwealth Caribbean, partly because it is not listed specifically as a right to privacy but is described or indeed, has been interpreted more in the nature of protection from search and seizure, specifically in the home. Further, even where privacy protection is located, it is easily circumscribed in the public interest.

The discrimination provisions in the various constitutions have also been weakened by the fact that it has been held in Trinidad and Tobago that malice is required to substantiate a claim of discrimination. Notwithstanding the above constitutional obstacles, any laws purporting to make provision for or against those living with HIV must be measured against the constitution and if found to violate the constitution, may be struck down as *ultra vires*. This may be a useful tool in countering the state action doctrine and in attempting to create checks and balances for restrictive, sanction based laws on HIV and AIDS. These include laws pertaining to immigration, work-permits, notification, and so on.

Judicial review as an alternative avenue for protection

Given the inadequacies in the Constitution and the almost total absence of legislation on HIV or on discrimination, we should look carefully at judicial review strategies which have proven more generous in anti-discrimination and further, are elastic enough to encompass wide notions of justice and fairness. On the question of discrimination on grounds of race and religion in Trinidad and Tobago, judicial review has been most useful. In *Rajkumar et al v Commissioner of Police*,[30] for example, a public servant of East-Indian ethnicity who had been denied promotion used this avenue successfully. Similarly, in the case of *Mohammed Morraine (religion)*, a schoolgirl who was prevented from attending school in Muslim dress, the hijab, turned to judicial review and not constitutional litigation for redress.[31] The route of judicial review is now further enhanced because the concepts of a public authority and an administrative act are now considerably widened. This means that the act or omission complained of need not emanate solely from a body established by the state. Any organization which has a significantly 'public' role may fall prey to judicial review. Indeed, recent cases demonstrate that HIV-vulnerable groups can, therefore, expect a wider umbrella of protection extending to non-State institutions which have important public functions, including the Church, university and even the cricket authority.

UNFAIR DISMISSAL LAW TO PROTECT PEOPLE LIVING WITH HIV

In the absence of comprehensive anti-discrimination legislation, unfair dismissal legislation and practice are useful in addressing prejudicial action against those persons with HIV. However, such protection is limited and can only address one such prejudicial act, dismissing or firing someone with the virus. It is not a holistic avenue for redress and cannot, for example, prevent discrimination at the hiring stage, or make adequate provision for accommodating persons with HIV.

The thrust of the unfair dismissal law is that no employee should be dismissed from employment without a valid reason. The court or tribunal will examine the dismissal to ensure that it is reasonable and not arbitrary or, as in Trinidad and Tobago, in line with unfair industrial relations practice. The assumption here is that dismissing someone simply because he or she is HIV-positive or has AIDS is a bad reason. This, indeed, is the approach that the courts have taken in a plethora of cases. This thesis has not yet been tested in the region's courts but it is likely that we will be in sync with unfair dismissal jurisprudence from elsewhere.

In determining whether a person who is HIV-positive or has AIDS should or should not be dismissed, the important question is whether that employee has the capacity to perform the job. This means that the stage of the disease is taken into account. Where a person merely has HIV and is not a real health and safety threat to anyone, there is *no valid reason* for terminating employment.[32] This situation may be contrasted to that of a person who has a clinical diagnosis of AIDS and is weak and extremely ill to the point of incapacity. However, the notion of incapacity is to be approached in similar vein to any other sick person.

Unfair dismissal law will impose a similar duty to accommodate the person with AIDS to that under disability/ discrimination law. Thus, the employee's ability to perform will be linked to the employer's attempts to assist him in performing. Home working, for example, should be given if possible, where it will be too difficult to travel to work or where he or she will be too humiliated to work at the place of employment.

Nonetheless, as with anti-discrimination law, what is reasonable will be adjudged taking into account the undue hardship and burdens placed on the employer, although we have noted in the discussion on anti-discrimination that the courts have placed high thresholds on employers for justifying prejudicial treatment to persons with AIDS. In addition, the notion of accommodation is not identified precisely in unfair dismissal law, unlike in discrimination law, and the reasonableness concept may fall short of this standard.

A more difficult question arises where a person who has HIV has to do different types of work because of illness or has to miss many days at work. In such circumstances, is there a valid reason for dismissal? As discussed above, the question of sick leave absences will be measured against the duty to accommodate and the undue hardship placed on the employer. The law, while it imposes strict standards in relation to dismissal does not, as a blanket rule, prohibit employers from dismissing someone with HIV, if it is reasonable taking into account all of the circumstances.

A difficulty with the unfair dismissal approach is that not all countries in the region have implemented unfair dismissal legislation. A few countries, such as Barbados, Jamaica and Saint Lucia still operate under the common law doctrines of employment at will, where the employer has complete freedom to hire and fire.[33]

Issue of constructive dismissal

Even in the absence of unfair dismissal legislation, however, an employee may utilize dismissal law for protection against discriminatory treatment, on the ground of HIV. Under the common law, where the employer's conduct is such that a worker cannot be reasonably expected to continue employment, that employee may unilaterally terminate the employment and claim that he or she has been constructively dismissed and is thus entitled to compensation. The principle can easily come into play where HIV is an issue. For example, where the employer's conduct is so discriminatory or prejudicial because of the worker's HIV status, or even where the co-workers are discriminatory, thereby creating a hostile working environment which is not ameliorated by the employer, an HIV infected employee may have a good cause for action.

IMPLIED TERMS

Courts have been willing to interpret contracts of employment to encompass unwritten terms where it is accepted that such unwritten terms are obvious inclusions to the contract, albeit unexpressed. This is an expanding and dynamic jurisprudence and can give considerable protection to persons living with HIV. While our law is still playing 'catch up' with HIV issues, some progress has been made in relation to more traditional labour law concepts, with discrimination likely being viewed as violating implied terms of the contract etc. For example, the jurisprudence has expanded to embrace other issues of inequity such as sexual harassment. It is suggested that non-discrimination on the ground of HIV may be viewed as such an implied term of the contract of employment.

In addition, more familiar implied terms may be interpreted expansively to include protections relevant to people living with HIV. Thus, rights to confidentiality may be inferred as an aspect of the duty toward trust and confidence. Other useful established implied terms include 'the duty not to create a hostile environment' (including a stressful environment) and to provide a 'healthy and safe workplace'. Health here can include mental health, in this case, of the employee to confront situations where he or she is ostracized and humiliated at the workplace.

IMMIGRATION – FREE MOVEMENT OF WORKERS AND HIV

As the goal of regional integration is strengthened within CARICOM, a number of new issues pertinent to HIV and AIDS come to the fore, in particular, in relation to the free movement of labour initiative. The most obvious concerns immigration and the compulsory testing of non-nationals. Non-nationals may not only be required to test for HIV but may be denied entry into a Caribbean neighbour country, whether for work or otherwise, if he or she is HIV-positive. The question arises whether this is in sync with Caribbean integration and the free movement of labour?

Other issues to consider include the question of which government has responsibility for the care and treatment of migrant workers who have AIDS or are HIV-positive. How do we deal with different standards in different countries in the region where they concern migrant workers or non-nationals? Does this militate toward the harmonization of work benefits and worker protections, obligations, and laws on public safety?

In addition, if workers have certain benefits in their home country, can they transfer these when they migrate to another Caribbean country for work purposes, what may be referred to as the 'portability of benefits'? For example, some countries, such as Barbados, have more generous social benefits such as medical insurance, NIS benefits or even unemployment benefit. Will the person living with HIV automatically lose these upon migration? What responsibilities does the State guarding the border have toward the person wishing to enter?

It is also important to question how HIV issues intersect with immigration policy and gender concerns. Curiously, the initiative toward the free movement of skilled workers under CSME assumes that it is a male, healthy worker who will move across borders. This assumption exacerbates gender inequities in immigration, citizenship and other related laws. For example, in The Bahamas, citizenship and nationality are not gender neutral and women cannot transfer these upon marriage although a man can. Implications from this inequity include the situation that the husband who comes into the country cannot work. More general concerns include the family functions of women who move. For example, no provision may be made for children.

These are all important questions to consider as Caribbean nationals take full advantage of the more liberal trade and work arrangements within CARICOM. Groups already vulnerable to HIV will be at greater risk if these issues are not addressed.

CONSTITUTIONAL LEEWAY ON GROUNDS OF NATIONALITY

It should be noted too that both our constitutions and administrative law jurisprudence under the common law give the State much leeway in its treatment of non-nationals or non-citizens, imposing a much lower threshold for the protection of rights than for other subject areas. It is not clear that in signing onto the CSME and related initiatives that Caribbean sovereign nations have abrogated these privileges and prerogatives in any way.

Often, it is seen as legitimate legal policy to put up barriers against non-nationals because of social factors which have obvious economic implications, such as health. EU cases on movement and immigration, refugee and asylum status as they relate to HIV are instructive. Such cases are now being examined within the context of cruel and inhuman punishment, torture and a host of other 'rights' variables. Denying an asylum seeker who is HIV-positive permission to remain may result in that person being sentenced, in effect, to inhuman punishment.

In some cases, persons from countries with poor HIV health benefits are attempting to migrate to more developed countries where they can access such treatment freely. In *R (On the Application of B and H) v The London Borough of Hackney*,[34] a Jamaican national sought asylum in the UK. The basis of the application was that his removal to Jamaica would be incompatible with Article 3 of the European Convention on Human Rights, because the unavailability of adequate medical treatment in Jamaica would result in his painful death.

In another case, *D v UK*,[35] a St Kitts national who was convicted of drug possession fared better. He was diagnosed with AIDS while in custody and successfully applied for asylum. The European Court of Human Rights found that while contracting states had the right to control the entry and residence of persons, the prohibition against torture or inhuman or degrading treatment or punishment under Article 3 was an absolute one, which applied regardless of the conduct of the individual concerned (to whom we will refer as D) and had to be respected when a state was considering an expulsion. Article 3 could apply to a situation which did not directly or indirectly concern the responsibilities of the public authorities. Withdrawal of the care, support and treatment D was currently receiving in the UK would have serious consequences for him, and, while the conditions in St Kitts did not themselves breach the standards demanded by Article 3, D's removal there would expose him to a real risk that he would die in distressing circumstances, which would amount to inhuman treatment contrary to Article 3. Although released alien prisoners did not normally have the right to remain so as to continue to received medical or welfare services, D's case was exceptional and involved compelling humanitarian factors.

However, the threshold to establish likelihood of inhumane treatment is high and most applicants fail.[36]

We are also beginning to see artificial arguments on rights when, really, the issue is about dollars and cents or, indeed, prejudice. However, constitutional 'rights' jurisprudence is being used for justification of these decisions. What this means is that there is, in essence, a whittling away or watering down of the relevant rights principle. One case suggested, for example, that the fact that the HIV person who was also homosexual lived 'in secret' meant that he did not need the protection on grounds of sex orientation.[37] The court was also concerned about the burden to be imposed on a host state.

It is apparent that the question of risk and vulnerability is applicable not only on an individual level, but speaks also to the vulnerabilities of small, poor, developing states such as those in the region. The issues of HIV and AIDS, considered particularly in the context of immigration and asylum, highlights the imbalances between rich and poor nations.

COMPULSORY TESTING AND PRIVACY

As yet in the region, there is no definite legal position on compulsory testing for HIV. The exception is in relation to immigration. Further, insurance companies will require such testing and many workplaces require or provide insurance. This presents interesting dilemmas. Should insurance companies be prohibited from requiring compulsory testing? Should they be required to protect any information on HIV from disclosure? Should insurance companies be prohibited from refusing coverage to persons living with AIDS, particularly where insurance coverage is required for the person to get the job? The well-known doctor-patient privilege of confidentiality appears easily subjugated in this context.

The issue of compulsory testing clearly invokes rights to privacy. However, we have already seen that the right is not adequately protected under the constitutions. Further, neither do labour laws nor other laws address any abuses in this context. As a general principle, since HIV involves complex social issues, there must be a balancing of conflicting rights, such as individual privacy rights versus public safety; confidentiality versus freedom of speech or the right to information. Such rights can easily succumb to the public interest or meet the usual constitutional threshold of justification in a free and democratic society.

We have noted previously that there is a 'culture of silence' surrounding HIV. This has implications for privacy, strengthening the need for privacy protection and assurances.

The cases on privacy, compulsory testing and HIV are inconsistent as is the legislation from around the world. On the one hand, the insurance company is in the business of assessing risk and HIV is just another such risk (and there is a much higher likelihood of death). On the other, there is the argument that persons living with HIV are not treated in the same manner as other persons with terminal illnesses such as cancer. It is to be noted, as an alternative approach, that the route to protection on the ground of HIV under the American Disability Act prohibits denial of employment on the ground of projected high insurance, medical, health care costs in the future.

Compulsory testing with a view to excluding persons living with HIV clearly exacerbates the vulnerabilities of those groups already at risk.

CONCLUSION

In charting a legal response to HIV and AIDS in employment, taking into account the question of existing vulnerabilities and risks, the law must first address gaps in relation to broad areas of inequity which fuel such vulnerabilities. The legal framework must also speak directly to protection of persons living with HIV and those at risk of contracting the disease. This should encompass specific legislation on discrimination, contextualizing existing employment law norms and generally infusing ideas central to HIV policy into the law, both domestic law and laws which will cross Commonwealth Caribbean borders.

NOTES

1. *Jones v Bico* (unreported) Magistrate Court, Barbados, decided February 16, 1995, affirmed in *Bico Ltd v Jones*, No. 3 of 1995, decided August 2, 1996, C.A. Barbados); (1996) 53 WIR 51.
2. See, e.g. *Chalk v USDC*, (CA) 840 F. 2nd 701, 1988.
3. See, e.g. *RG (Colombia) v Secretary of State for the Home Department* C5/2005/0977 [2006] EWCA Civ 57: 'However, I must assess the risk to the appellant on return that he will be targeted as a homosexual. Such risk must be a real risk to this appellant and not merely a probability. Simply because he is a member of a social group, it does not mean that he will necessarily be ill-treated or persecuted. The appellant is not suffering from AIDS and he does not have to draw attention to himself and his lifestyle as a gay man, consequently I find that whilst a possibility

exists that he may be ill-treated there is no real risk that it is likely to happen if he takes one or two elementary precautions.' Ibid. Para 7.

4. Rights theory is grounded in the naturalist school of legal thought which emphasized morals in the law.

5. Nowhere is this more apparent than in the constitutional jurisprudence surrounding the death penalty issue. See, e.g. Rose-Marie Antoine, *Commonwealth Caribbean Law and Legal Systems*. 2nd ed. (UK: Routledge-Cavendish, 2007).

6. (Unreported) No 371 of 1985, decided December 17, 1986 (Saint Lucia HC). See also the appeal judgment: (Unreported) Civil Appeals Ns 12 and 13 of 1986, 25 January, Court of Appeal, Saint Lucia.

7. The court also relied on the general principle of a presumption of constitutionality finding, consequently, that the relevant statute, regulation 23(3) of the Teaching Service Commission Regulations, was not in contravention with the Saint Lucia Constitution. See also *Surratt v AG of Trinidad and Tobago* TT 2004 HC 37, discussed below.

8. (CA) 840 F. 2nd 701, 1988.

9. See J.L Peterson and O.A. Grinstead. 'Correlates of HIV risk behaviours in black and white San Francisco heterosexuals: The population-based AIDS in multiethnic neighborhoods (AMEN) study.' *Ethnicity and Disease,* 2 (1992): 361–70; C. Harcourt, and B. Donovan, 'The Many Faces of sex work.' *Sexually Transmitted Infections,* 81 (2005): 201–206.

10. Marilyn Carr and Martha Alter Chen, *Globalisation and the Informal Economy: How Global Trade and Investment Impact on the Working Poor*. (Sussex: Institute of Development Studies. 2001).

11. L. Dunn, *Child Labour Study* (ILO, 2000).

12. For example, under *Notification of Diseases* Acts.

13. Information taken from an interview in Georgetown, Guyana, 2001 done by Rose Cadogan with the Minister of Labour of Guyana, for a Caribbean regional Discrimination Study carried out by the present author as ILO consultant.

14. The 1992 CARICOM Report recommended such laws for the region and this was accepted by the Heads of Government in 1992 and a Model Law subsequently drafted. See R. M. B. Antoine, *The CARICOM Harmonisation of Labour Laws Report* (Georgetown, Guyana: CARICOM Secretariat, 1992).

15. See also the Equality of Opportunity Act 2000 in Trinidad and Tobago which suffered a constitutional hurdle and which the Privy Council ruled must be implemented.

16. Either through case law or statute. See, for example, the American Disability Act of the US, 1992, (ADA).

17. See, e.g. *Couture v. Belle Bonfils Memorial Blood Center*, 151 Fed. Appx. 685, where the court found no discrimination when an employer who felt 'uncomfortable' that the applicant who was HIV-positive, was training for a doctor-technician position, was reassigned to a position not involving blood work. The court concluded that

Couture had suffered no adverse employment action when he was reassigned from the donor technician position to the product management technician position. See also the case of *Taylor v Condoleeza Rice* [2005] WL 913221, where the court accepted the argument that the State Department could refuse an HIV-positive applicant employment in a diplomatic post on the ground that he would not be able to satisfy a test of 'worldwide availability' for work.

18. 20 ILLR 63.
19. The ILO estimates that 60 per cent of new AIDS patients are women and the numbers are growing, 'Women, Girls, HIV/AIDS and the World of Work' ILO/AIDS Brief, Geneva, December 2004, p.1.
20. Ibid, quoting from the ILO Code of Practice.
21. Carr and Chen, *Globalisation and the Informal Economy.*
22. Equal remuneration demands that comparisons be made between women's work and men's work in real terms, using objective criteria. What is labeled as 'women's work' is typically undervalued. Such comparisons should, therefore, be done not only in relation to identical jobs between men and women, but also similar jobs in terms of effort and skill, even if cross-sector jobs.
23. In Barbados – 37 per cent, S. Adomakah and J. Sutherland. *HIV/AIDS Related Stigma, Discrimination and Denial – Overview of Key Findings from a Baseline Review of Forms, Context and Consequences in Barbados* (Trinidad: UWI, Cave Hill, 2002).
24. The latter is based on research findings by the University of the West-Indies. Adomakah and Sutherland, ibid.
25. Cf *Selgado v. Attorney General et al* BZ 2004 SC 7.
26. TT 2004 HC 37.
27. TT 2004 HC. … homosexual acts even between consenting male adults is still a criminal offence carrying serious penal consequences... at the time of the Independence Constitution of Trinidad and Tobago (1962) ….the Offences Against the Persons Act was an existing law which was preserved even if inconsistent with the Constitution … the framers of the Constitution … would have been aware that, buggery was a serious criminal offence by virtue of an existing law and therefore, they could not have intended to expand the prohibition of discrimination on the basis of sex to include sexual orientation when homosexuality was, after all, a criminal offence.' (Para 65). A rare glimmer of hope was seen in the Belize case of *Selgado v AG of Belize BZ*, above, n. 25.
28. *Girard v AG of St Lucia*, discussed above, n.3.
29. Civ Appeal No 5 of 2004, decided March 9, 2005.
30. (Unreported) No. 945 of 1998 (H.C.) Trinidad and Tobago, decided October 26, 1999, (Lucky, J.).
31. (1995) 49 WIR 371. Judicial review was also the avenue in the case of *Selgado.*
32. For example, in the *Chalk case,* a teacher had AIDS but his duties were not affected by this handicap. He was well qualified to continue to perform the job.

33. There have been some case law deviations from this in Jamaica and Barbados.
34. [2003] EWHC 1654 (ADMIN).
35. (1997) 24 E.H.R.R. 423.
36. See, e.g. *N v. Secretary of State for the Home Department (Terrence Higgins Trust intervening)*[2005] UKHL 31: 'article 3 of the Convention did not impose an obligation on a contracting state to provide aliens indefinitely with medical treatment which was unavailable in their home countries, even if the absence of such treatment would significantly shorten their lives; that article 3 could be extended to apply only in very exceptional circumstances . . .that N's present state of health was not critical and she could live for many decades with the right treatment, and she was fit to travel; that therefore her case was distinguishable from that of a person whose illness had reached its terminal stage so that he was beyond the reach of medical treatment and was unfit to travel; that N's case was no different from that of many AIDS sufferers who arrived in the United Kingdom from countries where medical treatment for AIDS was not available or was not of the standard freely available in the United Kingdom …' Ibid, paras. 11–19, 23–25, 30–36, 48–55, 6271, 80–81, 86–99).
37. *RG (Colombia) v Secretary of State for the Home Department.*

CHAPTER 4
SOCIAL EXCLUSION, CITIZENSHIP AND RIGHTS
Grappling with Vulnerability in the Epidemic of HIV

ROBERT CARR

Almost universally...the epidemic has disproportionately affected individuals and communities who are marginalized or discriminated against for reasons of sex, age, ethnicity, race, sexuality, economic status, and cultural, religious or political affiliation.
UNAIDS

[Across the globe] hundreds of millions of new urbanites must subdivide the peripheral economic niches of personal service, casual labour, street vending, rag picking, begging and crime. This outcast proletariat ... is a mass of humanity structurally and biologically redundant to global accumulation and the corporate matrix.
MIKE DAVIS

The need [for recognition] is one of the driving forces behind nationalist movements in politics. ... Due recognition is not just a courtesy we owe people. It is a vital human need.
CHARLES TAYLOR

A nation's greatness is measured by how it treats its weakest members.
MAHATMA GHANDI

PARAMETERS AND BEGINNINGS

As in most countries of the world where HIV and AIDS are concerns, the initial response in the Caribbean was managed by doctors and institutionalized in ministries of health, which focussed on risk reduction (prevention) and impact mediation (treatment). Further, what became increasingly clear and important, if still controversial, were the distinctions between AIDS as a medical condition requiring antiretroviral treatment, and HIV as an as yet incurable and panic-inducing sexually transmitted infection. Nevertheless, research shows that after more than 20 years of responding to HIV and AIDS, the Caribbean remains the region with the second highest infection rates among the general population (UNAIDS 2007).[1] While countries, such as Haiti, have experienced a decline in average prevalence rates, for most, progress has been measured only in terms of rates that have stabilized over time (CAREC 2007).[2] This means that success in HIV prevention is marked by increases in condom sales, and other proxy measures for changes in behaviour. Some countries have also relied on the results from Knowledge, Attitudes and Practices surveys (KAPs) both of the general population, but also among groups considered 'high risk' such as taxi drivers, informal commercial importers, and adolescents or, more infrequently, sex workers or men who have sex with men (CAREC 2004).[3] Notwithstanding the use of these markers, the general picture is worrying. Even where KAPs show high levels of knowledge, and where qualitative research shows that people know HIV is a risk, infection rates have not been brought down. To understand why this is so requires digging deeper into issues of human interaction and sexual exchanges, which points to the limits of disciplines such as psychology, particularly in relation to the psychology of behaviour change, which had hitherto made strong claims to truth, for example behaviour predictability based on increased knowledge.

In recognition of the fact that many traditional approaches and theories have proven inadequate to the task, the Joint United Nations Programme on HIV/AIDS (UNAIDS), the intergovernmental agency charged with guiding the global response, began looking more deeply into the complexity of country and population dynamics. A critical objective was to understand why certain groups who were already cast out as society's pariahs — whether in Eastern Europe, the Caribbean, Asia, or more controversially, Africa[4] — demonstrated higher than average infection rates. The analysis was made against the backdrop of famous if unevenly documented success stories, such as those of Uganda, Kenya, Zimbabwe,

Thailand, Cambodia, and South India, as well as the turnaround in infection rates among white, middle-class gay men who first demanded the attention of the global media and the Centres for Disease Control (CDC) as men infected with 'Gay Related Immune Deficiency' (GRID), in the 1980s United States. That introspection resulted in the *UNAIDS Policy Position Paper: Intensifying HIV Prevention* (2005), the *UNAIDS Action Plan on Intensifying HIV Prevention 2006–2007* (2007) and the *UNAIDS Practical Guidelines for Intensifying HIV Prevention Policy Guidelines* (2007). There, UNAIDS identifies three pillars — risk, impact, and vulnerability — as the core 'drivers' of the HIV epidemic. The analysis raises questions about structural factors related to social exclusion and marginalisation, as well as impact, and the consequences of both on those affected and infected by HIV and AIDS. It is with this last pillar — vulnerability — in mind that this chapter is written. I focus on vulnerability as it is the element in the model that is new to the Caribbean, although, in context, it is as old as the Caribbean encounter with Europe.

In the Caribbean, as elsewhere, it is necessary to identify the reasons that groups who are already marginalized, and in some cases criminalized, consistently show higher levels of HIV infection. The questions at the core of this investigation are whether the concentrated epidemics among these groups mean higher failure rates on the part of programmers to understand how to respond to the spread of HIV among them, and what role vulnerability plays in the equation. In this process, I wish to delve into what vulnerability means not as an abstraction — that has its own debates — but more as a concrete phenomenon. In this regard, I will examine it in relation to the way we speak about sex workers as one particular marginalized group, and what that tells us about our ideas about purity and danger. I will also examine how a particular set of representations of the members of this group becomes emblematic of our discourses on imagined communities and nationalism.

Wrestling with the concept of vulnerability in the context of the spread of HIV in the Caribbean means drawing on issues from two distinct, and equally complex, worlds. In one, there is a rich mosaic of Caribbean people living in poverty and subject to inequality and social exclusion.

They make moment to moment sexual decisions within complex personal and structural contexts of morality and (mal)functioning societal institutions, all the while struggling with issues of risk. In the other, removed from the streets of Caribbean cities, in meeting rooms in developing and developed countries alike, technical professionals are developing, manipulating and applying theoretical frameworks and institutional policies that police what is viable — what can be included, spoken, allowed — in nationally and regionally funded programmes.

To better understand the dynamics of the sexual exchanges in the Caribbean within which HIV is nested requires bridging these two worlds. To do this requires, in turn, that one dives into the wreckage of Caribbean history, sociology, political economics, jurisprudence — disciplines, which when worlded, are far from their *doppelgangers* in technical meeting rooms, university hallways, and government policy documents. To date, these dynamics have not been visible. Instead what has happened has been a marriage of biomedical approaches to psychology that has gained hegemony in the responses to HIV. The task now is to speak back to the empire created by that marriage and ask questions from the impolite and unruly realities of everyday life, that may help us to unmask the realities of these 'MARP's[5] — those socially excluded family outcasts, like gay and bisexual men and sex workers, who are nevertheless historically woven into the warp and woof of Caribbean societies.

In what follows, I want to explore 'vulnerability' in the Caribbean context, with a focus on those groups experiencing concentrated epidemics, in particular sex workers, and the way that their humanity is debated among the local elite, in the name of establishing social order and justice. In order to contextualize this exploration, we first have to appreciate some of the ways in which our present is embedded in our history, both our colonial past and our post-independence present. Throughout I will try to trace, in the short space allowed, the thread of the notions of justice and the social pact between the leadership, the citizenry, and those on whose exclusion citizenship is defined. In closing, we can look at a debate between the leadership and a local intellectual over sex work in Barbados, and a similar implicit debate over sex work in Jamaica. These debates, as we will see, were debates using the media as a forum for 'nation-building' and drawing the boundaries among and between people and citizens, debates sparked by stymied attempts to address human rights in the context of reducing vulnerability of sex workers to HIV. At stake, I will argue, is a fundamental challenge of governance and the logic of the modern Caribbean state, a logic that will come to question founding principles in the Enlightenment of Europe, minority rights, and the place of individual freedoms.

UNPACKING CARIBBEAN VULNERABILITIES

From the establishment of Caribbean societies through to Independence, modernity, enlightenment, and individual rights were reserved for the European elite; the political and legislative frameworks, the education system, and the teachings of the religious sector reflected that. Marronage notwithstanding, domination and exploitation by an elite was the natural order, sanctioned by religion as by the administrative structures of the colonies. The Independence movements were based on the principles that each person, regardless of skin colour and economic circumstance, deserved equal and full citizenship.[6] The basic principles in the charter of human rights — right to life, right to free association, right to freedom from torture, the right to speak, and so on — are in fact central to our most fundamental beliefs about the obligation of the state and the nation to the citizen in the Caribbean. Each of us deserves 'respect'.

Yet, while we hold to the fundamental belief in respect, we accept the routine violation of this right as part of everyday life. The protection and value of children is important here as a cultural norm — our reliance on corporal punishment notwithstanding. Yet this reliance points to our own ambivalence. On one hand we believe children have the right to be free from physical abuse (torture) yet we also believe that beating children is good for them.[7]

What this ambivalence suggests is that on the one hand we appreciate the ideals of rights and freedoms traditional to liberal democracies, but on the other we are blind to the ways in which we have internalized, and then in turn institutionalized, social norms that work to preserve colonial regimes and which are in conflict with those ideals. This ambivalence comes back when we look at issues like respecting diversity, minority and individual rights — issues at the core of reducing stigma and discrimination against people living with HIV, for example, or providing safe spaces, or safe societies for youth from slum communities, children living with HIV, prisoners, sex workers, or men who have sex with men.

One of the benefits of using the prism of vulnerability is that it reveals linkages between our mosaic of HIV epidemics, what we observe when we research patterns of Caribbean sexual behaviour, and our history. Grappling with vulnerability also requires us to look at the challenges we know we have in our institutions — our public education systems, our health systems, our judicial and security systems, and so on. It also asks us to understand how these systems are all linked to our expectations and the choices we make that constitute Caribbean cultural norms and what is considered inimical to these norms. These choices include our gender and power behaviour which, then, also shows up in our sexual behaviour, in our behaviour labelled 'crime', in our performance in the school system, and many other behaviours labelled in different ways. Grappling with vulnerability allows us to recognize the role(s) that our embeddedness in social, security and economic systems plays in setting the stage for our behaviour. This embeddedness also points to the role played by the breach of citizenship rights in fuelling the epidemic, linking effective governance and respect for human rights to reducing structural vulnerability to HIV. We come back to the idea that HIV is a disease of inequality, and expresses itself most intensely where inequality is entrenched.

EXPLORING CARIBBEAN MODELS OF GOVERNANCE AND SOCIAL EXCLUSION THROUGH THE LENS OF SUBALTERN STUDIES

The work of the Subaltern Studies Group — and more famously, Gayatri Spivak's 'Can the Subaltern Speak' (1988)[8] — was an historic intervention in understanding nationalism's relationship to the underclasses created by colonialism and the link between the systems created by that colonialism and nationalist movements, at least in the British Empire. Like Partha Chatterjee's *The Nation and Its Fragments* (1993)[9] these critiques gave rise to a powerful set of debates on key issues of how we read agency and represent the marginalized or excluded — the vulnerable — in understanding post-colonial social processes with an interest in justice, and out of many, becoming one people. Spivak's intervention in bringing subaltern studies to the attention of the West, and from there the wider world, was all the more powerful because it fuelled an internal dialogue over the terms on which nationalism had constituted the relationship of the state to the nation between the fathers of Independence and their successors among the post-colonial intelligentsia.

The South Asian Subaltern Studies project thus raises critical questions for understanding vulnerability in Caribbean contexts. It triggers us to ask: how is citizenship constituted? What is the relationship of that constitution to power, its domestic history and dynamic? What does this say about the complexity of the social pact subtended by the rhetoric of the elite — government and private sector — invoked at election time, or embodied in the behaviour of social and political institutions?

Over the decades of the twentieth century, the Creole elite that inherited state power from the colonial masters, in partnership with a mass democratic base, seemed the appropriate and inevitable repository of 'progress', understood as the guarantor of ever greater justice and security.[10] Subaltern studies in a Caribbean context asks to what extent nationalist movements dismantled, or simply inherited, colonial structures of oppression from which the Creole elite were exempt. This is the point made by Bogues (2002), Obika Grey (2002), and cultural analysts like Carolyn Cooper (2004); however, there is a strong debate now on the extent to which the 'counter' elite structures and philosophies reproduce the brutal authoritarianism of the elite apparatuses.[11] What makes the stakes of the pact between the elite and the masses so high are promises of inclusion over exclusion, and struggles over power and legitimacy, definitions of nation, and, fundamentally, overdevelopment and expanded access to resources and choices as freedom.[12] It is this context that makes it possible in traditional HIV programming for the debate on law, ethics and human rights to take place. Accordingly, it provides a framework for the push for reform of legislative and policy structures towards more enlightened approaches, often more consonant with public health than the status quo, and which pave the way, broadly, for more just societies. At the same time, however, there is an absence of respect for individual rights, and a deep ambivalence among the public — mass and elite alike — regarding whether 'progress for the nation' means an increasingly tolerant society, and whether sex workers, gay men, or drug users even have rights. Thus, the decriminalization of sex work, like that of consensual sexual acts between adult men, while a cornerstone of addressing the vulnerability for those who sell or buy sex, remains *verboten*.

At the heart of the political struggle over whether progress means tolerance are the exponents of religious strictures which define the public-political universe in which these issues are debated. The public sphere, understood under democratic regimes as the space in which ideas of progress, national belonging, public good and citizenship rights are debated, is both framed and policed by contentious faith-based discussions managed by the elites in dialogue with the mass base. Jamaican Prime Minister Bruce Golding's adamant claims on the BBC television programme HARDtalk that no gay man would be welcome in his Cabinet, combined with his appeal to Christian virtues, is a clear example of this, topped only by the accolades he received from his mass base in Jamaica.[13] In this situation, poor attempts at biblical exegesis substitute for debates on the ethics of minority rights.

The role of the church in providing education to newly-freed slaves — including the use of religious primers and hymnals as reading texts and the link, still often unbroken, between churches and the public and private education system — means that the ideas of the world inculcated in the public psyche always come back to religious fundaments, themselves imported from Europe or the United States. Discussions about the appropriate response to the presence in our societies of sex workers, people who use drugs, gay and bisexual men, and so on, often flounder on these beliefs, with hostile repudiations of human rights for such

Caribbean citizens both as individuals and as groups. This refusal of basic rights and assertion of the importance of rescinding such rights are somehow constructed as deeply 'Caribbean'. Progress as tolerance for the individual comes to be seen as inimical to the Caribbean psyche and its own 'natural' cum 'national' identity.

As we move deeper into the twenty-first century, despite being embedded in larger, global multi-state and post-state structures in which Enlightenment ideals and individual liberty are seen as fundamental to neoliberal capitalism under globalisation, Caribbean societies respond to civil rights as alien to a 'natural' culture and national identity to which the leadership clings. Human rights, previously central to the abolition of slavery and to anti-racist socio-political and legislative movements such as anti-colonialism, become a sign of our Caribbean world losing its way.

The sexual economy of the Caribbean is deeply embedded in this environment, as the analyses of Hilary Beckles (1999) and Kamala Kempadoo (2004) have shown, and it is this environment in which multiple and overlapping HIV epidemics are thriving.[14] One area where this is most clearly played out is that of the sex work. Sex work has long been an important feature of Caribbean life. This has taken several forms, from the letting of female slaves to visitors to the plantation, to the privileging of certain non-white women where colour (black versus mulatta vs quadroon) and status (bound versus free) determined a woman's value in plantation sexual economies. This sexual exchange and control of women's bodies have been central to the underside of the social system. Yet, as has been demonstrated by the offence expressed by Lady Nugent and other travellers of her ilk to the West Indies, it was always framed by shame. The role of the media as a public sphere in which debates are managed and controlled in Caribbean societies and which structure one sphere in which Caribbean national and regional communities imagine themselves will provide important parameters.

Subalternity and citizenship — Framing sex work in the Barbados and Jamaica print media

Benedict Anderson's *Imagined Communities* (1991) opens with an extended analysis of the role of communication in creating and cohering communities, with the necessary complement of outsiders and barbarians. In mediaeval Western Europe, as much as in the Islamic and Chinese traditions, communication shaped the culture's understanding of the place of its people in the wider universe through a culture of writing. This role for communication, Anderson argues, continued with the emergence of the modern nation state, even if the mechanism changed from ancient elite texts to modern mass media (11–36).[15] With the coming of capitalism, he argues, print media emerged to bind the people as a nation based on the creation of 'common' values, even where, subsequently, that value was premised on the right to disagreement and the freedom to speak.

One school of thought in communication and media studies would argue that the ownership of the media, especially under media monopolies, sets the structure for the content of the media by how the world or nation is framed and by its editorial policies. Audience studies, a subdiscipline of communication studies, tells us that readers, in turn, make their own meanings in a complex mix of resistance to, and compliance with, the media content that they consume. For the purposes of this brief analysis of media coverage of female sex work in Barbados and Jamaica, undertaken below, the key theoretical references are framing, agenda setting and priming. Intimately interconnected, these theories argue that the media sets the terms on which debates are waged, and sets the 'frames' for the discussion. By the repeated use of certain loaded words and images, the media conditions the consuming public to read with or against the grain of a terrain already primed by prior editorial and journalistic policies, positions taken by the elite and by editorial decisions about how those positions should be understood.[16] As Chong and Druckman (2007) write:

> virtually all public debates [in the mass media] involve competition
> between contending parties to establish the meaning and

interpretation of issues. When citizens engage an issue — be it social security, foreign aid, a hate-group rally, affirmative action, or the use of public funds for art — they must grapple with opposing frames that are intended by opinion leaders to influence public preferences (100).[17]

Van Gorp (2007) argues that the framing process is also, inevitably, embedded in cultures, and that we also have to understand the role that power is playing, and so examine 'framing processes within wider political and social contexts' (61). Entman (2007) also reminds us that within all these debates is an un- or ill-theorized notion of power that is missing, and that he proposes to organize under the rubric of 'bias' (163). He defines content bias operationally as 'consistent patterns in the framing of mediated communication that promote the influence of one side in conflicts over the use of government power' (166).[18]

I want to look at examples of coverage of debates in two important national newspapers over who sex workers are and what is their place in the national framework, and the appropriate role of government and other elites in defining and securing the nation. The first is the Barbados daily the *Nation*, and second is the Jamaica *Gleaner*. These brief forays analysing the way sex workers and sex work are framed will provide an opportunity for us to delve more deeply into the analysis of the implications of addressing structural vulnerability. In each case, the text is dialogic, and reflects deeply conflicted reactions to the central challenge — the humanity of women who sell sex. It is also important because the national debates that take place in the pages of these newspapers are, in part, a reflection of the attempts by national HIV control programmes to stimulate national debate to address structural drivers of the epidemic through policy and legislative reform. In this case, the structural driver is the underground nature of sex work and subsequent difficulties in attaining 100 per cent condom use among sex workers and their clients. As we shall see, these attempts to address rights-based and public health policy frameworks founded on the principles of the rational, secular state, with individual rights and tolerance extrapolated from the Enlightenment, run afoul of the religious framework embedded into Caribbean cultural nationalism at the moment of Emancipation and after as the basis for ethics and therefore the law and justice. Tracy Robinson's chapter shows that while repressive laws are seen as holdovers from the British colonial era, in fact, modern day legislative reform has resisted the ideas of individual freedoms and human rights as the basis of progress, creating crimes and criminals at the end of the twentieth century where none existed before (Robinson, 5).

The *Nation*

The arrival of the World Cup Cricket (WCC) competition in the Caribbean brought with it debates in the media about the management of Caribbean territorial boundaries, rethinking regulations, economic opportunities, and the movement of people between sovereign Caribbean states. In anticipation of the WCC, many among the elite saw the occasion as an important opportunity to move agendas. Such was the context for the Minister of Health of Antigua and Barbuda, when, at a regional health ministers meeting in Barbados, he raised the possibility of legalizing sex work. This set off a fire-storm in Barbados.

One story, with a headline 'Prostitution "not an option"' reported on a press briefing by the minister of state in the Barbados Prime Minister's Office (September 13, 2006).[20] The article begins with a categorical statement: 'Government has emphatically said no to legalizing prostitution for World Cup Barbados 2007 or thereafter.' The combination of attributes signalling a univocality of the government elite — the minister of state, his role in the Prime Minister's Cabinet, his speaking on behalf of the entire government — is reinforced by the statement that the government called the press conference for the explicit reason of 'dispel[ling] rumours that "the registration and licensing of prostitutes was part and parcel of the marketing package of World Cup 2007".'

The minister of state's words are clearly a counter-frame to the framing of sex work as work. This frame that has been promoted by national and global sex work organizations and advocates in an attempt to set the discussion of sex work on the path of the humanity of sex workers and their right to work as consenting adults selling a skill (here the skill is good sexual services) to another consenting adult. In this frame, sex workers are business people and workers, and as such deserve workers' rights. Taken further, this approach leads to (sometimes problematic) discussions about 'regulation' of 'the market' including health checks for sexually transmitted infections and policies of 100 per cent condom use. This approach frames the issue squarely as a matter of the rights of workers, the freedom of the marketplace, of sellers and buyers/consumers, and a matter of public health.

For the Barbados minister of state in the Prime Minister's Office, however, the purpose of the press conference is to reframe the issue away from marketing packages for a tourism boom, attributed to the Antiguan health minister. The terms on which he counterframes the debate are important: an issue of 'public morals' that is the proper jurisdiction of the Royal Barbados Police Force. The minister then inflects this affirmation of the role of the state in policing sin by linking sex work to transatlantic slavery, a foundational moment in Caribbean national history. 'I would go on to suggest that Government' he states, 'does not see the matter of trading in human flesh as legitimate sectoral activity or some specialized industry.'

Framing 'sex work' as 'human trafficking' targets especially sex workers who rely on mobility — if we refer to the frame of sex work as labour to access better markets as part of their own financial planning. For this, the minister is also clear that 'anyone coming to the island to engage in prostitution would be arrested.' In a context where the free movement of people within a Common Caribbean Market is agreed as urgently needed to take advantage of the opportunities presented by the WCC, sex workers are exempted from the free movement of labour towards which the regional market reforms aim. Moreover, this rejection of the framing of sex work as work is tied to the historical role the ruling party intends for the Barbadian nation, with metaphors rife with the romanticism and social exclusions of Creole nationalist rhetoric based on

Democratic Parliamentarianism: "'Barbados will be left with a glorious legacy," he stated, "and to decriminalize prostitution would not be the kind of legacy the Government wants….'" The statement clearly frames sex workers as outside the national borders as people, as citizens and as workers.

While the language of this battle over framing is absolute in its terms, the minister stops just short of a Thai-style war on the marginalized: 'We have to lament the fact that the police, as diligent as they are and as stretched as they are…have far more sinister issues to deal with.' The double-play of this frame, which stops just short of sending the police to the night streets of Bridgetown, is not lost on the reporter who juxtaposes both elements as the lead for the story; although the reporter is clear in detailing how emphatic the minister's statement was in the name of the government. The dominant frame, as emphasized by the Prime Minister's Office, is that sex workers are outside of the nation and are non-citizens, a frame predicated on:

- the unacceptability of both sex work and the licensing of sex workers as workers;
- the role of the police and immigration officials in securing the borders of the nation from those who would undermine national public morals;
- the reframing of sex work in terms of transatlantic slavery; and
- the place of the government's stand in ensuring an appropriate legacy from the government to the nation proper.

This statement is countered strongly by a reframing of the issue and the minister's statements by Barbadian activist Robert Best in his column, Best on Tuesday. Best calls his column that week (September 19, 2006), 'Who wants sex workers?' in a pun that reframes the debate over who is inside and who is outside the nation, and whether those boundaries can even be policed.[21]

The column is written from the vantage point provided by knowledge of and access to the frames that have come with rights debates in the wake of policy and legislative reform to address vulnerability to HIV.

Best (2006) reframes the minister of state's denunciation by locating the government's response within an ongoing debate about the illogic of anti-sex work legislation. For, Best counters, 'What we all know is that for generations prostitution has prevailed long before any talk about having it legalized and it will continue to do so if only because there is a demand created for prostitutes.' Best thus switches the frame back to markets, buyers and sellers in a globalizing economic environment, but then disentangles the persistence of that market from the framing wars, in order to take the debate to another level, where those who sell sex are people earning a living from people who have an interest in buying what they are selling: 'This is why it is amusing that when prostitutes refer to themselves as "sex workers" and others cry shame of them, it makes no difference to the "sex workers" since they know they will be in demand in many places.'

Best (2007) engages in an astute strategy of switching the frame of the sex worker as 'criminal outsider' and the government as 'protector of the moral nation,' as well as its notion of and legacy to that 'moral nation.' In the process of undoing those distinctions he points to the fact that the 'sex workers' under discussion are Caribbean citizens crossing borders bearing legitimate passports, and in so doing turns inside out the notion that sex workers are somehow discernable as sex workers, just as those to whom they sell sex are not discernable as 'whoremongers':

> It is the "games people play" that create the demand and the sex workers move to provide the supply. That is how they see and do their business as they travel around, and their passports do not say they are sex workers. (...) It is one of the ironies in our society that we are most tolerant of whoremongers but are prepared to go to extremes when dealing with the whores, sex workers or whatever.

The boundaries between the insiders and outsiders are reversed, as Best reframes the language of the state with the language of a nation and its people selling and buying in a market that is embedded within cultural norms that counter-frame the people-nation. Best's best efforts notwithstanding, sex work remains illegal in Barbados.

The Jamaica *Gleaner*

The debate in the *Nation* is marked by a diversity of frames and vantage points on the role of decriminalizing sex work as a public health issue and in defence of sex workers' right to health. By contrast, the debate in the Jamaican print media is marked by a preponderance of appeals to interpretations of Biblical text. These are used by those who perceive themselves as Christian guardians of a nation under siege to counter any attempt to foster social inclusion of marginalized groups. Thus, tolerance of excluded groups in the name of rights, evidence-based programming, public health and/or the control of HIV becomes seen as the path towards destruction of the nation.

In the Jamaica *Gleaner* of April 16, 2006, the editors print a letter which lambastes Lascelles Chin, a member of the financial elite, for proposing the 'Thai model' of regulating sex work which is famous for having drastically reduced the prevalence of HIV among sex workers and the general population.[22] The letter writer's response is predictable, but the terms on which the attempt by Chin to reframe the place of sex work is attacked is telling. He begins by condemning 'someone of Lascelles Chin's prominence and privilege' for 'pushing the Thai prostitution model on Jamaica.' Reverting to the history of oppression from which the nation is struggling to free itself, he then poses a question: 'For the love of God, have not the Jamaican people, in history, suffered enough from poverty, exploitation and degradation already?' This serves as the framework within which the country would be saved from the desire of Chin to 'impose that degradation on Jamaica and its people'. Framed thus, the question, though purporting to be a contribution to a rational debate on state policy and the leadership of the elite who should know better reflected the mandate of state policy to adhere to Biblical morality. The nation is thus to be rescued from the morass symbolized by 'the Thai model', all proven public health value notwithstanding. The writer, like the minister of state in Barbados, in keeping with Van Gorp's (2007) prediction of the embeddedness of frames in culture and the distribution of power, collapses governance with religious dogma. In another instance of the same frame, the writer reinforces the borders of the nation against those who would sully its inner sanctity: 'He obviously has no respect for Jamaica ... or for his fellow Jamaicans', the pause underlining the affront to national decency embodied in proposing the regulation of sex work, not even in the name of sex worker rights but in the name of public health and HIV control.

Prominent Roman Catholic priest and commentator in the Jamaica *Gleaner*, Father Richard Ho Lung (March 1, 2004) captures the frame of the Caribbean nation under siege and the battle for the salvation of its soul against the onset of a modernity based on Enlightenment liberalism rather than the Bible:[23]

> In the name of liberalism we have removed the underpinnings of our country and our nation.... Whether it be flexi-week, abortion, drugs, rape, stealing, gambling, drunkenness, prostitution, loud and offensive music it doesn't matter; it is permitted. ... I pray that we will not become like Europe, which has lost its soul.

The erasure of distinctions between rape and drunkenness, between playing loud music and stealing, are made in the name of protecting the morality of the nation and in so doing urging Jamaica to 'return' to its 'true self' (Ho Lung, ibid). The degraded present, in which sex workers are embedded, is a betrayal of a timeless national character, linked to the Bible as the touchstone of identity and the future, and in direct contrast to Europe, which is presumably damned for its liberalism.

CONCLUSIONS — VULNERABILITY AND SOCIAL INCLUSION

In the epigraphs that open this chapter, I invoke and imply an interrelationship between four main concepts: the power of the politics of recognition and tolerance of difference, the idea that a nation is judged by the place it makes for those at the bottom of the social structure or excluded from the mainstream, the economic and other dislocations caused by increasing 'ghettoisation' of the poor, and the pattern that has shown itself in many societies, where the marginalized experience the effects of HIV and AIDS most brutally. By way of closing, I want to pull together these strands that have signalled central concerns in this chapter on the place Caribbean societies make for accommodating the meek.

The measure of respect for civil liberties and citizenship rights of a society is in the way it handles those it despises, and in the norms it establishes for those who are minorities. In this sense, the question of difference and minority status are wrapped up in ideas of the proper function of government. It is a central irony of our history in the Caribbean that we have adopted political structures such as parliamentary democracies, yet cling to the colonial models of social exclusion embedded in our everyday lives, and in our assumptions about the value of the human lives around us.

To align the passage from Ho Lung to the press conference called by the minister of state in the Office of the Prime Minister in Barbados may seem like an extreme comparison, but both are based on the same premise: the dehumanization of entire strata of the citizenry in the name of the virtue of the nation, and its purity. The copula of purity and danger has its own complicated history, but for our purposes, it has come to occupy the place where the nation is linked to the state in the concept of the nation-state, and to characterize the very nature of that bond implied by the hyphen that connects. The example of sex workers may also seem extreme, but the same processes play out when it is legally impossible for a man to rape his wife — the category of wife having lost its human content. In this, the esteemed 'ghetto priest' of a Father Ho Lung takes his place next to the political elite, not as an extremist, but as an accessory to that elite comfortable in the dehumanisation of women seeking to earn a living by selling sex. This is not to romanticize those on the structural underside of the social order — the pathologies and complex internalisations and resistances are everywhere evident, for example in the political, economic, social and academic debates over violence in anti-gay dancehall music. The same pathologies have held as true for those who are politicians, priests or scions of Caribbean industry.

What we need is to replace the logic that requires the dehumanization of large swathes of Caribbean humanity, rather than rotating those who occupy that space, and stay true to the logic of tolerance and individual rights as progress. This is at the root of the Abolitionist logic, and at the root of the Enlightenment logic that led to Independence in many nation-states in the Caribbean. The brutal conflicts which have marked Haiti's political history become a case in point, not so much a world apart from the orderly elections of the English-speaking Caribbean, as much as laying bare the logic of political systems that refuse to transform fundamental institutions in the name of the rights of the collective to recognition and to the promise of citizenship held out by the independent nation-state.

In its stead, human rights, including individual and minority rights, become central to the role of state, and to addressing the structural inequities that feed on subalternity in order to constitute the citizenry. Addressing vulnerability means addressing this failure of the social pact. The epidemic of HIV, just like the consistent pattern of persons with AIDS presenting so late in the progression of their illness they can barely survive, is a symptom of a larger societal illness because HIV drives citizens into black hole/hull of subalternity through the failure of key institutions to fulfill the social pact extended by the state and to premise social order on justice and the protection of minority rights.

The question remains, however, of how our societies can move to address such embedded inequalities. I believe an important step is in supporting and listening to social movements of the oppressed, based on principles of social justice, equity and citizenship not only by escaping the strictures of subalternity, but by dismantling the structures that feed subalternity itself. The social movements that evolved into nationalism in the 1930s English-speaking Caribbean had the promise of moving the social order to another level. Such movements are not inevitably more just, but they open up important conversations about justice — consider the move from the brutalization of Rastafarian communities to making social, economic and political spaces for those who choose to follow that path.

What makes such movements possible, however, are some fundamental principles that we need to agree on which tie our struggles together: respect for the inherent dignity of *all* human beings rather than only those who are like us or who are in the majority; understanding that the role of charters of rights and of constitutions are to embody those core values; leadership taking responsibility for problem solving based on normalising such values; and therefore revisiting concepts of freedom and citizenship, and the proper function of the state in relation to the nation. I believe that the only way we can address symptoms like epidemics of HIV — or crime, or brain drains, or other issues that underdevelop our societies — is by addressing these fundamental failures of governance, justice, and the social pact that connects us to one another.

To do that we have to challenge head-on the stranglehold colonial models of social order have on our societies, and begin to admit that stranglehold exists. From there, as Caribbean people, we need to engage these structural issues through interventions with multiple points of entry premised on social justice; holding key social institutions accountable; expanding resources for community-based justice movements; and embracing participation, social inclusion and choice as fundamental premises of development as freedom in twenty-first century Caribbean societies.

NOTES

1. Joint United Nations Programme on HIV/AIDS, *2006 Report on the global AIDS epidemic*, (Geneva: UNAIDS, 2006).
2. CAREC Special Programme on Sexually Transmitted Infections, *The Caribbean HIV/AIDS Epidemic and the Situation in Member Countries of the Caribbean Epidemiology Centre (CAREC)*, (Port of Spain: PAHO/CAREC, 2007).
3. Caribbean Epidemiology Centre, *Status and Trends Analysis of the Caribbean HIV/AIDS Epidemic 1982-2002*, (Port of Spain, Trinidad: CAREC/PAHO, 2004).
4. See Cary Alan Johnson, *Off the Map: How HIV/AIDS Programming is Failing Same-Sex Practicing People in Africa*, (New York: International Gay and Lesbian Human Rights Commission, 2007).
5. 'Most At Risk Population'.
6. There is a strong Caribbean intellectual interrogation of this. See, for example, Perry C. Hintzon, 'Rethinking Democracy in the Postnationalist State', in *New Caribbean Thought: A Reader*, eds Brian Meeks and Folke Lindahl, (Barbados, Jamaica, Trinidad and Tobago: University of the West Indies Press, 2001), 104–24. Many of the chapters in that volume interrogate these issues, from a range of perspectives.

7. See, for example, Hyacinth Evans and Rose Davies, 'Overview of Issues in Childhood Socialization in the Caribbean', in *Caribbean Families: Diversity Among Ethnic Groups*, eds. Jaipaul L. Roopnarine and Janet Brown, (London: ABLEX Publishing Corporation, 1997), 1–24. See also Christine Barrow, ed, *Children's Rights: Caribbean Realities*, (Kingston: Ian Randle Publishers, 2002).

8. Gayatri Chakravorty Spivak, 'Can the Subaltern Speak?' in *Marxism and the Interpretation of Culture*, eds Cary Nelson and Lawrence Grossberg, (Urbana, IL: University of Illinois Press, 1988), 271–313.

9. Partha Chatterjee, *The Nation and Its Fragments: Colonial and Postcolonial Histories*, (Princeton, New Jersey: Princeton University Press, 1993).

10. This process has been the subject of a great deal of analysis, for example by Anthony Bogues, Brian Meeks, Ralph Premdas, and others. See Anthony Bogues 'Politics, Nation and Post Colony: Caribbean Inflections,' *Small Axe* 11, (March 2002): 1–30; Brian Meeks and Folke Lindahl, eds, *New Caribbean Thought: A Reader*; Selwyn Ryan, 'Caribbean Political Thought, From Westminster to Philadelphia, 248–273, as well as the other papers published in *Contending with Destiny: the Caribbean in the 21st Century*, eds. Kenneth Hall and Dennis Benn, (Kingston: Ian Randle Publishers, 2000); also Robert Carr, *Black Nationalism in the New World: Reading African-American and West Indian Nationalisms*, (Duke UP, 2002).

11. See Amartya Sen, *Development as Freedom*, Oxford University Press, 1999.

12. See Obika Grey, *Demeaned but Empowered: The Social Power of the Urban Poor in Jamaica*, (Mona, Jamaica: The University of West Indies Press, 2004); Stanley Niah; Ramesh Deosaran, *Psychonomics and Poverty: Towards Governance and a Civil Society*, Mona, Jamaica: The University of the West Indies Press, 2000); and Carolyn Cooper, *Sound Clash: Jamaican Dancehall Culture At Large*, (New York: Palgrave Macmillan, 2004).

13. See Amartya Sen, *Development as Freedom*.

14. See BBC.com coverage retrieved May 27, 2008 at http://news.bbc.co.uk/1/hi/programmes/hardtalk/7410382.stm

15. See Hilary McD Beckles, *Centering Woman: Gender Discourse in Caribbean Slave Society*, (Kingston: Ian Randle Publishers, 1999); Kamala Kempadoo, *Sexing the Caribbean: Gender, Race and Sexual Labor*, (New York and London: Routledge, 2004); The Pan Caribbean Partnership Against HIV/AIDS, *Caribbean Regional Strategic Framework 2008–2012*, (Georgetown, Guyana: PANCAP, 2008).

16. Benedict Anderson, *Imagined Communities: Reflections on the Origins and Spread of Nationalism*, rev edition, Verso, (London, 1991).

17. See the special issue of the *Journal of Communication* Vol. 57, Issue 1 (March 2007) on Framing, Priming, and Agenda Setting. For an explanation of these concepts, see the introduction to the special issue, Dietram A. Scheufele and David Tewksbury, 'Framing, Agenda Setting, and Priming: The Evolution of Three Media Effects Models', *Journal of Communication* 57 (2007), 9–20.

18. Dennis Chong and James N. Druckman, 'A Theory of Framing and Opinion Formation in Competitive Elite Environments', *Journal of Communication* 57 (2007), 99–118.

19. Robert M. Entman, 'Framing Bias: Media in the Distribution of Power', *Journal of Communication* 57 (2007), 163–173.

20. Prostitution 'is not an option', September 13, 2006, Brief, Nationews.com. Retrieved March 17, 2008 at:*http://bararchive.bits.baseview.comarchive_ detail.php?archiveFile=./pubfiles/bar/archive/2006/September/13/ LocalNews25938.xml&start=0&numPer=20&keyword=Prostitution+is+not+an+option& sectionSearch=&begindate=1%2F1%2F1994&enddate=12%2F31%2F2008&authorSearch= &IncludeStories=1&pubsection=&page=&IncludePages=1&IncludeImages= 1&mode=allwords& archive_pubname=Daily+Nation%0A%09%09%09*

21. Robert Best, 'Who wants sex workers?' *The Nation*, September 19, 2006, Retrieved March 17 at: *http://bararchive.bits.baseview.com/archive_detail.php?archiveFile=./ pubfiles/bar/archive/2006/September/19/Editorial/26250.xml&start= 0&numPer=20&keyword=who+wants+sex+workers&sectionSearch=& begindate=1%2F1%2F1994&enddate=12%2F31%2F2008&author Search=&IncludeStories=1&pubsection=&page=&IncludePages=1&IncludeIm ages=1&mode=allwords&archive_pubname=Daily+Nation%0A%09%09%09*

22. Anthony G. Gumbs, Letter to the Editor, published Sunday April 16, 2006. Retrieved March 17, 2008 at: *http://www.jamaica-gleaner.com/gleaner/20060416/ letters/letters4.html*

23. Father Richard Ho Lung, 'Civil war: In Jamaica or Haiti?' published: Monday March 1, 2004, Retrieved March 17, 2008 at: *http://www.jamaica-gleaner.com/ gleaner/20040301/cleisure/cleisure3.html*

RETHINKING
COMMUNICATION

CHAPTER 5

SPEAKING SEXUALITY

The Heteronationalism of MSM

ANDIL GOSINE

In the nearly three decades since HIV and AIDS have been named, policy makers, researchers and workers in the field have broadened characterization of the virus and disease from a condition affecting individual bodies to one that threatens communities, nations and, quite possibly, the world itself. This shift is demonstrated by contemporary analyses of the disease which more often emphasize social economic costs — especially to states — as well as by the organization of responses to it, operated and coordinated at community (NGOs), national (state commissions on HIV and AIDS) and global (UNAIDS) levels of governance. One simple demonstration of this globalized construction of the epidemic is the 'We All Have AIDS' campaign, which debuted on World AIDS Day in 2005. The campaign features celebrities like Elizabeth Taylor, Elton John and Harry Belafonte, as well as political statesmen like Archbishop Desmond Tutu and Nelson Mandela, appearing alongside this phrase in posters and on T-shirts. Their mission, campaign literature explains, is to fight stigma, 'because if one of us has AIDS, we all have it' (*http://www.weallhaveaids.com*). More than ethical humanitarianism, this doctrine is meant to convey the far-reaching social costs of the disease.

The most valiant efforts calling for recognition of HIV and AIDS as social phenomena draw attention to this truth of its production (as many of the essays in this collection point out, it *is* socially constituted and experienced), and attempts to hold various actors accountable for its spread and impact. HIV and AIDS prevention and care advocates, researchers, health practitioners and policy workers now more regularly point to data illustrating the relationship between poverty, discrimination, provision of social services, education and the spread of the disease, and its broader social and economic costs, in mobilizing public support. For the most part, this articulation of the epidemic is considered to be a welcome and effective approach. Evidence of its threat to economic and social stability has moved governments, as well as global policy regulators like the World Bank, to be more vigilant in taking action. While still falling far short of what most experts have suggested is needed to effectively treat and combat the disease, worldwide AIDS spending has increased significantly over the time that it has become articulated as a social phenomenon. Global spending on HIV and AIDS increased 28-fold from US$300 million in 1996 to just under US$8.3 billion in 2005 and is expected to have reached US$10 billion by the end of 2007 (UNAIDS 2006). This growth has happened in conjunction with demonstrations of stronger political support from a broader set of actors, ranging from presidents to pop stars. On May 30, 2007, even the once sceptical US President George W. Bush was widely praised by AIDS activists for committing to a five-year US$30 billion plan to fight AIDS.

While this mobilization around AIDS care and prevention is surely welcome, it is also deserving of more careful and necessary consideration. It is important to ask: What rationales have been advanced in the construction of HIV and AIDS as a social phenomenon? What are the implications of this articulation? How do we begin to map and make sense of some of the contradictions engendered through this approach? How, for example, do we weigh Bush's funding commitments to HIV and AIDS programmes against his administration's simultaneous heteronationalism and religious fundamentalism? What makes it possible for both homosexual and homophobic actors to champion a social framing of the disease? In this chapter, I begin to think through some of these questions by consideration of one component of contemporary HIV and AIDS discourses: the figure of the MSM — 'men who have sex with men.' Consideration of the discursive production of MSM in the Anglo-Caribbean is especially instructive in contemplating some of these questions.

In many Caribbean states, as in other countries across the world, references to MSM appear in National HIV and AIDS Plans and other documents related to HIV and AIDS prevention and care research, policies and programmes. This acknowledgement of sex between men exists alongside virulent political rhetoric that denunciates homosexuality as 'unnatural' and foreign and punitive anti-sodomy laws. In this context, many health advocates and activists working in the Caribbean have viewed (and used) MSM both as the only possibility to ensure some attention to this constituency's needs, as well as an opportunity to engage and possibly advance sexuality rights and well-being agendas. Many hope that attention to the particular vulnerabilities of MSM to HIV and AIDS will route supporting resources to gay and lesbian communities, and lead to a critical examination of homophobia and the revision of statutes that have been used to undermine sexuality rights. This outcome is possible. However, as I argue below, current discursive productions of MSM do not necessarily encourage realization of this radical potential. In dominant HIV and AIDS analyses and policies in the Anglo-Caribbean, MSM is primarily intended to facilitate, rather than challenge, heteronationalism (the processes through which citizenship is premised on racialised and gendered heterosexuality). In framings of HIV and AIDS as social phenomena, MSM constructs men engaged in homosexual acts as infecting agents who threaten the welfare of communities, states, peoples. They are presented as a *pox* on nations in all senses of the word: a curse on and an indication of the national body's illness. MSM are a temporary, toxic presence — outsiders in the nation who, by virtue of their non-heterosexuality, threaten its reproduction and survival.

The discussion that follows describes how the figure of the MSM is constructed in dominant discourses on HIV and AIDS so that it works to facilitate, rather than challenge, the heteronationalist intent of anti-sodomy laws and other measures used to strip homosexual actors of citizenship and human rights in many Anglo-Caribbean states. Following an explanation of the term and description of some forms of 'heteronationalism' in the region and a brief introduction of some genealogies of MSM discourse as used in HIV and AIDS care and prevention work, I begin to demonstrate how the latter may be complicit with, or even work to support maintenance of, the former. Although heteronationalist objectives are not always fulfilled — many activists creatively pursue a more liberating re-articulation of the discourse — it powerfully informs how HIV and AIDS is constructed as a social disease and, in part, explains how efforts to build support for action on HIV and AIDS may simultaneously leave commitments to heteronationalism intact.

HETERONATIONALISM IN THE CARIBBEAN

M. Jacqui Alexander uses the term heteropatriarchy to refer to 'the twin processes of heterosexualization and patriarchy' that underpin colonial and neocolonial state formations, and which are maintained through state laws and social regulations that deny the erotic autonomy of its subjects (2005, 22–23). Alexander explains that

Erotic autonomy signals danger to the heterosexual family and to the nation. And because loyalty to the nation as citizen is perennially colonized within reproduction and heterosexuality, erotic autonomy brings with it the potential of undoing the nation entirely, a possible charge of irresponsible citizenship, or no responsibility at all (2005, 22–23).

She further argues that 'at this moment in the neocolonial state's diffusion of sexualized definitions of morality, sexual and erotic autonomy have been most frequently cathected on the body of the prostitute and the lesbian' (23). Revising Alexander's analytic, I use the term 'heteronationalism' to include racism and ethnocentrism with heteorsexism and patriarchy as foundational imperatives of neocolonial nation-building, privileging 'hetero' in this instance because it is the primary focus of this chapter, not because it the most important component of nationalisms. Nations must always be heterosexualized to ensure the reproduction of citizens, just as they must also be racialized and gendered to ensure the construction of national boundaries and bodies.

As Alexander points out, women's bodies — including prostitutes and lesbians — have been primary sites of moral regulation since, at least, the colonial era. However, men's bodies have also been implicated in this process. In recent years nationalist anxieties in Anglo-Caribbean states have been especially fixated on the threat posed by male homosexual subjects, in no small part, due to growing popular consciousness of gay culture and of HIV and AIDS. Demonstrations of these anxieties have been expressed through homophobic violence, organising against the landing of gay cruise ships and of attempts to achieve sexuality rights, as discussed later in the chapter. These anxieties are indeed a production of a patriarchal power that collapses gender with sex and inscribes male and female bodies with fixed functionalities. I think it is important to shift attention to nationalism not because I object to Alexander's analysis but, rather, to insist on problematization of the nation itself. As a critical response to the positioning of homosexuality outside nations, the production of new forms of potentially more inclusive nationalism has only very limited promise. Even though it may be necessary in the short term, and for a number of strategic purposes, to demand the inclusion of homosexual subjects in nations (e.g. to assert citizenship rights), certainly the structure of the nation is no panacea for injustice and provides no assurance of erotic autonomy.

In 2007, a number of events across the Caribbean showcased heightened moral panic over homosexuality. Demonstrations against the docking of cruise ships carrying gay and lesbian passengers and of a performance by a gay music icon, outrage expressed over the inclusion of materials on gay and lesbian families in high school textbooks, reggae and dancehall acts calling for the murder of gay men, physical assault of gay men and the states' vigilant maintenance of homophobic anti-sodomy laws were pursued, all in the name of nationalism. Incidences of homophobic violence in Jamaica were widely reported by various news outlets over the last year. In February 2007, a mob of at least 200 people gathered outside a pharmacy calling for three men inside to be beaten to death because they were believed to be gay. On April 2, a crowd threw stones and bottles at a group of costumed men dancing in the carnival procession in Montego Bay. According to a report entitled 'Anti-gay attack,' in the *Jamaica Observer* published April 3, 2007, the crowd was angered because 'the men were gyrating in a sexually suggestive manner'. Six days later, in Mandeville, attacks were directed at mourners whom the crowd believed to be gay. And, on April 27, a mob at Falmouth was photographed beating up a cross-dresser (Hines). These events followed the murder of gay activist Brian Williamson in Kingston in 2004 and Steve Harvey in 2005 (Padgett 2006). A homophobic climate, some argue, has been exacerbated by the performance of 'murder music' by dancehall artists such as Buju Banton, Beenie Man, Vybz Kartel, Elephant Man, Sizzla, Capleton, T.O.K. and Shabba Ranks (Kinsella 2007). Speaking about the acceptance of his claim for asylum in the US, Jamaican national Van Messam stated:

> My life in Jamaica was constantly in danger, with angry mobs carrying machetes, stones, knives, and guns, threatening to kill me because I am gay. When I tried to contact the police for help, the police instead threatened to arrest me and told me to leave the country if I wanted to stay safe (Schmalz 2007).

Summing up the situation, the newspaper *Jamaica Observer* in 2002 published a letter headlined 'It's hell to be gay in Jamaica', (C. P. Creary), while the British *Guardian* went further to declare 'If you're gay in Jamaica, you're dead' (Taylor 2004). *Time* magazine asked, Is Jamaica 'the most homophobic place on earth?' (Padgett 2006). Sensing no improvement in the situation faced by gay men and lesbians in Jamaica, Human Rights Watch reissued a call for police protection on February 1, 2008. 'Roving mobs attacking innocent people and staining the streets with blood should shame the nation's leaders', said Scott Long, director of the Lesbian, Gay, Bisexual and Transgender Rights Programme at Human Rights Watch. 'Gays and lesbians in Jamaica face violence at home, in public, even in a house of worship, and official silence encourages the spread of hate' (Human Rights Watch accessed at *http://hrw.org/english/docs/2008/02/01/jamaic17957.htm*).

Events in Jamaica garnered the most media attention, but it is certainly not the only Caribbean state where moral panics about homosexuality are being played out. St Vincent and the Grenadines and The Cayman

Islands have blocked gay and lesbian cruise ships from docking on the islands, and campaigns have been organised to pressure others, such as Grenada and Bermuda, to follow suit. Protests in Bermuda were sufficient to cause cancellation of the planned landing of the popular 'r family' cruises associated with American television personality Rosie O'Donnell. Even in islands that have notably relaxed laws on sexuality, like St Maarten, there have been movements calling for a ban on gay cruise ships (*Le Journal d'un Terrien*, accessed at *http://caraibes.wordpress.com/2007/06/02/homosexual-cruise-in-st-maarten/*). In Trinidad and Tobago, lawsuits were filed against police charged with harassing men who appeared to be gay (Swamber 2007), and election platforms staged there in September 2007 also featured notably gay-bashing singers like Beenie Man as star attractions. In Tobago, a local pastor's (failed) efforts to stop British pop singer Elton John's performance also provided a rallying point for homophobic anxieties. And, in Guyana, the Society Against Sexual Orientation Discrimination (SASOD) failed to stop the performances of Kiprich and Buju Banton at the Guyana Music Festival. Despite assurances that they would not sing homophobic tunes, they performed 'Boom Bye Bye', which calls for the killing of batty boys (gay men).

Throughout, these various forms of moral panic construct non-heterosexual subjects — for the most part, gay men — as a dirty infringement upon the national body. This rhetoric was promoted by many participants attending Advocates International, a 'Christian Lawyers' conference held in Tobago on the weekend of July 27–29, 2007. One presentation, explaining the 'ideological attack' on families and God, highlights three focal issues: Comprehensive Sex Education (which, according to the presenter, is 'teaching children about birth control, abortion, masturbation, homosexual behaviour and other evils'); sexual and reproductive health, (a 'euphemism used to introduce all the foregoing deceitfully into legislation'), and GLBT rights, 'part of the Culture of Death that seeks to destroy marriage and its Godly participation in the unitive life of the Trinity and carry out Satan's hoped-for triumph over God's plan for the human race to bring love and life to mankind.' Similarly, vitriolic sentiments were unleashed by some religious leaders in St Maarten, an island which has, until recently, been known for its relaxed attitudes toward sexual regulation. According to one report, pastors from the Kingdom Come Ministries Church claimed that the cruise ships would 'bring destruction and calamity on the island,' '[send] a negative message to our youth,' and encourage violence (*St Maarten Private Eye*, reported at *http://sxmprivateeye.com/*). Pastor Elijah Singer argued that the gay lifestyle 'is destroying the fabric of the society where they impose their way of life on the community' (Ibid.).

In this climate, violence levelled at gays, lesbians and others who are seen to dissent from acceptable social norms is then seen as a 'cleansing' exercise. In Fall 2007, the Columbia Law School clinic helped win asylum from the US Department of Homeland Security for Jamaican national Van Messam, by contending that 'rampant rumours that hostile groups are plotting the *social cleansing* of hundreds of gay people by year's end have forced countless GLBT people into hiding' (emphasis mine). This view is echoed in dancehall compositions which similarly call for a cleansing of the population through the murder of gays and lesbians. Commitments to protect national bodies from homosexuality have in some cases even appeared to trump economic interests. Speaking about St Vincent Prime Minister Ralph Gonsalves's banishment of gay cruise ships from the Grenadines, trade unionist Chester Humphrey explained, 'People have said that St Vincent will lose money and he has said we are not losers we are winners. We have won the moral question and the moral question is far more valuable than money' (Titus 2007).

The furore over the landing of cruise ships of gay and lesbian passengers is especially illustrative of this representation of the national body as heterosexual. Attempts to forbid entry to identifiable gays and lesbian passengers on cruise ships mirror, in important respects, the attempts by Euro-American states to keep out people from the global south through strict immigration controls: both measures rest on the assumption that the outsiders will sully the national body. Just as immigration policies in North America and Europe are at least partly predicated on a racialisation of geography that cannot imagine non-white people as citizens, so, too, do the demands to refuse gay cruise ship passengers force the imagination of Caribbean peoples as heterosexual only. The rationalization of homosexuality as an affront to the national body is made clear in the opening lines of an article published in the Grenadian paper *CMC*, credited to Grenadian journalist Rawle Titus:

> When American soldiers invaded Grenada in 1983 they carried guns and explosives to quell political upheaval on this tiny Caribbean island nation. If an invasion of gay tourists is allowed in the next few months, they will bring revenue and as such trigger further growth in cruise tourism. But that's not all that could be brought to St George's if the concerns of those contributing to Grenada's hottest topic of debate these days are anything to go. A gay lifestyle flaunted across the country as a threat to local cultural and religious values, seems to be a main bone of contention by many a caller to radio talk shows and social commentators here (November, 2007).

Practising 'gay lifestyles', whatever they may be, is akin to military invasion of the nation.

Staying with this theme, one lawyer attending the Advocates International conference noted:

> Bureaucrats within the United Nations (UN) and the European Union (EU) have been carrying out policies within their International programmes to pressure Developing Countries to reduce population growth and to legalise some actions normally considered immoral, e.g. same-sex copulation, prostitution – both male and female, explicit sex education (aka. pornography) and preeminently, abortion ('The Gender Agenda in Trinidad and Tobago').

Making a pitch for mobilization against sexuality and reproductive rights, Shirley Richards declared, 'Caribbean people must not submit to this neo-colonization. We were colonized once before let us vow — never again!' (Notably, the Advocates International forum was primarily financed and led by Canadian branches of the organization).

ENTER 'MSM'

In the Caribbean, HIV and AIDS troubled the construction of homosexuality as a foreign vice. Responses to the high rate of incidence in the region have had to, in some way, take into account male-to-male sexual contact, especially in view of the early and still powerful articulation of HIV and AIDS as gay diseases. Thus, in national HIV and AIDS plans and other policy documents, many Caribbean states have followed what has become an institutionalized global practice and included references to 'men who have sex with men,' or by the more popular, more used acronym, MSM. Expectations by the United Nations and other organisations are that all states will pursue specific strategic responses to curb the spread of HIV and AIDS among MSM.

References to MSM in national AIDS plans and other government documents would appear to recognize the existence of homosexual acts within the nation. Even if the references have suggested male homosexuality is responsible for the spread of the virus (and, as I argue below, this has often been the case) in these documents, the very recognition that homosexual practices took place among Caribbean men, in Caribbean states, would appear to, at least in part, rebuke some important aspects of the homophobic rhetoric of conservative religious organisations among others. The mention of MSM as a 'high risk' or 'vulnerable' group has also been viewed by some as a boon to sexuality rights campaigns, particularly in light of the considerable financial resources that are being made available for HIV and AIDS care and prevention work (cf. Wright 2000). Following this recognition of sex between men, many hope that more effective HIV and AIDS prevention and care strategies, as well as opportunities to move forward in securing sexuality rights for all people engaged in homosexual acts, will come. However, even a cursory review of how MSM functions discursively raises some cautionary questions about the impact of this approach.

MSM and, later, WSW (women who have sex with women) emerged as ways of talking about homosexuality without committing subjects to fixed sexual orientation identities, and to break away from narrow culturally-specific configurations of 'gay', 'lesbian', etc. According to Young and Meyer, arguments for MSM and WSW are driven by the convergence of epidemiological and social constructionist perspectives. 'By using identity free terms', they explain, 'epidemiologists sought to avoid complex social and cultural connotations that, according to a strict biomedical view, have little to do with epidemiological investigation of diseases' (2005, 1,144). MSM thus put attention on how 'behaviours', not identities, place individuals at risk for HIV infection. This distinction was significant since early on 'gay identity' was identified as a risk for HIV and AIDS, resulting in the stigmatization of queer communities and undermining prevention efforts. MSM, like WSW, also appeared to support a social constructionist view of sexuality. While the epidemiological perspective reduces sexualities to bodily behaviours, social constructionist critiques, as Young and Meyer also point out, sought to do the opposite: 'more textured understandings of sexuality that do not assume alignments among identity, behaviour, and desire' (1,144).

Reflecting on the globalized use of the term over the last two decades, Young and Meyer now see several problems with the conceptualization and use of MSM/WSW. In particular, they are concerned that the 'ubiquitous use' of *WSW* and *MSM* 'undermines the self-determined sexual identity of members of sexual-minority groups, in particular people of colour'; 'deflects attention from social dimensions of sexuality that are critical in understanding sexual health'; and 'obscures elements of sexual behaviour that are important for public health research and intervention' (1,144). In *'Race', Culture, Power, Sex, Desire, Love: Writing in Men who have Sex with Men* (Gosine 2006), I also argued that the term's racialising imperatives, easy conflation of specific cultural practices, oversimplification and sometimes negation of sexual desire, pleasure and love, deflection away from women engaged in same-sex relationships, and failure to contest dominant, heteronormative power relations, raise serious doubts about its universal application across health and development fields. A review of how MSM is conceptualized, articulated and materialized in one organization in Trinidad and Tobago, 'MSM No Political Agenda', and in relation to popular media discourses on gays and lesbians, and homosexuality, reveals some of the term's contradictory uses and exposes how it may in fact serve to support forces of heteronationalism in the region.

'MSM No Political Agenda'

'MSM No Political Agenda' grew out of a study of MSM conducted by Geoffrey Stanford between 1994 and 1998 in Trinidad. The group was founded in 1999 and set out to work toward related objectives, including production and circulation of *FreeForum*, a newsletter for MSM in Trinidad and Tobago; provision of education tools on HIV and AIDS, STDs and Safe Sex Information; development of research and analysis on local MSM issues and concerns; reduction of HIV and AIDS. As of December 2007, the newsletter was still being produced and the group maintained an online presence. Three aspects of the group, I suggest, demonstrate how MSM discourse may function to uphold heteronationalism in the region: the rationale for its foundation; its differentiation of MSM from 'gay' as a behaviour versus identity marker; and, as so clearly suggested by its name, its intended apolitical or 'politically neutral' convictions.

A note titled '*Project Research and Justification*' featured on the group's website, posits that the high incidence of HIV and AIDS is the main basis for the group's existence:

> An important challenge for Trinidad and Tobago is the higher rate/ likelihood of men to contract HIV and AIDS. A sobering statistic is the estimated 45 per cent of total reported cases in which transmission of the virus is surmised to be through *male-to-male sexual contact* …Epidemiological data estimates that 67 per cent (1996/97 statistics) of all AIDS cases are male. The social and health impacts on the gay community, the community of men who have sex with men (MSM), and by extension the society as a whole, are already tremendous. If we can reduce the rates of HIV transmission within the 'community', we can effectively lower the national incidence of HIV and AIDS.

The argument expressed here is similar to that espoused in most other parts of the world where this work is done, investments in HIV and AIDS care and prevention among MSM is good for the nation. This is not necessarily because this population is a valued part of the nation — dominant heteronationalist discourses, as discussed, render the contrary — but because of the risk they pose to heterosexual men and women. As put in one World Bank Report, 'MSM are not an isolated group, but are in fact intensely and extensively sexually linked with the heterosexual members of African society' (World Bank 2004). The AIDS Alliance International 'Key Population' report, *Between Men* is even more blunt in making the connection clear:

Sex between men — in particular, anal intercourse without a condom — is one of the primary ways in which HIV and other sexually transmitted infections are passed on. In every society some men have sex with other men, and some of these men have many sexual partners, including women. This means that anal intercourse without a condom between men also places the men's female partners and the future of their future children at risk of infection (2003, 3).

In other words, health care interventions directed at MSM are justified toward protection and preservation of the heterosexual nation.

This position offers no guarantee of disrupting heteronationalist frameworks, but it provides a basis for its further entrenchment. Consider the identification of MSM as a 'high risk' or 'vulnerable' in this framework. In employing these terms, health advocates no doubt mean well in exposing the ways in which they experience marginalization. In the same World Bank report, its authors note:

A prerequisite for an effective public health response is the recognition that MSM represent a high-risk group for spreading HIV. The inclusion of MSM in HIV and AIDS programming, however, may lead to wider acceptance of the group and may also help to lift some of the wider cultural taboos and stigma associated with HIV and homosexuality or same-gender sex (vi).

Yet, what the recognition of MSM as a 'high risk' or 'vulnerable' group also offers is the sustained marking of them as a polluting influence and weak component of the nation. This argument has been pitched in many Caribbean media forums over the last few years. Writing in the *St Lucia Star* of March 2004, Benoit makes a call for further repression of homosexuals upon the premise that they engage in dangerous activities that are linked to and threaten heterosexuals in the nation:

> Homosexuals are sexually disturbed individuals who are engaging in dangerous activities. The society cares about them and those tempted to join them, therefore it is extremely important that we neither encourage nor legitimize such a destructive lifestyle.

If protection of heterosexual reproduction is the primary objective for intervening on sexual rights issues, then, it can also be the same grounds from which to launch opposition to rights' claims. Writing in response to the publication of calls to consider decriminalization of homosexuality in Barbados as a means of fighting HIV and AIDS, Hoyos (2003) suggests:

> If the object is really to deal with HIV and AIDS, it would seem more useful and practical to establish treatment and counselling centres in strategic locations where homosexuals and prostitutes would know via public relations, that they may discreetly attend and be counselled, treated, given access to prophylactics.

Making protection of the heterosexual nation the main grounds for delivering services and offering support to MSM offers no certainty of the meaningful social transformation that health advocates suggest is necessary in the long term.

Indeed, the use of MSM over 'gay' in HIV and AIDS care and prevention programmes also appears to rebuke challenges to heteronationalism in significant ways. Calling men MSM is an exercise in not naming them 'gay'. While there are compelling reasons for doing so, the practice is deserving of more careful, critical evaluation. For example, as earlier noted, MSM is understood to work as a technical term that recognises many different kinds of sexual identification practices and traditions. However, in practice, MSM appears to function to similarly universalise sexual cultures. Functioning in the same way as 'gay', MSM is used as a broad descriptor of men leading very different lives in very different contexts. *Kothis* in Bangladesh, *Ibbi* in Senegal, *yan daudu* in Nigeria, African-American and Latino men on the 'down low', and *hijra* in India are all collapsed, in Oriental fashion, as MSM — despite speaking different languages, holding different religious beliefs, living in different social conditions and participating in different sexual cultures (cf. Gosine 2006). As Young and Meyer note, 'with this usage, the rich information on identity is lost, with *MSM* conveying transactional, decontexualized same-gender acts.' Consequently, applying *MSM* in this way universalizes a culturally specific phenomenon in much the same way that critics say does the term *gay* (1,146).

The issue is further complicated in the Caribbean. Unlike the examples from India, Senegal, Nigeria and Bangladesh noted above, evidence of 'indigenous' (or indigenized) markers of sexual preferences or behaviours are less available in the Caribbean. Important work has been conducted about same-sex relationships between women (e.g. Wekker 2006), but less is known about those between men. Euro-American terms 'gay', 'bisexual', 'queer' etc. resonate deeply with a great number of men engaged in sexual relationships with other men. This is hardly surprising given the overwhelming impact and hegemonizing influence of Euro-American culture in the region. As evidenced by the existence of many organisations and social networks for gay men (e.g. the various 'Friends of Lesbians, [All-sexuals] and Gays' in several countries and region-wide), very many men see themselves as 'gay men'. Whatever its many faults and flaws (cf. Gosine 2004, Sinfield 1998), 'gay' and 'bisexual' are identifiers of choice for many Caribbean men engaged in same-sex relationships. In fact, it is only in response to the considerable pressure of HIV and AIDS health interventions that have resulted in the formation of groups like MSMNPA, that groups have used the 'MSM' tag in their title. This process is not one of health policy makers recognising the erotic autonomy of Caribbean people by respecting the names they give themselves, but, rather, of directing them to fit particular policy plans. It is, in this sense, an act in support of heteronationalism as it disregards the choices men have made to name themselves 'gay'.

As research on gay/queer/MSM communities in the Caribbean is only just emerging, it might be informative to think through some of these issues as they have played out in other places. In the United States, Malebranche et al. studied Black men to assess the impact of a social environment characterized by prejudice on health services provided to these men (2004). In interviews, respondents were asked to discuss some of the challenges they faced as gay men. One interviewee said: 'When I go to a physician's office, and when I identify myself as a gay person, part of that is looking for acceptance from them, because I haven't gotten it from my family you know?' (2004, 100). His social identification was important. Young and Meyer note that in studies of how HIV and AIDS impact non-white gay men in the United States, the men's value of their social identification practices are commonly disregarded. In the Malebranche study, the authors refer to their respondents as *BMSM* (Black men who have sex with men), despite the fact that most reported that they used an identity term to describe themselves (53 per cent *gay*, 12 per cent *bisexual,* 12 per cent *same-gender loving,* 12 per cent *homosexual*) (2004). Young and Meyer point out, 'It is an ironic commentary on the pervasiveness of *men who have sex with men* and *MSM* that the authors… provided a nuanced cultural analysis but resorted to a deliberately anticultural term in describing the groups of men they studied' (2005, 1,146). Labelling as *MSM* men who describe themselves as gay, they argue, denies their self-determination (1,146). Indeed, as Munoz-Laboy has noted, 'The problem with the *MSM* category is that many men do not identify with the label, which leads to their increased alienation from HIV prevention strategies' (2004, 58). Young and Meyer warn that 'ignoring identity in HIV prevention efforts can be perilous, because sexual identities may provide important clues for public health prevention efforts'; for example, they note,

'top' and 'bottom' to denote sexual roles, and 'bareback,' to denote sex without condoms, are part of a sex culture and connote meanings as well as behaviors that are associated with HIV risk and are relevant to HIV prevention. These terms and others could be more useful than *MSM* in public health research and intervention in that they reveal more nuanced information about sexuality, identity, and risk for HIV infection (2005, 1,147).

Through the broad labelling of all Caribbean men engaged in homosexual practices as MSM, heteronationalism is asserted by both denying the self-identification practices men already use, and the failure of investment in historical research on sexual cultures in the region, which could result in a more nuanced reading of sexual practices than the prescriptive MSM model and, ultimately, better prevention efforts.

Given the importance of social and cultural analysis, it is difficult to accept claims that the de-politicization of sexuality issues is really in the best service of prevention and care objectives. Following a global trend, the Trinidadian organization 'MSM No Political Agenda' is forthright in declaring its apolitical outlook. Indeed, 'MSM' appears to have become a way of speaking about sexuality without forcing (although still making available) an examination of the ways in which sexual practices and identities are regulated and repressed, and without holding various actors accountable for sexuality-based marginalization. As explained in trend-setting Naz Foundation (India) Trust's 2004 manual, 'MSM'

> recognizes that many men may have sex with other men, but do not necessarily consider themselves to be homosexual or gay. They do not consider their sexual encounters with other men in terms of sexual identity or orientation.

Conversely,

> being gay is more of an identity or "lifestyle." They see their gay identity as a determining or defining characteristic for making certain lifestyle choices. These may include not getting married, living with a male partner, etc. In some cases the gay man may be "out," or open to family, friends, work colleagues and others about their sexuality.

'Some men who identify as "gay"', the authors also submit,

> do so as a means of politicizing homosexuality. They are interested
> in increasing the visibility of the homosexual men and the struggle
> for their rights. In this sense, the term "gay" is increasingly being
> adopted as a social and political identity (Naz 2004, 8–9).

'MSM' is thus articulated as a politically 'neutral' term, operating as a
tacit agreement between the larger development agencies and states that
the identification of 'MSM' as a key target group for the purposes of
controlling HIV and AIDS will not commit either party to a broader
conversation about their 'lifestyles' or rights — those are seen as issues
that relate to gay men, *not* 'MSM'. Thus, references to MSM can
comfortably appear in national AIDS plans of countries with anti-sodomy
legislation, like Saint Lucia, Trinidad and Tobago, and Barbados. MSM
offers a way to speak about sex without speaking of rights or welfare,
providing a way for governments to respond to the HIV and AIDS crises
and access the new resources made available, without committing them
to any serious reconsideration of dominant heteronationalism.

The availability of more funding opportunities for groups focused on
sexual health work directed at 'MSM' may have also blunted the political
agendas of NGOs and activist groups. As they redefine work programmes
around funders' primary interests in HIV and AIDS control and
prevention, questions about rights, power and justice may be lost, or less
strongly emphasized. If, as the name of 'MSM No Political Agenda' so
unabashedly conveys, HIV and AIDS work is best conducted as an
'apolitical' or 'politically neutral' project, how are we to evaluate its pursuit
in a context where heteronationalist imperatives dominate? Indeed, how
can any project be considered 'politically neutral' if it acts to mediate a
form of organisation that is oppressive — particularly to those very groups
it claims to 'protect'? The appeal of MSM as a 'neutral' category that
does not incite as much controversy or public attention as 'gay' or other
terms must be seriously reconsidered.

Hope in the Contradictions?

The objective of this discussion of MSM is neither to denounce it, nor to encourage any project that would seek out 'the right' language for carrying out HIV and AIDS work in the Caribbean. Rather, it serves a cautionary note that compels consistent critical attention to discourse in the way HIV and AIDS care and prevention mandates are carried out. As I have argued above, although it is presented as an unproblematic epidemiological category, the employment of MSM discourse has profound implications for not just the implementation of sexual health objectives, but also the rights and welfare of Caribbean people, and the organisation of power relations in Caribbean societies. I have pointed to some important ways in which I believe the discourse of MSM serves to maintain heteronationalism in the region. But it is also important to recognise that whatever the mandates of UNAIDS, the World Bank, national governments, international NGOs and other actors who shape HIV and AIDS projects, the creative agency of individuals and communities give rise to more interesting and radical possibilities.

References

AIDS Alliance. 2003. *Between Men*, Brighton: Internaional HIV/AIDS Alliance.

Alexander, M. J. 2005. *Pedagogies of Crossing: Meditations on Feminism, Sexual Politics, Memory, and The Sacred.* Durham and London: Duke University Press.

Benoit, M. 'Homosexuality: Natural or Unnatural?' *St. Lucia Star,* March 10, 2004.

Creary, L.P. 2002. 'It's hell being gay in Jamaica.' *The Jamaica Observer,* October 30. Accessed at http://www.jamaicaobserver.com/letters/html/20021029t230000-0500_34394, January 30, 2008.

Gosine, A. 2004. *Sex for pleasure, rights to participation and alternatives to HIV/AIDS: Placing sexual minorities and/or dissidents in international development.* Sussex: Institute for Development Studies.

————. 2006. 'Race,' Culture, Power, Sex, Desire, Love: Writing in Men who have Sex with men. *IDS Bulletin* 37, no. 5: 27–33.

Hines, H. 2007. 'Mob beats crossdresser'. *The Jamaica Observer.* April 28. Accessed at *http://www.jamaicaobserver.com/news/html/20070428T020000-0500_122324_obs_ mob_beats_cross_dresser.asp*, January 30, 2007.

Hoyos, D. E. 2003. 'Back to basics'. *The Nation,* October 27.

Human Rights Watch. 2008. 'Jamaica: Shield gays from mob attacks,' *http://hrw.org/english/docs/2008/02/01/jamaic17957.htm*, accessed February 10, 2008.

Jamaica Observer. 2007. 'Anti-gay attack'. April 3. Accessed at *http://www.jamaicaobserver.com/news/html/20070402t230000-0500_121276_obs_anti_ gay_attack.asp*, January 30, 2008.

Kinsella, W. 2007. 'Jamaican murder music does not belong in Canada.' *The National Post.* September 22. Accessed at *http://www.nationalpost.com/opinion/columnists/story.html?id=450ece5d-d24e-4258-a3e1-9b5b822934c9&k=54493*, January 30, 2008.

"Le Journal d'un Terrien," web blog accessed at *http://caraibes.wordpress.com/2007/06/02/homosexual-cruise-in-st-maarten/*, January 30, 2008.

Malebranche, D. J., RW Stackhouse et al. (2004). 'Race and sexual identity: perceptions about medical culture and healthcare among black men who have sex with men'. *J Natl Med Assoc.,* 96: 97–107.

Munoz-Laboy, M. 2004. 'Beyond "MSM": Sexual Desire among Bisexually-Active Latino Men in New York City'. *Sexualities,* 7, no. 1: 55–80.

Naz Foundation (India) Trust. 2004. *Training Manual: An Introduction to Promoting Sexual Health for Men Who Have Sex with Men and Gay Men,* New Delhi: Naz.

Niang, I. C., et al. 2004. 'Targeting Vulnerable Groups in National HIV/AIDS Programs: The Case of Men Who Have Sex with Men – Senegal, Burkina Faso, The Gambia'. African Region human development working paper series no. 82. *World Bank Report.*

Padgett, T. 2006. 'The most homophobic place on earth?' *TIME* April 12: Time Warner. Accessed at *http://www.time.com/time/world/article/0,8599,1182991,00.html,* January 30, 2007.

Reid, T. 2007. 'Same-sex lessons – Ministry recommended textbook lists homosexual unions as family option'. Jamaica *Gleaner ,* Oct. 31. Accessed at *http://www.jamaica-gleaner.com/gleaner/20071031/lead/lead1.html,* January 30, 2007.

Schmalz, E. 2007. 'Sexuality and Gender Law Clinic Secures Asylum for Gay Men'. Press release. Columbia Law School.

Sinfield, A. 1998. *Gay and After.* London: Serpent's Tail.

Swamber, Keino. 2007. 'Gay man seeks compensation'. *Trinidad Express,* August 30. Accessed at *http://www.trinidadexpress.com/index.pl/article_news?id=161196478,* January 30, 2008.

St Maarten Private Eye, reported at *http://sxmprivateeye.com/,* accessed January 30, 2008

Taylor, D. 2004. 'If you're gay in Jamaica, you're dead'. *The Guardian,* August 2. Accessed at *http://www.guardian.co.uk/g2/story/0,,1274067,00.html,* January 30, 2008.

Titus, R. 2007. November 20. Gay cruise ship 'invasion' ignites debate in Grenada. *CMC,* accessed at cananes.net, January 30, 2008.

UNAIDS 2006, Report on the Global AIDS epidemic. Geneva: UNAIDS.

Wekker, G. 2006. *The Politics of Passion: Women's Sexual Culture in the Afro-Surinamese Diaspora.* New York: Columbia University Press.

World Bank Group. 2004. *Issue Brief: HIV/AIDS. South Asia Region (SAR) India,* March, 15. Retrieved October 1, 2007 from World Bank. Website: *http://www.worldbank.org/in*

World Bank. 2004. *Targeting Vulnerable Groups in National HIV/AIDS Programs. The Case of Men Who Have Sex with Men-Senegal, Burkina Faso, The Gambia.* Africa Region Human Development Working Paper Series, September. World Bank. Website: *http://www.worldbank.org/in*

Wright, T. 2000. 'Gay organisations, NGOs and the globalization of sexual identity: the case of Bolivia'. *Journal of Latin American Anthropology* 5, no. 2: 89–111.

Young, R. M. and I. Meyer, 2005. 'The Trouble with "MSM" and "WSW": Erasure of the Sexual-Minority Person in Public Health Discourse'. *American Journal of Public Health* 95, no. 7: 1144, 1149.

CHAPTER 6

POSITIVELY LIMITED

Gender, Sexuality and HIV and AIDS Discourses in Barbados

DAVID MURRAY

In the call for papers for this volume, Barrow, De Bruin, and Carr note how responses to HIV have recognized the importance of vulnerability, a term that captures larger structural determinants of choices and behaviours in which risky practices occur. Vulnerability thus speaks to larger-scale inequities that can produce social exclusion and increase risky behaviour. Many researchers have, rightly, noted that these inequities can only be understood through research that takes into account socio-cultural contexts: But, we must first ask what exactly is a 'socio-cultural context'; how are cultural contexts defined? Are they local practices and structures that interact to produce particular forms of inequality? How do we define 'local' in the Caribbean? Is culture nationally bounded, ethno-racially bounded, or more global in scope and nature? While this may appear to be an academic and abstract question of definitions, I think it has important ramifications for policy development and actions aimed at reducing the spread of HIV, especially now that bodies like UNAIDS are acknowledging that understanding cultural (as well as political and economic) factors are critical to understanding ways in which gender and sexuality are key components of determining vulnerability. In the Caribbean, as elsewhere in the world, when we speak of cultural determinants of structural inequalities, we must be careful not to forget the ways in which they are produced in and through multiple local and transnational discourses and materialities. Localities are produced in a world of globalizing capital, communications and mobile populations; in the case of gender and sexuality, this means that while we must carefully scrutinize how masculinity and femininity are produced in local contexts in ways that privilege some individuals and groups and marginalize, or silence, others, we must also and always explore how privileging discourses and practices are reinforced through their links to transnational economic and political interests. This is, of course, a point made by Alexander (2005) and others.

In this chapter, I engage with the local-transnational dynamic of gender and sexuality through an exploration of how the state has become involved in the sexuality of its citizens (an involvement which is also and always gendered) through activities and statements related to HIV, a virus that knows no national boundaries. The fact that most HIV treatment, prevention and education efforts in the Caribbean are managed and/or funded at least in part through international (as well as national) health organisations requires any analysis to acknowledge transnational influences on state policies and actions. My focus in this chapter is on the nation state of Barbados and the National HIV and AIDS Commission, established in 2001, whose mandate is 'To coordinate effectively the national expanded response to reduce the incidence and spread of the epidemic in Barbados' and whose mission is to 'advise the government on plans and policies and to build strategic partnerships to effectively manage, control and reduce the spread of HIV in Barbados'. (www.hivaidsbarbados.com).

Numerous scholars analysing the global HIV pandemic have observed the ways in which government and international health organisations' efforts to control and manage the spread of the virus have often perpetuated moral agendas which in turn perpetuate gendered, sexual, race and/or class inequalities. Researchers like Cindy Patton (1997, 2002), Paula Treichler (1999) and Thomas Yingling (1997) have demonstrated how, in the early years of the epidemic, media representations, government policies and health organisation interventions often stigmatized already marginalized social groups, ranging from 'Africans', 'female sex workers', and 'homosexuals' to struggling immigrant populations. In many cases, these forms of viral-based discrimination also reproduced transnational inequalities established during periods of colonization which are reflected today in ongoing political and economic inequalities between so-called developed and developing nations. Within national borders of developing nations whose policies are influenced, if not dictated, by supra national organisations who control the purse strings of these nations' health and welfare programmes, state-level HIV discourses often reproduce these problematic moral agendas, and become a way of talking about or constructing threats to the national body. That is, talk about how to ensure public health through prevention education conveys moral agendas in which certain bodies are privileged as model citizens of the nation state while others are labelled dangerous through their association with improper gendered and sexual behaviour which renders them diseased and deadly.

In this chapter, I focus on the ways in which gendered and sexual citizenship has been produced through statements made by Barbadian government officials and in publications of the National HIV and AIDS Commission (NHAC) in the early years of the new millennium. Much of what I am arguing builds on Andil Gosine's research on the ways in which sexuality rights and international development have been related through the AIDS epidemic. Gosine (2004) notes that while HIV has resulted in recognising the importance of understanding sexual practices and customs in all aspects of international development, and that, at the very least, sexual diversity is now recognized as a universal fact, there are still significant problems in the ways in which sexual minorities are perceived or represented in international development policies. For example, studies have noted that in many societies, men have sex with men as well as with women but in few societies is male-male sex widely acceptable. These studies often argue that in states where homosexual practices are illegal, laws must be revised so that there is less stigma attached to these practices, allowing state health organizations to better access this high-risk group in order to protect the wider society, as women are also at risk from these men. However, Gosine notes that in places where same-sex sexuality is only publicly discussed in relation to an HIV framework, sexual minorities come to matter only in terms of causing or alleviating HIV (Gosine 2004, 5–6). This creates or perpetuates a reductive understanding of these groups' sexual identities to something that is primarily associated with a dangerous disease, and therefore also elides numerous other social and economic issues they must deal with. The end result is perpetuation of heteronormativity in development policy and planning, which, once again, means that gender roles for men and women are constructed within narrow confines (Gosine 2004, 10). In other words, HIV policies, which are now integral components of both national and international development programmes, often reproduce dominant heteronormative frameworks which are also and always colonially inflected racial and gendered frameworks, and thus contribute towards the privileging of a delimited gendered and sexed citizen of the state. Limiting discussions of same-sex sexual behaviour to an HIV framework leaves no room available for thinking about sex in other, more productive and pleasurable frameworks, nor for recognizing the rights of men and women engaged in those practices.

Building on these observations, I argue that in Barbadian public and institutional contexts, same-sex sexual minorities are, for the most part, unmentioned or unmentionable, and that when they are visible their visibility tends to be only in association with HIV as 'risk' groups whose sexuality ends up being represented as a problem or threat. HIV talk in Barbados, while opening up new avenues of dialogue about sexual behaviour and morality in Barbadian society, has thus far reinscribed normative gender/sex roles.

HOMOSEXUALITY IN BARBADOS: A BRIEF OVERVIEW

Before going any further, a few words contextualizing the place of homosexuality in Barbados are necessary. Over the past ten to 15 years the Caribbean has come to be identified as a 'homophobic' region (Human Rights Watch 2004; Atluri 2001). In another paper, I have reviewed media coverage on homosexuality in Barbados, and found that it concurs with these claims; that is, I found a general pattern of negative representation in media discussions of homosexuality (Murray 2007). However, over the course of three research trips in Barbados between 2002–2005 exploring the purported rise in homophobia, I heard both gay and straight identified Barbadians in the community where I was working (a working-class neighbourhood in the Cheapside section of Bridgetown) claim that homosexuals are not discriminated against in terms of employment, housing or general treatment — as 'everyone knows' there are homosexuals in positions of power and influence and no one is forcing them to quit their jobs.[1] A number of my gay interviewees[2] stated that there are members of their family, friends and associates in the workplace who are supportive and/or have no issue with their sexual orientation. At the same time, I collected stories of harassment and violence from other interviewees. Furthermore, there is evidence that the situation in Barbados is not improving for these men — the majority of them said they felt that there is an increasing amount of hostility towards them compared to 15–20 years ago.

Based on these findings, to claim that Barbados as a society or the Caribbean as a region is homophobic or discriminates against homosexuals is both correct *and* incorrect. I would argue that this claim glosses over a complex set of attitudes and differing values; it becomes a misleading appellation that obliterates the sexual diversity and acceptance of that diversity by many. Clearly, there are widespread opinions and beliefs that say otherwise, but to claim that there is no diversity of perspective on this problem is misrepresentative and forecloses further discussion of it.

Nevertheless, governmental departments and units like NHAC must develop policy in tandem with the laws of the state. Currently, there are laws in the Criminal Code of Barbados which are interpreted as anti-homosexual. These laws refer to acts of 'sodomy' — strictly speaking, this means that heterosexual sodomy is outlawed as much as homosexual. As some legal analysts have pointed out, it could, therefore, be argued that homosexuality is not illegal in Barbados, only certain sexual positions are, but, in almost all contemporary discussions, these laws are utilized as primary examples of the state's criminalisation of homosexuality. The HIV crisis has been the catalyst for a recent parliamentary discussion on the decriminalization of laws which are interpreted to be anti homosexual, which, in turn, has generated a media frenzy.

MIA MOTTLEY'S STATEMENT AND PROFESSOR WALROND'S REPORT

In 2003, Mia Mottley, then deputy prime minister and attorney general of Barbados, spoke of the 'cancer of discrimination' that was preventing 'highly at risk' segments of the population from benefiting from HIV prevention programmes. The threat posed by male-to-male sexual transmission of HIV to whole communities — a threat exacerbated by social discrimination against men who have sex with men (MSM) — compelled a review of the state's approaches to sexual regulation. A year later, the Attorney General's Office requested a consultation on the legal, ethical and socioeconomic issues relevant to HIV and AIDS in Barbados from Professor E.R. Walrond, former dean of the School of Clinical Medicine and Research at UWI, Cave Hill and chairman of the National Advisory Committee on AIDS 1987–1994. This report recommended numerous revisions to Barbadian legislation relevant to HIV which were 'intended to remove the social barriers to the spread of HIV' (Walrond 2004, 6). Once again, Professor Walrond recommended changes to the criminal code that would assist in the 'process of destigmatizing marginalized groups such as homosexuals, prostitutes and sexually active adolescents who are at high risk of HIV infection in order to diagnose them earlier and reduce the prevalence of HIV' (Walrond 2004, 7). Following publication of this report NHAC held a series of public forums in which they sought feedback on this report's recommendations. I attended three of these forums in 2004–05. Most of the comments at these forums focused on Walrond's recommendations to decriminalize laws against 'homosexuals and prostitutes' and were vehemently opposed. These forums received a great deal of coverage on local television and in the two daily newspapers, the latter publishing a steady stream of letters to the editor expressing, for the most part, similar points of view on these recommendations on HIV and homosexuality in Barbados

Mottley and Walrond's statements about homosexuality, HIV and discrimination were not just idle thoughts; they were based on studies of HIV conducted by various groups throughout Barbados and the rest of the Caribbean. We need to keep in mind that Barbados has an HIV prevalence rate of approximately 1.8 per cent (United Nations General Assembly Special Session on HIV and AIDS, Country Report Barbados 2006), which translates to approximately 5,080 people living with HIV out of a population of 280,000 (2007 Estimate, US Census Bureau, International Programs Center; *www.census.gov*). This is a relatively high rate compared to countries like Canada, where the prevalence rate is between 0.2–0.5 per cent, but significantly lower than other Caribbean countries like Trinidad and Tobago (2.6 per cent) or Haiti (3.8 per cent) (Joint United Nations Programme on HIV and AIDS 2007: *http:// www.unaids.org/en/Regions_Countries*).

I found it difficult to obtain information on the modes of transmission of the virus for Barbados: One NHAC document stated that from December 1984 to March 2001, 86.8 per cent of HIV infections had been transmitted via heterosexual sex, and only 5.7 per cent through homosexual/ bisexual (NHAC 2001) (the remainder were perinatal and blood transfusions) but, as the authors note, these figures may underestimate the rate of homosexual/bisexual transmission due to stigma associated with these sexual practices. A more general statement about transmission can be found in the UNAIDS epidemic update report for 2006 which states:

> The Caribbean's largely heterosexual epidemics occur in the context of harsh gender inequalities and are being fuelled by a thriving sex industry, which services both local and foreign clients. Sex between men, a hidden phenomenon in the generally homophobic social environments found in this region, is a smaller but important factor, and unsafe sex between men is believed to account for about one tenth of reported HIV cases in the region (UNAIDS 2006).

The Caribbean Epidemiology Centre's 2007 Report on HIV in member countries makes a similar observation:

> As in the wider Caribbean, the primary mode of HIV transmission in CAREC member countries is through unprotected sexual intercourse. In the early years, surveillance data revealed that transmission of HIV was primarily homosexual; current data reveals

a mosaic of homo/bi and heterosexual transmission with a current male-to-female ratio of almost one-to-one. (CAREC 2007)

These and other reports go on to note that most Caribbean nations are homophobic, and their governments unwilling to change discriminatory laws. Official indifference or hostility means that there are few prevention and care programmes for men who have sex with men which, in turn, means that these groups are not being reached and thus continue to pose a risk for the spread of the virus among themselves and to others (i.e. female partners).

Mottley's statements and Walrond's report are clearly influenced by this framing of sexual alterity in HIV research. These positions argue that the rights of homosexuals must be assured in Barbados primarily in order to contain HIV from spreading throughout the nation. This is a limited representation of homosexuality as it (a) focuses primarily on men (there is no mention of women) who are (b) constructed primarily through sexual practices which works to reinscribe an old stereotype — the homosexual defined through deviant sexual acts — and adds another, more threatening layer — that these sexual acts are dangerous and may kill women and children. Thus, we see an argument for the rights of homosexuals constituted primarily through devious and dangerous sex acts which not only reproduces a problematic stereotype but also works to reproduce racialising colonial narratives about the 'natural' proclivities of non-white men, and undermines the complex negotiations they make in expressing sexual choices.

THE FRAGILE ANUS

Evidence of the ways in which these official recommendations worked to reinscribe discriminatory attitudes towards homosexuality could be found in media coverage, particularly in letters to the editor sections of the Barbadian daily newspapers, The *Advocate* and The *Nation*. One letter writer was quite explicit in her critique of the recommendation to decriminalize homosexuality:

It was the former United States Surgeon General, Dr Benjamin Koop, who cautioned that the anal canal is not intended for use as a sexual orifice, given its very thin and fragile lining. This, together with the disease profile and early death of homosexuals through hepatitis, liver disease, gastro-intestinal parasites, sexually transmitted diseases...should be of particular concern to Professor Walrond who should oppose homosexuality on purely medical grounds...We must not forsake our enduring Christian morality for the bigotry of secularism...It will be tyrannical of the government to support (this recommendation). (The *Nation,* January 12, 2005*)*

Other letters, similarly, spoke of 'the abuse of the gift of sexuality' and/or the danger of legislating support for something that 'goes against the laws of nature'. In these comments, homosexuality is reductively defined or discussed primarily in relation to a specific sexual act, anal intercourse, which comes to stand for a particular type of person or personality type. The metonymic value of a sex act — standing for a deviant kind of person — illustrates how this public debate over changing a couple of Barbadian laws is about more than just decriminalization of a sexual activity; it is about how the state should legislate the gendered and sexual identities of its citizens, or, more generally, how the terms of inclusion of citizenship are set in the Barbadian nation state. The problem here lies in the conceptual framework in which the terms of inclusion are negotiated and how particular sexual practices and identities are organized to operate as the limits of inclusion/exclusion (Alexander 2005). In this context, there is one primary sign, anal sexual intercourse, which represents and frames both sides of the debate over the homosexual's place in the Barbadian nation; the effect of this limited representation simultaneously reinscribes long established discriminatory attitudes towards those who are believed to engage in this act and now connects them to a deadly virus which threatens to infect the 'good' (heterosexual) citizens of the state. The result may further objectify the category of the homosexual while simultaneously trying to 'normalize' it through decriminalization.

The first steps to awareness + social change is teaching gender queer individuals about sexuality. That it's not THIS or THAT.

Furthermore, as noted above, the articulation of 'homosexual rights' only in relation to HIV prevention obscures a more complex understanding of the implications of sexual regulations on the lives of Barbadian men and women. In other words, by only focusing on HIV prevention, other consequences of repressive or negligent state laws are overlooked such as issues of sexual harassment in public spaces, including workplaces, verbal and physical violence both at home and in the public, police harassment, employment discrimination and other areas in which sexuality may be significant.

'HOMOSEXUALS' AND UNDESERVED SEXUAL 'RIGHTS'

Mottley's and Walrond's recommendations and the public reactions to them were framed in terms of 'the rights of 'homosexuals': both 'rights' and 'homosexuals' are culturally specific and historically loaded categories which need to be critically interrogated for the ways in which their meanings circulate in particular ways in Barbados. The 'homosexual' is a term with a Euro-American etymology: in most popular contexts, it is a sexual identity category in which particular sexual acts are tied to essentialist identities, and those identities are presumed to share certain personality or behavioural traits. However, scholars of Latin American and Caribbean sexuality have demonstrated that using the label 'homosexual' to describe a wide range of behaviours and values associated with those behaviours is problematic, and ethnographic research in this region clearly demonstrates the fluidity of sexual behaviours and their categorizations (See Kulick 1998; Lancaster 1992; Murray 2002; Padilla 2007; Prieur 1998; Wekker 1999). While I met numerous Barbadian men who identify as 'gay' or 'homosexual', most of them noted that there were many men who had sex with other men in Barbados who did not identify in this way for a variety of reasons, ranging from associating 'gay' with a metropolitan, middle-class and white male identity located mostly in Euro-American cities, to stating that they were primarily interested in women sexually, which, therefore, meant they could not be 'homosexual'. Much more could be said on this issue in terms of how gender and sexuality roles and

125

identities are combined and developed in Barbados, but, suffice it to say, that government and health officials advocating rights for and outreach to 'homosexuals' may be only partially representing the sexual landscape in Barbados, and, thus, only partially successful in their desired social and health objectives.

I have addressed the complexity of using 'rights' as a discourse to promote social justice for a sexual minority in another article where I argue that framing justice and equality through rights talk may have deleterious effects for its advocates, as there is no 'clear' or transparent universality as to what rights means and that particular interpretations may be used to further marginalise already stigmatized groups (Murray 2006). For the purposes of this chapter, I will only highlight the point that we must recognize there is more than one way of understanding what 'rights' means. One way of understanding rights is, as Mottley and Walrond frame them — that is — as a demand for political and legal equality of all citizens of a state. Their statements reflect a basic liberal understanding of rights as guarantors of *individual* liberal freedom based on the *natural* equality of all human beings. However, in NHAC's public forums gauging community response to the Walrond Report, another interpretation of rights emerged: one audience member said that she could not understand why the Commission was supporting the idea of 'giving rights' to a group who engaged in activities that most Barbadians do not approve of. Another person spoke passionately about the need to protect Barbados against the 'gay agenda', which is apparently being promoted by a highly organized, secret group with members in positions of political and economic power around the world who are trying to force all nations to accept their 'gay rights manifesto'. These comments interpret rights as 'special rights', that is, as a demand by a particular minority group to be granted protected status or to be treated in some special way that will prove prejudicial to the majority. There are additional ways in which rights may be interpreted in different contexts (see Murray 2006), but at the very least we can begin to recognize that it is problematic to speak about 'the rights of homosexuals' in a place where Euro-American sexual identity categories and models of social justice may be interpreted in relation to distinct local values pertaining to individuality, sociality and sexuality.

CONCLUSION

During the media melee following Mottley's statements and Walrond's report, I noticed that there were no comments or official response by any member of NHAC. I was not surprised: When I interviewed a member of the executive board of NHAC in 2003 and asked what programmes were planned or in place targeting gay men or MSM, I was first reminded that in Barbados, the vast majority of transmissions are caused through heterosexual sex, but, more significantly, the Commission's 'hands were tied' when it came to outreach to groups like homosexuals and sex workers due to the laws of the Criminal Code. Members of the Commission were well aware that outreach to these groups was critical[3] but they could not make any public statements supporting more controversial proposals like changing legislation as this was a political hot potato, and since they were funded through the Prime Minister's Office, they could not risk controversy.

Four years later, when I visited to the NHAC website (*http:// www.hivaidsbarbados.com/* accessed August 2007) I saw their motto, 'Stay Safe, Love Life' written around a red ribbon on every page. While the website contained information on how the virus is transmitted, how to protect oneself, and where to go for testing or further information, there was no mention of sexual diversity, except for one line which stated that:

> men who have sex with men and commercial sex workers are examples of groups...(where) there is a higher prevalence of the virus because of their sexual practices and therefore having unsafe sex with someone from one of these groups places you at a higher risk of contracting the virus.

As one can probably surmise from this kind of statement, the Criminal Code of Barbados remains unchanged at this point; Mottley's and

Walrond's recommendations have not been implemented. More important, however, is the perpetuation of the reductive representation of a sexual minority to a (dangerous) sex act and the deleterious effects of this representation on the place of homosexual men or MSM in discourses of citizenship in the Barbadian nation state, not to mention the perpetuation of absolute invisibility of lesbians or women who have sex with women. It would be wrong to blame the Barbadian health and HIV authorities for constructing and circulating this representation on their own — as I have tried to demonstrate in this chapter, the Barbadian position on the relationship between sexual minorities, HIV, and the state has been constructed in and through transnational discourses positing a particular set of values about the relationship between health, sex, gender and the nation. While we cannot, and should not, dismiss the importance of targeting groups who are at higher risk of contracting HIV in public health programmes, a more meaningful public conversation about sexual diversity must be developed in order to recognize, guarantee, and protect the place of sexual minorities as equal citizens of their states. Much more could be said about this but suffice it to say that until this conversation takes place, the Barbadian state's interventions (and those of numerous other states both North and South of the equator) in the sexual health of its citizens will continue to perpetuate a message of heternormativity which will in turn perpetuate the exclusion, marginalization and dangerous silencing of significant numbers of men and women from effectively participating in their own health and well being.

NOTES

1. I also heard similar comments from some UWI faculty when I presented a paper on homophobia and sexual rights at the UWI Cave Hill campus in January 2005, indicating that these views are not limited to a particular class.
2. I conducted formal taped interviews with 15 gay identified men in this community, and had informal discussions focusing on topics similar to those in the interviews with another 12 men.
3. Based on this comment, it was not clear whether gay and bisexual men were viewed by the Committee as vectors of disease or as having a right to health.

REFERENCES

Alexander, Jacqui. 2005. *Pedagogies of Crossing: Meditations on Feminism, Sexual Politics, Memory and the Sacred.* New York. Durham.

Atluri, Tara. 2001. *When the Closet is a Region.* Cave Hill, Barbados: Centre for Gender and Development Studies. University of West Indies.

CAREC. 2007. Annual Report Trinidad and Tobago: CAREC. Accessed March 2008 at: *http://www.carec.org/*

Gosine, Andil. 2004. 'Sex for Pleasure, Right to Participation, and Alternatives to AIDS: Placing Sexual Minorities and/or Dissidents in Development'. Working Paper no. 228.

————. 2007. *Reading Mia Mottley's Statement on (homo)sex: An Interrogation of HIV/AIDS Scripts on Sexuality (and a call to engage alternate strategies for sexual autonomy).* Unpublished manuscript.

Human Rights Watch. 2004. *Hated to Death: Homophobia, Violence and Jamaica's HIV/AIDS Epidemic.* Accessed at *http://hrw.org/reports/2004/jamaica1104/*.

Kulick, Don. 1998. *Travesti: Sex, Gender and Culture among Brazilian Transgendered Prostitutes.* University of Chicago Press: Chicago.

Lancaster, Roger. 1992. *Life is Hard: Machismo, Danger and the Intimacy of Power in Nicaragua.* Berkeley: University of California Press.

Murray, David A. B. 2002. *Opacity: Gender, Sexuality, Race and the 'Problem' of Identity in Martinique.* New York: Peter Lang Press.

————. 2006. 'Who's Right? Human Rights, Sexual Rights and Social Change in Barbados'. *Culture, Health and Sexuality* 8 no. 3-4.

————. 2007. *Homo hauntings: Spectral Sexuality and the Good Citizen in Barbadian Media.* Unpublished Manuscript.

National HIV/AIDS Commission of Barbados. 2001 *The HIV/AIDS Epidemic: An Update.* Bridgetown.

Padilla, Mark. 2007. *Caribbean Pleasure Industry: Tourism, Sexuality and AIDS in the Dominican Republic.* Chicago: University of Chicago Press.

Patton, Cindy. 1997. 'From Nation to Family: Containing African AIDS'. In *The Gender/Sexuality Reader*, eds. R. Lancaster and M. DiLeonardo. New York: Routledge Press.

————. 2002. *Gobalizing AIDS.* Minneapolis: University of Minnesota Press.

Prieur, Annick. 1998. *Mema's House, Mexico City: On Transvestites, Queens and Machos.* Chicago: University of Chicago.

Treichler, Paula. 1999. *How to have Theory in an Epidemic: Cultural Chronicles of AIDS.* Durham: Duke University Press.

United Nations General Assembly Special Session HIV/AIDS 2006 *Country Report: Barbados. http://www.unaids.org/en/Regions_Countries* (accessed December 8, 2007).

Walrond, E. R. 2004. *Report on the Legal Ethical and Socio-Economic Issues Relevant to HIV/AIDS.* Bridgetown.

Wekker, Gloria. 1999. 'What's Identity Got to do with it? Rethinking Identity in Light of the Mati Work in Suriname'. In *Same Sex Relations and Transgender Practices Across Cultures*, eds. E. Blackwood and S. Wieringa. New York: Columbia University Press.

Yingling, Thomas. 1997. *AIDS and the National Body.* Durham: Duke University Press.

CHAPTER 7
COMMUNICATION AND HIV
Multi-Dimensional Frustration

MARJAN DE BRUIN

INTRODUCTION

Experts in HIV prevention in the Caribbean are beginning to realize that their efforts, in which communication planning and interventions play crucial roles, have not been very successful. Although studies show some achievement, important groups of people are still not responding as expected. In 2006 the Caribbean's average HIV rate was one per cent but prevalence in individual countries varied considerably. While Cuba's adult HIV prevalence was among the lowest in the world at 0.1 per cent, rates in The Bahamas and Haiti were among the worst — as high as 3.3 per cent and 3.8 per cent (UNAIDS 2007). Particularly vulnerable communities such as commercial sex workers — mobile groups, in-country as well as intra-regionally — inhabit a range from 3.5 per cent in the Dominican Republic to 31 per cent in Guyana. With such disparities, it is more appropriate to speak of a region with multiple epidemics — some of which have stabilised while others are still growing.

HIV in the Caribbean is transmitted primarily through unprotected sex with an HIV-positive partner — much more commonly than through use of needles or contaminated (transfused) blood and hardly at all through mother-to-child transmission (MTC), the rate of which is falling rapidly. Recent data reveal a 'mosaic of homo/bi and heterosexual transmission with a current male-to-female ratio of almost one-to-one.' (CAREC 2007, 4).

This chapter will examine the role of communication in HIV-prevention strategies. Assuming that HIV-prevention interventions in the field are guided by national and regional strategic planning, I intend to identify precisely what role is ascribed to 'communication' by policy frameworks in the region, generally, and specifically in three countries — Barbados, Jamaica and Trinidad and Tobago. I will do this by analysing the recent policy frameworks in this area: the relevant National Strategic Plans (NSPs) and PANCAP's (the Pan Caribbean Partnership against HIV and AIDS) Regional Strategic Framework (RSF) and Regional Action Plan. In my analysis, I will try to identify the models and strategies of communication approaches to which these policies refer and raise questions on the underlying, apparently implicit, assumptions.

Before presenting the results of this analysis, I will point to some of the puzzling data in Caribbean research on sexual behaviour: contradictions and gaps in the quantitative data, mainly coming from knowledge, attitude, practice and behaviour (KAPB) surveys. In trying to understand these gaps, I will return to data from qualitative research which seems to give the surveyed realities more depth. These 'puzzling gaps' may indicate the need to revise some of the concepts and assumptions employed in HIV prevention and the role communication may usefully play.

I will show that the Caribbean is not the only region in which there are serious questions about the foundations of communication interventions in HIV prevention. International debates, over the last decade, have focused on similar issues. I will conclude my examination by identifying the need for conceptual revision and reorientation of policy and proposing suggestions for follow-up action.

HIV AND SEXUAL BEHAVIOUR IN THE CARIBBEAN

To develop a better understanding of sexual behaviour in the Caribbean, studies in the '80s, and certainly up to the mid- '90s, tried to map out the more salient issues such as risky sexual behaviour, partnership status, median age at first sex, knowledge of HIV-prevention methods and use of condoms. Later additions were stigma and discrimination — all explored through regular, large-scale KAPB surveys. These studies were mainly descriptive, providing important baseline information and enabling the tracking of changes in sexual behaviour. Although we see the occasional qualitative study exploring the reasons and motives behind what seemed to be behaviour patterns (Chevannes 1994; Chevannes and Mitchell-Kernan 1993), it was only more recently that the 'why' questions would be raised on a more regular basis (Bailey et al. 1998; Chevannes 2001; Kempadoo and Dunn 2002; Leo-Rhynie and Pencle 2002; Parry 2000; Senderowitz et al. 1998; The Policy Project 1999; Williams 1999).

Most of the KAPB studies over the years show puzzling findings on the issues of knowledge and practice behaviour. For instance, in Jamaica, the most populous English-speaking country in the Caribbean, the latest national KAPB study (2004) shows a 'significant growth' in knowledge of prevention methods — between 75 per cent and 79 per cent of the population answered correctly when questioned on this. But, at the same time, one out of 12 adolescents (15–24 years) is not able to adequately assess their own risk (Hope Enterprises 2004). Or, another 'puzzle': recognition of the fact that inconsistent or no condom use is increasing risk-exposure among women from 39 per cent in 2000 to 48 per cent (Hope Enterprises 2004). Yet, 21 per cent of the grown-up women — the majority knowledgeable of HIV transmission modes — did not use a condom because they thought their partners didn't like them or might be upset if they suggested doing so (Hope Enterprises 2004). Or: in spite of high knowledge levels, 70 per cent of the women and 50 per cent of the men (both in the age group 25–49 years) engaged in high-risk sex and did not demonstrate consistent condom use (Ibid., 7).

Similar contradictions can be found in the Behaviour Surveillance Survey (BSS), describing 1999/2000 behaviour of youth in selected Jamaican parishes (FHI 2004). Of the in-school youth, of whom almost two-thirds had had sexual intercourse, 'general awareness' of HIV, STDs and condoms was 'universal', but only about one-third of students answered correctly to key questions about HIV prevention and transmission (FHI 2004, 17). Almost 30 per cent of the students who had used a condom also reported having had unprotected sex in the three months prior to the research (Ibid., 21). Data on the out-of-school youth — of whom more than 80 per cent had had sexual intercourse — showed a similar discrepancy between awareness of condom use (nearly universal) and the practice of unprotected sex. Of those who had had sex and who also had used a condom, almost 38 per cent reported engaging in unprotected sex in the three months prior to the interview (Ibid., 25).

This gap between HIV-prevention 'knowledge' and sound preventive 'practice' pervades the Anglophone Caribbean. In surveys done in Antigua and Barbuda, Dominica, Grenada, St Kitts and Nevis, Saint Lucia, St Vincent and the Grenadines, almost all youngsters between 10 and 14 years old had heard of HIV and AIDS and knew that the virus could be transmitted through sexual intercourse. The majority of in-school youth in these countries reported that they were still virgins (CAREC 2007a, 9) and only six per cent were sexually active (CAREC 2007a, 6). Yet, six out of ten of those who were sexually active had not used a condom at last sex (CAREC 2007b, 6).

Puzzling 'gaps' occur not only in data on youngsters; more than 80 per cent of the general population in the six Organisation of Eastern Caribbean States' (OECS) countries knew that consistent condom use was needed to protect against HIV, but less than half of the sexually active men and less than 20 per cent of the active women reported consistent condom use with casual partners (CAREC 2007b, 9).

The gap between knowledge and practice is not the only reason for concern; the confusion between knowledge and myth also puzzles researchers. In spite of the universal, or nearly universal, knowledge levels, myths about transmission remain persistent. In the Eastern Caribbean between 20 per cent and 40 per cent of those interviewed in the six countries believed that HIV could be spread by saliva, urine or sweat, mosquito bites, sitting on a toilet seat previously used by an HIV-positive person, sharing a meal, cutlery, plates, or cup with an HIV-positive person (CAREC 2007a, 6). Similarly, in Jamaica, between 14 per cent (females) and 17 per cent (males) thought that sharing food with HIV-positive persons would be risky (Hope Enterprises 2004). The mosquito-bite myth, although not as strong as in earlier years, is still alive. Knowledge of HIV and AIDS and misperceptions or myths on the same issue seem to co-exist without any problem.

Some of these gaps in Caribbean data were spotted earlier. Chevannes, almost 15 years ago, wrote about, what he called, an inferred gap between knowledge concerning the modes of transmitting HIV and attitudes towards people living with HIV (1994). Senderowitz et al. (1998) referred to a 'behavioural disconnect' in describing the knowledge on safe sex among young people and their translation of this knowledge into practice. Senderowitz claims that this disconnect, in part, results from traditional attitudes toward various features of sexual behaviour: multiple partners, early sexual initiation and non use of contraception. In reviewing a decade of studies on adolescents' reproductive health, de Bruin (2002) pointed to the existence of gaps and contradictions surfacing 'at various levels: within knowledge (the difference between prompted and unprompted knowledge of contraceptive methods), between knowledge and attitudes, knowledge and behaviour, or knowledge and beliefs.' (32). Up to that time, 2002, these gaps had not led to any follow-up research questions but only created a new concept: the KAP gap.

'OFF-SCENE' FACTORS

Factors well beyond the availability of information and level of knowledge seem to play important roles in decisions to engage in sexual activity. A slowly growing body of qualitative research begins to show more nuances among the surveyed realities. These studies show a range of benefits that girls derive from sexual activity and from becoming pregnant: improved status and social advancement, peer group approval, money and material things are some (Chevannes, 1994, 2001; Hope Enterprises 2000; Kempadoo and Dunn 2002; Parry 2000). The rules of the community may give them little choice when their 'dons' demand sexual favours, as we know happens in Jamaica and other countries. The slogan 'Use a Condom Every Time' must compete with the fear of what could be lost by saying 'no' to unprotected sex (for instance — a relationship; child support; lunch money; school fees; etc.). In many instances the economic reality in deprived communities appears to be the primary catalyst for 'risky' behaviour. These phenomena have also been observed in other regions of the world. All these conditions may have 'disabled volitional control over sexual activity and contribute to overall vulnerability to HIV infection.' (Parker 2004, 3).

On the other hand, some researchers warn that 'It is simplistic to conclude that young women are just forced into risky sexual relationships, either by coercive men or through poverty (although both of these scenarios are common)' (Rolfe and Hemmings 2007, 10). Rolfe and Hemmings' recent qualitative study is based on 126 in-depth interviews with young Jamaican women in inner-city Kingston. Although their data point to 'competition in a complex and hostile environment' with livelihood strategies 'as either high risk, high reward (generally through relationships with risky men), or low risk, low reward (domestic services, petty trading)' (Ibid., 10) the researchers also emphasize:

> We found young women to actively and consciously manage their relationships with different men, both to meet basic subsistence needs and to take part in the competitive life of the ghetto; to enjoy the material goods, status and experiences that successfully accessing resources brings.

The cultural wisdom of the community on what is needed for survival makes multiple partnerships the norm in many cases. Transactional sex enjoys 'a widespread acceptance' (Rolfe and Hemmings 2007, 40) and 'emerges as a series of rational choices made in response to socio-economic realities, rather than individual lifestyle decisions' (Ibid., 38).

The same study shows how HIV 'knowledge' may be adapted — prevention workers may say 'getting clouded' — into the discourse of the community. It becomes incorporated in the pertinence of laymen's knowledge, bending some of the facts and fitting others, or as the researchers describe — 'correct beliefs are typically mixed in with incorrect beliefs'. (Ibid., 58). This community knowledge is fed by the grapevine, absorbed by gossip and rumour and perpetuated by the majority of the community which strengthens its justification. From a prevention perspective, a 'large volume of street talk' supports a 'a great deal of misinformation and misunderstanding' (Ibid., 58). Beliefs, interaction and communication emerge as cornerstones of community culture, providing, what the researchers call, 'a local risk assessment framework'. Such a community-supported point of reference may often turn out to be stronger than the correct facts of transmission modes of HIV and the risks of unsafe sex.

In the context that multiple-partnership and its value for survival are approved of by the community, if not in words then certainly in behaviour, condom use has acquired additional meaning. Not only does it have a technical, instrumental value — preventing pregnancy and STDs — but it appears to carry additional and, perhaps, more important, layers of political and cultural meaning. It seems intrinsically related to symbolic values of trust and fidelity or, as in beginning relations, care and good intentions. Such meanings can be recognized when we read the major reason for not practising safe sex with non-regular partners: 'I know him well', women assured themselves (Hope Enterprise 2000). Their partners' likes and dislikes in using a condom outweighs women's safety concern — almost three times more often than for men (Hope Enterprises 2000 and 2004; McFarlane et al. 1994). Men's refusal to use condoms has more to do with their own dislike: 'it kills the vibes'; it kills their 'nature' — they simply 'don't like it'. (Hope Enterprises 2000, 2004; McFarlane et al. 1994; Rolfe and Hemmings 2007).

The community knowledge also guides the judgment of risk: immune from HIV are those with the right social profile (a background of a wealthy or well-known family), or those who represent proximity (knowing the person for a while) or are physically attractive (Bomberau and Allen 2007, 37).

Negotiating condom use in this context (of interactional dynamics, gender-determined inequality, access to resources, power and community norms) requires more than having good negotiating skills: it needs the ability to balance costs and benefits, 'gift' and 'counter-gift' (Barthelemy 2000, cited in Bomberau and Allen 2007), perhaps, also, favours and obligations, while at the same time enduring hard living conditions, keeping ambitions alive, coping with stress and having fun.

RE-DEFINING HIV PREVENTION

The initial behaviour change focus assumed that high-risk sexual behaviour could be changed into safer sexual behaviour by encouraging 'desired behaviours': abstinence, staying faithful with one partner or protected sex (condom use). These assumptions certainly did not do justice to HIV and AIDS as 'complex and multi-dimensional' challenges. This realization began to show up in international debates among and between major NGOs and donor agencies. In the late '90s, the Joint United Nations Program on HIV and AIDS (UNAIDS) published a new *Communications Framework for HIV and AIDS* that identified several weaknesses in the then popular theories and approaches and attempted to develop new directions (Airhihenbuwa et al. 1999).

The *Framework* continued the discussions initiated a few years earlier by the Rockefeller Foundation during two international think-tank conferences on the need to develop a new model of communication. This new model would need to be 'decentralized, pluralistic and democratic; … to empower rather than persuade people; it fosters debate among and between citizens, among and between communities, and between people and government. This model envisages increasingly horizontal communication allowing people to communicate with each other easily and inexpensively.' (Rockefeller Foundation 1999, 14). Referring to traditional media, the Foundation stated that this new model 'also involves the steady disintegration of traditional monolithic vertical lines of communication' (Ibid.), while, at the same time, not being too sure 'how to make it work' (Ibid., 23).

The new *Framework* captured many of the thoughts expressed in earlier thinking and criticized:

- 'the simple, linear relationship between individual knowledge and action;
- the emphasis on quantitative research;
- external decision-making catering to short term interests;
- overlooking the benefits of long term, internally derived, broad-based solutions;

- the assumption that individuals can or will exercise total control over their behaviour, disregarding the influence of contextual variables;
- the assumption that decisions about HIV and AIDS prevention are based on rational, volitional thinking with no regard to more true-to-life emotional scenarios.' (Airhihenbuwa et al. 1999, 22, 23)

The *Framework* hit the nail on the head. However, six years later, the approach, although 'widely acclaimed', was described as having had 'limited uptake' ... showing perhaps 'the difficulty in implementing complex and multi-layered communication programmes in resource-poor settings.' (Skuse and Power 2005, 10).

In the years following the publication of the new *Framework* a series of international conferences and roundtable meetings were held and several discussion papers and reports published, all trying to conceptualize communication for development strategies with HIV and AIDS as the particular focus.

The Nicaragua Round Table Conference in 2001 speaks of the failure of communication strategies in preventing the HIV pandemic: '... inadequate in containing and mitigating the effects of the academic' (United Nations Population Fund [UNFPA] 2002, 10). Its Declaration emphasizes the need for a 'multi-sectoral response' and the use of communication to respond to the epidemic at a behavioural as well as social political level. 'Collective behaviour change' is promoted and 'ideation' is introduced as 'the spread of new ways of thinking through communication and interaction' (UNFPA 2002, 10, 38).

The Panos Institute, which had characterised 20 years of HIV and AIDS response as 'entirely inadequate' (Scalway 2003, 57) concurs with the earlier critiques and underlines the need to focus on 'enabling communication environments', emphasizing more responsive and accountable local policy environments, local media that provide public debate and civil society with access to information and free speech.

NEW BUZZWORDS EMERGE

One of the major donor agencies in the HIV and AIDS arena — the World Bank — adopted the term 'integrated communication strategy'. Referring to 61 World Bank-funded projects in 36 African countries over more than 20 years, the Bank is critical of earlier communication strategies. It refers to its own failure 'to deploy strategic communication to support health reform projects'. (Elmendorf, et al. 2005, vii). It emphasizes the need to revise its approach to communication for behaviour change (BCC). Communication should be integrated at an earlier stage; BCC should become a 'management tool' and development communication is seen as the integration of strategic communication in development projects.

Other major international donors began to push for change. In the UK, the Department for International Development (DFID) makes a strong case for shifting from 'the often inappropriate and unrealistic targets for changing behaviour that are set at project or programme level, towards a stronger emphasis on rights to education and information, community participation and dialogue.' (Skuse and Powers 2005, 4). Perhaps this overlapped the earlier UNAIDS' critique of 'external decision-making catering to short term interests; and overlooking the benefits of long term, internally derived, broad-based solutions' (Airhihenbuwa et al. 1999, 22, 23). What is needed is: 'An integration ... of communication for HIV prevention, AIDS treatment and care' and 'a theoretical framework that aims to promote a broad based multi method approach to communications'. (Skuse and Powers 2005, 4).

Most of the discussions reflect the need to steer away from an exclusive focus on the individual: to include community, social political, economic and other factors. Similar sounds can be heard from other agencies: a stronger focus on the community; making communities the agents of their own change; community-based and community-owned dialogue, debate and negotiation.

UN agencies emphasize the need to approach communication from a human rights perspective — referring to the right to participation in decision-making, improved health and increased life opportunities (WHO, UNFPA, UNAIDS and IPPF 2002). UNAIDS is trying hard to analyse what this actually would imply. Its 2005 policy position paper on HIV prevention, emphasizes that effective prevention programmes must address 'deep seated causes of vulnerability' (UNAIDS 2005, 20). Against this background, principles of effective HIV prevention, it states, are: human rights, including gender equality; comprehensive, differentiated and locally adapted programmes with community participation of those for whom the programmes were planned; evidence-informed actions; requiring long-term and sustained effort; sufficient coverage, scale and intensity to make a difference (Ibid., 17). It also points to the need to link these initiatives with poverty-reduction strategies, and to provide 'more opportunities and greater equity in education and employment' (Ibid., 20). However, the policy limited this approach to 'key affected groups' and did not recognize any overarching need to link with national policies on education and employment (Ibid., 29).

The position paper on HIV prevention recognized the disconnect between knowledge and practice: 'despite high levels of awareness about the existence of AIDS, a large number of people feel that they are not at risk.' (UNAIDS 2005, 37). What it did not recognize was the complexity of this phenomenon. Without any further analysis it suggested an answer which encouraged more of the same: 'Information must be provided at all available opportunities'. (UNAIDS 2005, 37). Communication is interpreted firstly as 'utilizing all media', complemented by interpersonal communication, especially needed for 'increasing awareness', (Ibid., 27). What seems to be left unnoticed is the reality of 'communication' as a phenomenon that goes well beyond 'utilizing all media'.

The discussions at the level of international organisations cover, more or less, the same ground — a growing dissatisfaction with the limited approaches of the traditional theories which are criticised as too individual-oriented, too Western-founded and too committed to interpreting all behaviour as rational and planned; and requiring a stronger emphasis on communities and their specific context. They are all trying to come to grips with what Deane characterised as: 'a significant sense of strategic confusion related to HIV communication' (2004, 9).

GOVERNMENTS' INTERPRETATIONS OF HIV

How does Caribbean policy address this challenge? How does it define HIV and AIDS? And which role does it ascribe to 'communication'? Initially HIV and AIDS in the Caribbean — and worldwide — were seen as predominantly (public) health issues. For many years, governments and NGOs concentrated their attention on influencing the physical act of unprotected sex — aimed at changing copulatory etiquette rather than sexual behaviour. But, recently, most Caribbean governments have become familiar with the description of HIV as a 'multi-dimensional' issue. The National Strategic Plans (NSPs) of three Caribbean governments (Barbados, Jamaica, and Trinidad and Tobago) and PANCAP's Regional Strategic Framework (RSF) and Regional Action Plan included in this study all recognise the complexity of the 'disease'. The *2002-2006 HIV and AIDS National Strategic Plan of Jamaica* acknowledges that the HIV and AIDS epidemics are 'driven by a variety of behavioural, cultural, societal and economic factors', (Ministry of Health, Jamaica 2002, 3). Barbados's NSP states that HIV and AIDS as 'a disease … must be treated as a social and developmental issue' (Government of Barbados 2000, 16) and Trinidad and Tobago's NSP refers to 'the complex nature of the disease' (Office of the Prime Minister, Republic of Trinidad and Tobago 2003, 1). The challenge is now what to do with this relatively new insight.

Barbados wants to learn from the past and acknowledges that during the 1990s, the programmes instituted for HIV prevention and control had 'not been sufficiently broad-based to address the social, economic, cultural and behavioural aspects of the disease' (Government of Barbados 2000, 5). The solution is sought in a 'proactive response with a multi-sectoral approach'. The importance of the initiative is indicated by locating the implementing agency in the Office of the Prime Minister. Jamaica, too, recognizes that 'the complex nature of the epidemic necessitates the mobilization of adequate resources from all sectors in the society.' The

Plan is 'more than a plan for the health sector' (Ministry of Health, Jamaica 2002, 1); hence 'the involvement of the private sector, faith based organisations, political leaders, governmental organisations and community-based organisations including persons living with HIV and AIDS is an essential step towards mitigating the impact of AIDS on our society' (Ibid., 1). Trinidad and Tobago calls for national commitment in a response 'that goes beyond the health sector, to incorporate all other sectors of society including key organisations and all stakeholders' (Office of the Prime Minister, Republic of Trinidad and Tobago 2003, 1).

These NSPs seem to follow the direction set by the Caribbean Regional Strategic Framework which outlines HIV and AIDS as a 'development problem' (PANCAP 2002, 1), in need of an expanded 'multi-sectoral response' involving 'all sectors of society, including health, education, social welfare, finance and the highest levels of the executive … as well as the civil society and business sector' (Ibid., 2002, 9).

'Broad-based' and 'multi-dimensional' are the buzzwords in these new perspectives and their essence seem to be constituted by broadening the mobilization of resources from all sectors in the society — multi-sectoral approaches — and organisational restructuring at the government's national level, with, in some cases, coordination of the programme by the Prime Minister's Office.

In the early approaches risk-taking was interpreted as being caused by a lack of information and knowledge. The way to pass this obstacle was straightforward: if lack of information and knowledge were the problems, one of the answers had to be 'Providing knowledge' and 'Increasing awareness'. This design can still be seen in several of the National Strategic Plans (NSPs) in the Caribbean (de Bruin 2006).

POLICY DEFINITIONS AND INTERPRETATIONS OF 'COMMUNICATION'

The few times the word 'communication' is mentioned in the national and regional reports under review is when it is part of a phrase: Behaviour Change and Communication programmes, Behaviour Change

Intervention and Communication; communication materials; communication mechanisms; communication channels; Information, Education and Communication material or messages.

'Information and knowledge' are more easily used. The Barbados NSP, for instance, envisions 'a nation where every citizen is aware of the ways through which HIV can be contracted and the consequences of becoming infected, and is thus equipped with the information and knowledge to behave responsibly.' (Government of Barbados 2000, 17) The absence of information and knowledge is seen as the cause of not being able to act 'responsibly' Being aware is equated with being equipped 'with the information and knowledge to behave responsibly' (Ibid., 17). And being equipped with such knowledge appears to be seen as sufficient for behaviour change.

Similarly, the Trinidad and Tobago's NSP, in its 'Heighten Education and Awareness Strategy', also perceives behaviour change as a result of education and awareness: 'To promote healthy sexual behaviours, emphasis will be placed on intensifying HIV and AIDS education and awareness programmes' (Office of the Prime Minister, Republic of Trindad and Tobago 2003, 20). The understanding of communication as mainly information handling and storage is patent.

Jamaica's NSP describes behaviour change and communication as a 'technical component' with emphases on face-to-face communication, peer education, targeted community interventions and media awareness campaigns (Ministry of Health, Jamaica 2002, 8). It briefly outlines a strategy of producing and disseminating information and communication materials 'for the general and target population in order to heighten individual sense of risk perception and promote healthy and responsible sexual behaviours' (Ibid., 21). However, nothing can be found that goes beyond this limited notion of communication. The plan mentions other strategies, but fails to place them in a coherent context.

At the level of strategy, the Barbados NSP identifies raising awareness, behaviour change and social mobilization as its major 'communication strategies'. Although this listing seems to be a mix of objectives and strategies, the described components of these strategies do refer to a wide area of application: use of mass media, advocacy, inter-sectoral collaboration involving NGOs, research, training, and condom social marketing. This range clearly reveals a wider concept of communication; however, not in any coherent or consistent framework (Government of Barbados 2001, 45). At a tactical level the Barbados Plan chooses information, education and communication (IEC) as its main approach and shows high expectations: IEC will, hopefully, 'not only increase or enhance awareness of the disease and the means by which to prevent or reduce its spread, but will ultimately lead to the adoption of improved sexual practices' (Ibid., 22).

Similarly, Trinidad and Tobago's NSP has no systematic outline of how to use communication. Communication seems to be equated with media use: several references are made to the selection of channels, but, the challenges in terms of message production remain unnoticed. The media/advertising industry is identified as a 'strategic partner' (Office of the Prime Minister, Republic of Trinidad and Tobago 2003, 21). This narrow interpretation of communication to mean simply 'use of media' causes important areas to be overlooked.

Several of the guiding principles and central strategies mentioned in each country's National Strategic Plan contain such overlooked areas. For instance, Jamaica's NSP states that 'HIV and AIDS must be normalised so that it becomes a part of the customary public discourse' (Ministry of Health, Jamaica 2001, 4). But, how can public discourse be influenced without paying attention to a strategic communication plan? Barbados's NSP speaks about creating a supportive environment; development and implementation of appropriate public policies; an on-going anti-HIV and AIDS education and training programme; etc. At the same time, the plan does not address how this can be done in a systematic, strategic way. Communication planning itself is not addressed. In most of the plans stigmatization and discrimination as priority areas are mentioned. But, the fact that such social processes are rooted in communication seems to be left unnoticed.

In academic terms, stigmatization and discrimination are recognized as relational processes, taking place at interpersonal as well as group and community levels (Heatherton et al. 2000) — making them communication processes in themselves. Communication, as a multidisciplinary field, may have something to offer in achieving the desired support and empowerment of stigmatized and discriminated communities, but this goes well beyond media messages and campaigns.

AGREEMENTS

Several of the debates over the last decade mention the necessary connection between socio-cultural, economic and political factors and seem to agree on the failures of behaviour change communication. In the context of HIV and AIDS, it does not work as well as it should; it does not change behaviour in any significant way. Academics also seem to agree on what may contribute to this shortfall: for the larger part of the world the approaches are not indigenous, but imported. They have a limited focus — on the individual only and on the sexual act exclusively — and function from the top-down, assuming rational and volitional sexual behaviour (Melkote 2003; Parker 2004; Servaes and Malikhao 2005a, 2005b; Waisbord 2005). In the discussion, there seems to be agreement on principles: developing a broad-based, multi-method approach to communications at multiple levels, including enabling environments, taking into account socio-cultural context, emphasising communication production by target groups, integrating prevention, support and care. Scholars articulate the need to 'address enabling environments and contextual factors' (Parker 2003, 3) and underline the necessity for participatory approaches, to include communities as agents of change. However, Melkote (2003) noted how tricky the encouragement of participatory approaches could be by observing that 'the outcome in most cases has not been true empowerment of the people, but the attainment of some indicator of development as articulated in the modernization paradigm'. (138).

Recently, UNAIDS has been trying to blow new life into the concept of 'social change communication'. Years ago the Rockefeller Foundation encouraged this approach with a strong emphasis on 'participatory communication' (Dagron 2001); some see this concept as not sufficiently addressing the structural and political issues (Skuse and Power 2005). Now that UNAIDS has put social change communication back on the agenda, it is supposed to address the societal drivers of the epidemic. The challenge, however, will be how to address the societal drivers; how to ensure that the 'range of macro level, structural, environmental and policy factors' is addressed sufficiently and how to achieve 'going to scale' with what are essentially community based and highly localised communication responses (Skuse and Power 2005, 11). For communication researchers, the 'going to scale' may even be more challenging. Many of them have been used to the traditional focus on mass media — not necessarily comprehensive — as 'communication'.

What has become clear, through practise and research from a variety of viewpoints and disciplines, is that HIV and AIDS appear to be intricately connected with social change and development issues; not only by the impact of the pandemic in taking away the most productive layers of the society, but as a consequence of the enabling conditions and underlying factors of 'power inequality, rights-based issues, social injustice, gender imbalances, disempowerment and apathy' (Tufte 2005, 4).

WHERE DOES THIS LEAD US?

Factors contributing to what was called earlier the 'strategic confusion' seem to be at least threefold: blind spots in some national and regional policies (de Bruin 2005); insufficiently documented practices and an inadequate theoretical framework.

Policies

National and regional policies defining HIV and AIDS as 'multi-dimensional' issues remain silent on what multi-dimensionality may mean. In addition, in these policies, communication *strategy* seems to be poorly conceptualized and in need of revision. There is no sign of any attention given to the actual depth of these concepts, their meaning being taken for granted. No thought is spent on the width of 'communication'.

The need to not only understand the drivers but to effectively address them through inter-disciplinary approaches, including unemployment, income inequality, community disintegration and lack of educational opportunities — in short, social and economic policy promoting sustainable human development.

Practices

Documented practices are, more often than not, tailored to donor-dictated specifications. This creates a vacuum of critical and honest analyses of current prevention and communication strategies and the underlying assumptions, models and theories that serve as points of departure for designing these strategies. The Caribbean's only best practice document in this area, for instance, relates to the regional structure of the Pan-Caribbean Partnership Against AIDS (PANCAP) — a special project of the Caribbean Community (CARICOM), the regional political structure in which 15 full member states and five associate members participate.

Theories

Many of the communication approaches in HIV prevention used over the years, up to the late '90s, were borrowed from, or applied by health communicators in health promotion and disease prevention practice: the health belief model, the theory of reasoned action, the AIDS risk reduction model, and theories of social learning, diffusion of innovation ... The origins of several of these theories were rooted in health promotion, later also health communication, aimed at solving behaviour problems — implicitly bypassing solutions based on creating opportunities for social change. However, there is no thorough review of traditional and emerging theories which could serve as an informed basis for the development of alternatives more suited to the culture, needs and experience of a resource-poor reality.

The community of scholars and practitioners seems to be hobbled when it comes to articulating a coherent new approach for Communication and HIV and AIDS when faced with the challenge of innovating an appropriate conceptual framework. Even the *Lancet Infectious Diseases*, emblem of the medical establishment, addressed in its opinion columns the need to critically review the current definition of the problem, governing ideologies and assumptions about drivers (Barnett and Parkhurst 2005).

Even what seems to be obvious and transparent terminology may mean different things by different authors, representing different institutions and disciplines. For instance 'the social and cultural factors that drive the HIV epidemic in the Caribbean' by Bombereau and Allen (2008), representing the Caribbean Health Research Council (CHRC), refer to 'behaviours that drive the epidemic, which 'are mainly sexual'. Consequently, fighting the epidemic means addressing 'private behaviours, including behaviours that are illegal in most of the countries (such as homosexuality and forced sex); economic behaviours (such as transactional sex) and cultural norms (such as approval of men with multiple partners)' (Ibid., 4). The analysis remains at the level of 'behaviours' — contextual conditions are mentioned, but not examined.

It is not only the problem of HIV and AIDS that seems to be in need of re-definition, 'communication' with all its strengths and weaknesses is in need of clarification. Is it to be seen as a tool, a conduit for information? Or, also as a field of inquiry which will take us far beyond media and audience studies?

Other conceptual weaknesses are encapsulated in research traditions: the terms knowledge, attitude, practice and behaviour have become clichés with, perhaps, no commonly agreed meaning. What constitutes 'knowledge'? How do we conceptualize attitude? What do we assume to be the connections between practice and behaviour? The connection between those concepts is not in any way problematic, in spite of obvious questions that may be drawn from the wealth of, often, conflicting data.

There is work to be done: epistemological and theoretical thinking; transcending traditional disciplinary boundaries; cutting across compartmentalized policy preparations — all without the pressure of short-term outputs to fit external donors' agendas.

REFERENCES

Airhihenbuwa, Collins, Bunmi Makinwa, Michael Frith and Rafael Obregon. 1999. *Communications Framework for HIV/AIDS – A New Direction.* Geneva, Switzerland: UNAIDS.

Bailey, Wilma, Clement Branche, Gail McGarrity and Sheila Stuart. 1998. *Family and the Quality of Gender Relations in the Caribbean.* UWI, Mona: ISER.

Barnett, Tony and Justin Parkhurst. 2005. 'HIV/AIDS: sex, abstinence, and behaviour change'. *Lancet Infectious Diseases* 5: 590–93.

Bomberau, Gaelle and Caroline F. Allen. 2008. *Social and cultural factors driving the HIV epidemic in the Caribbean: a literature review.* Trinidad and Tobago: CHRC.

Bruin de, Marjan. 2002. *Teenagers At Risk. High-risk Behaviour of Jamaican Adolescents in the Context of Reproductive Health – Observations and Impressions.* Kingston, Jamaica: Ministry of Health, Youth Now.

———. 2006. 'Blind spots and wasted effort in Caribbean HIV/AIDS policy making. Communication and Behaviour Change. *Glocal Times, Globala Tider* 2, no. 4: http://www.glocaltimes.k3.mah.se/viewarticle.aspx?articleID=59&issueID=6.

CAREC. 2007a. *Behavioural Surveillance Surveys (BSS) in Six Countries of the Organisation of Eastern Caribbean States (OECS). Round 1: 2005. Antigua and Barbuda; Grenada; St Lucia; Dominica; St Kitts and Nevis; St Vincent and the Grenadines. Executive Summary.* CAREC, PAHO, WHO.

———. 2007b. *The Caribbean HIV/AIDS Epidemic and the Situation in Member Countries of the Caribbean Epidemiology Centre* (CAREC). CAREC, PAHO, WHO

Chevannes, Barry. 1994. *Sexual Decision-Making Among Jamaicans 1990–1994.* UCLA Report. Submitted to FHI /UCLA/ISER. Final report, Part I, II, III (unpublished manuscript).

———. April 1996. *The Women's Centre Foundation of Jamaica: An Evaluation.* Commissioned by UNICER/UNFPA.

———. 2001. *Learning To Be A Man; Culture, Socialization and Gender Identity in Five Caribbean Communities.* Barbados, Jamaica, Trinidad and Tobago: The University of the West Indies Press.

Chevannes, Barry and Claudia Mitchell-Kernan. 1993. *'How we were grown': Cultural aspects of high-risk sexual behaviour in Jamaica.* Appendix C2 In-depth Interview Report.

Dagron, Alfonso Gumucio. 2001. *Making Waves, stories of participatory communication for social change. A report to the Rockefeller Foundation.* The Rockefeller Foundation.

Deane, James. 2004. *The Context of Communication for Development.* Report 9th United Nations Roundtable on Communication for Development, September, 6–9. Rome, Italy: FAO.

DFID. 2006. *The importance of secondary, vocational and higher education to development.* A DFID practise paper. UK: DFID (Department for International Development).

———. 2006. *DFID's medium term action plan on aid effectiveness – Our response to the*

Paris Declaration, by Donor Policy and Partnerships Team, Policy Division, Department for International Development.

Elmendorf, Edward, Cecilia Cabañero-Verzosa, Michele Lioy and Kathryn LaRusso. 2005. *Behavior Change Communication for Better Health Outcomes in Africa. Experience and Lessons Learned from World Bank-Financed Health, Nutrition and Population Projects.* Washington: World Bank.

FAO. 2005. *Communication for Development Roundtable Report. Focus on sustainable development (2004).* Rome, Italy: FAO, with the Government of Italy, UNESCO, World Bank, IDRC, CTA.

FHI. 2004. *HIV/AIDS Behavioural Surveillance Survey, Jamaica, 1999–2000* BSS Round 1–Final Report, FHI, Impact, USAID.

Office of the Prime Minister, Republic of Trinidad and Tobago. 2003. *Five-year National HIV/AIDS Strategic Plan, 2003–2008.* Trinidad and Tobago.

Government of Barbados. November 2000. *Action plan for a comprehensive programme on the management, prevention and control of HIV/AIDS 2001–2006.* Ministry of Health Barbados.

Heatherton, Todd F., Robert E. Klerck, Michelle R. Hebl and Jay G. Hull (eds.) *The Social Psychology of Stigma.* New York, London: The Guilford Press.

Hemer, Oscar and Thomas Tufte. (Eds.) 2005. *Media & Global Change; Rethinking Communication for Development.* Goteborg: CLASCO and NORDICOM.

Hope Enterprises. 2000. *Report of National Knowledge, Attitudes, Behaviour & Practices Survey Year 2000.* Prepared for the Ministry of Health. Kingston, Jamaica.

———. 2004. *Report of National Knowledge, Attitudes, Behaviour & Practices Survey Year 2004.* Prepared for the Ministry of Health. Kingston, Jamaica.

Kempadoo, Kamala and Leith Dunn. 2002. *Factors that Shape the Initiation of Early Sexual Activity among Adolescent Boys and Girls. Meeting Adolescent Development and Participation Rights. The findings of Five Research Studies on Adolescents in Jamaica.* Kingston: UNICEF, UNFPA.

Leo-Rhynie, Elsa and Carmen Pencle. 2002. 'Gender Stereotypes: Perceptions and Awareness of a Sample of Jamaican Adolescents'. In *Gendered Realities; Essays in Caribbean Feminist Thought,* ed. Pat Mohammed, 201–18. Mona, Jamaica: UWI Press and Centre for Gender and Development Studies.

McFarlane, Carmen P., Jay S. Friedman, Leo Morris and Howard I. Goldberg. 1994. *Contraceptive Prevalence Survey Jamaica 1993. Volume III: Sexual Experience, Contraceptive Practice and Fertility.* Atlanta: National Family Planning Board, US Department of Health and Human Services, CDC.

Melkote, Srinivas R. 2003. 'Theories of Development Communication'. In *International and Development Communication – A 21st-Century Perspective,* ed. Bella Mody. Thousands Oaks, London, New Delhi: Sage.

Ministry of Health, Jamaica. 2002. *Jamaica HIV/AIDS/STI National Strategic Plan 2002–2006.* Ministry of Health, Jamaica.

Parker, Warren. 2004. *Rethinking conceptual approaches to behaviour change: The importance of context.* South Africa: Centre for AIDS Development, Research and Evaluation.

Parry, Odette. 2000. *Male Underachievement in High School Education in Jamaica, Barbados and St. Vincent and the Grenadines.* Barbados, Jamaica, Trinidad and Tobago: University of the West Indies, Canoe Press.

Rockefeller Foundation. 1999. *Communication for Social Change: A Position Paper and Conference Report.* Rockefeller Foundation.

Rolfe, Ben and Joanne Hemmings with Tricia Anne Morris and Veronica Samuels-Dixon. 2007. *'She sweet up the boopsy and him nu get nuh wine.' Young women and sexual relationships in Kingston, Jamaica.* Swansea: Options and Centre for Development Studies.

Scalway, Thomas. 2003. *Missing the message? 20 years of learning from HIV/AIDS.* London: PANOS.

Senderowitz, Judith, Elsie Le Franc and James Sitrick Jr. March 1998. *A Program to Address Adolescent Reproductive Health in Jamaica.* Prepared for USAID/Jamaica.

Servaes, Jan and Patchanee Malikhao. 2005a. 'Participatory Communication: the new paradigm?' In *Media & Glocal Change; Rethinking Communication for Development*, eds Oscar Hemer and Thomas Tufte, 91–103. Göteborg: CLASCO and NORDICOM.

———. 2005b. 'Communication strategies for the implementation of sustainable development'. In *Communication for Development Roundtable Report. Focus on Sustainable development.* 9th United Nations Communication for Development Roundtable September 6–9, 2004, Rome, Italy. Organised by FAO with the Government of Italy, UNESCO, World Bank, IDRC, CTA. 27–28 (summary of paper).

Shelton, James D., Daniel T. Halperin, Vinand Nantulya, Malcolm Potts, Helene D. Gayle and K. K. Holmes. *Partner Reduction in HIV Prevention: The Neglected Middle Child of 'ABC'.* Washington: United States Agency for International Development.

Skuse, Andrew and Fiona Power. 2005. *AIDS Communication. Information and Communication for Development.* London, UK: Department for International Development.

Theodore, Karl. 2001. *HIV/AIDS in the Caribbean.* Unpublished paper. Department of Economics, Health Economics Unit, St. Augustine Campus, UWI.

Tufte, Thomas. 2005. 'Communicating for what? How globalization and HIV/AIDS push the ComDev agenda'. In *Media & Glocal Change;Rethinking Communication for Development*, eds. Oscar Hemer and Thomas Tufte, 105–119. Göteborg: CLASCO and NORDICOM.

The Policy Project. November 1999. *Reproductive Health in Jamaica, Volume 1, Analysis of Current Reproductive Health Status, Gaps, Needs and Opportunities.* Prepared for the Ministry of Health. The Futures Group International.

UNAIDS. 2005. *Intensifying HIV Prevention–UNAIDS policy position paper.* Geneva, Switzerland: UNAIDS.

UNFPA. 2002. *Communication for Development Roundtable Report. Focus on HIV/AIDS communication and evaluation. Communication for Development Roundtable.* Managua, Nicaragua: UNFPA.

Waisbord, Silvio. 2005. 'Five key ideas: coincidences and challenges in development communication'. In *Media & Glocal Change;Rethinking Communication for Development,* eds Oscar Hemer and Thomas Tufte, 77–90, Göteborg: CLASCO and NORDICOM.

WHO. 2005. *HIV/AIDS Epidemiological Surveillance Report for the WHO African Region.* 2005 Update, WHO Regional Office Africa.

———. UNFPA, UNAIDS and IPPF. 2002. *Linking Sexual and Reproductive Health and HIV/AIDS–an annotated inventory.* Geneva, Switzerland: WHO and UNAIDS.

Williams, Sian. 1999. Sexual Violence and Exploitation of Children in Latin America and the Caribbean: The Case of Jamaica. Kingston, Jamaica: Caribbean Child Development Centre, University of the West Indies, Mona.

World Bank. July 4, 2006. http://web.worldbank.org/WBSITE/EXTERNAL/TOPICS/ EXTDEVCOMMENG/

CHAPTER 8
TACKLING THE SOCIAL COMPLEXITIES OF HIV AND AIDS

Understanding the social roots of the epidemic and learning from developments in HIV communication

ROBIN VINCENT

INTRODUCTION

There is an urgent need to tackle the social drivers of HIV and AIDS if global HIV infection rates are to be reduced, and the current targets — for universal access to prevention, treatment, care and support by 2010, and the Millennium Development Goal of halting or starting to reverse the spread of HIV by 2015 — are to be realized. It is particularly urgent that effective HIV communication approaches are developed to tackle key social challenges underpinning vulnerability to HIV — such as stigma and discrimination, gender inequity, and socio-economic inequality — given the challenges of preventing emerging epidemics in Eastern Europe, South Asia, and the Caribbean, and the increasing 'feminization' of the pandemic identified in recent epidemiological trends. ' The need to address social, political and economic factors that structure differential vulnerability to HIV is increasingly recognized, yet, policy relevant research that renders these complex social factors amenable to intervention is lacking. This chapter reviews a range of recent international developments in HIV and AIDS communication theory and practice, which attempt to address its social dimensions more effectively: to look beyond narrow, short-term interventions focused on individual behaviours, and understand some of the social and structural underpinnings of an effective public health response to HIV and AIDS. The chapter draws on developments in participatory communication for social change thinking and practice, lessons from the dynamics of HIV social movements, and recent attempts to apply the theory of complex systems to understand social change. Together, these suggest the need to work to support and facilitate a range of broader social capacities and capabilities that underpin health and well-being, rather than the predominant narrow focus on changing the sexual and 'risky' behaviour of individuals in HIV and AIDS programmes. Such approaches connect with the present concern to move from a focus on individual risk to the way vulnerability to HIV is structured by a range of social factors, and the need to address these factors for effective HIV programming.

Recent initiatives aimed at addressing stigma and discrimination and gender inequity — identified as key social drivers of HIV by UNAIDS in 126 country consultations during 2005/6 (UNAIDS 2006) — confirm the need for multileveled and integrated approaches which go beyond the more discrete project interventions common in HIV and AIDS responses. By reflecting on a range of such examples from around the world, and from Africa in particular, the paper offers a range of lessons learned and productive questions, which may inform the ongoing development of responses to HIV and AIDS in the countries of the Caribbean.

Addressing the social dimensions of
HIV and AIDS

The need to address the social dimensions of HIV and AIDS has been driven partly by lessons learned from previous experiences in HIV and AIDS responses, and also by developments in the fields of HIV and development communication. A number of factors, present to varying degrees in different countries, have been prominent in successful responses to HIV and AIDS, and have been reviewed elsewhere in detail (Panos 2006a).[1] Factors which contribute to a successful response include: political leadership; civil society mobilization; open dialogue and discussion and knowledge-sharing in personal communication networks (Panos 2003, 11); media promoting dialogue and debate; country-driven responses (Green 2003); multisectoral responses to prevention and care (Sittitrai 2001, 5); matching the response to the stage and character of the epidemic;

targeted large-scale interventions; effective monitoring and evaluation fed back into programmes.

The importance of social factors and elements of public communication — particularly participation, ownership and accountability — in relatively successful responses has added impetus to the need to question the prevailing focus on individual behaviour change in HIV policy and practice (Panos 2003). The fact that the early success in reducing HIV infection rates in Uganda was achieved largely without the external intervention of development initiatives (Green 2003), has also raised humbling questions about the scope and impact of development interventions and the importance of understanding the relatively independent dynamics of civil society, including social movements, cultural practices and the contours of interpersonal communication (Epstein 2007), something returned to below.

The rise of social change communication approaches

A growing recognition in HIV and development communication that individual behaviour is intimately intertwined with broader social norms and social change has driven innovations in HIV and AIDS communication to look beyond focused interventions targeting individuals and their particular behaviours, to a broader concern with facilitating social change. The UNAIDS communication framework for HIV and AIDS, developed through global consultation in 1997–99, draws attention to the importance of social context in the response to HIV and AIDS (UNAIDS 1999). It criticises the 'methodological individualism' of the behaviour change tradition of health communication, with its assumptions of voluntary change on the part of rational individuals (Airhihenbuwa and Obregon 2000). In responding to HIV and AIDS, the framework highlights several aspects of context that need to be addressed to sustain changes in behaviour: spirituality, gender, socio-economic status, policy frameworks and culture. Communication for Social Change (CFSC)[2] is an approach that puts people at the centre of their own change process, in common with more established participatory communication approaches such as REFLECT.[3]

Communication for social change in practice

In Ethiopia, CFSC/UNICEF have drawn on a human rights-based approach to programming,[4] to work through a large network of youth clubs in a dialogue and decision-making process that sets the agenda for the HIV and AIDS response. The voices and concerns of young people and their communities were amplified through a variety of media to stimulate discussion at district and national levels (Byrne et al. 2005). Linkages with government partners and development agencies sought to create channels for them to respond to the issues raised and improve services and policy. The process built on the 'community conversations' developed by UNDP and UNICEF which have promoted dialogue around previously taboo subjects such as female genital mutilation, early marriage and sexual violence and built the capacity of communities to reflect on their own priorities and find their own solutions. They have also creatively addressed religious and traditional practices that may heighten risk of HIV transmission.[5]

The emphasis on dialogue and reflection on social realities to promote social change, is also a key feature of an emerging 'third generation' of entertainment-education approaches. The prime time Nicaraguan television soap opera, *Sexto Sentido* (The Sixth Sense), for example, aims to consciously address the root causes of the everyday social problems and power inequalities faced by its young protagonists, stimulating debate and ultimately collective action and structural change (Tufte 2005). *Sexto Sentido* is part of a combined communication for social change approach by feminist NGO 'Puntos de Encuentro' that includes empowerment and training with young people, and broader networking of community initiatives and social movements.

Operationalizing approaches that aim to tackle several social factors at once remain a challenge as the slow progress in translating the UNAIDS communication framework into practice and concrete programming highlights (Obregon 2004). However, the need for communication approaches that can address social complexity remains (DFID 2005), and in 2007 UNAIDS convened a timely technical consultation on

Communication for Social Change, bringing together a range of practitioners and experts to develop guidance to support countries to develop national communication for social change programming.[6]

COMBATING STIGMA AND DISCRIMINATION AND GENDER INEQUITY — THE NEED FOR MULTILEVELED ACTION

The challenge of addressing a range of social factors simultaneously is echoed in recent initiatives to address stigma and discrimination and gender inequity. A review of contemporary approaches shows that in both cases such complex social issues demand concerted action at a range of different levels in order to realize sustainable change. There is a need to combine interventions in community and interpersonal settings with initiatives in institutions such as schools and workplaces, and changes in legal and policy frameworks (Panos 2006a).

Tackling stigma and discrimination

Stigma and discrimination are still everyday experiences for people living with HIV and AIDS around the world (Panos 2006). Numerous studies have shown that stigma and discrimination are major obstacles preventing effective HIV and AIDS responses; they make people less likely to participate in prevention activities, less likely to get tested for HIV, and less likely to enrol for treatment even where it exists. People may be fearful of disclosing their status, and may postpone seeking care, and they may also suffer violence, particularly gender-based violence, related to their HIV status (ICRW 2007). Once seen as being about individual behaviour, awareness and prejudice, stigma and discrimination are now more usefully recognized as a broad social process that 'maintains power inequalities' (Parker et al. 2002). Stigma and discrimination can be seen to actively sustain boundaries between those in power and those without, and justify and support social patterns of exclusion and inequality, thus perpetuating differential vulnerability to HIV infection.

Despite being a central obstacle, there is a shortage of well documented and evaluated interventions to tackle stigma and discrimination. This is partly due to their complexity, with stigma being found everywhere, from everyday beliefs and actions to institutional settings, to legal and economic frameworks, and societal attitudes around gender, illness and sexuality. It is increasingly recognized, however, that tackling stigma and discrimination requires approaches that promote action at several levels together (UNAIDS 2005):

- Working with individuals, households and affected communities to engage and challenge their own stigmatising assumptions, understandings and practices;
- Non-discriminatory policies and procedures in institutional contexts, such as schools, workplaces and health care settings; and
- Legal and national policy frameworks that uphold human rights and do not perpetuate discrimination.

The involvement of people living with HIV and AIDS in designing, facilitating and delivering anti-stigma initiatives has also been vital to their effectiveness.

A recent review of initiatives conducted by the International Centre for Research on Women (ICRW 2007) has confirmed the need for interventions addressing stigma and discrimination at all the above levels, through a range of approaches, with different 'target groups' in an integrated way. The review highlights the success of participatory education approaches, but also concludes that initiatives that tackle the broader legal and structural underpinnings of stigma and discrimination are relatively few and tend to focus on the individual legal redress, rather than broader social infrastructure.

In addition to these formal development interventions, it is important to recognize the initiative and relatively independent dynamics of civil society, through social movements and alternative cultural and public action. Social movements of people living with HIV and AIDS have generated solidarity and mutual support and sometimes developed 'resistance identities' to challenge their marginalization and to redefine their allotted position in society. Gay men, women, sex workers and injecting drug consumers have refused to accept their discredited status and developed a variety of innovative responses to HIV and AIDS in different settings, as well as organizing to challenge stigma and discriminatory institutional practices and laws (Stoller 1998). At the same time, at a more everyday level, cultural beliefs and practices affect people's capacity to accept or stigmatize PLWHA, their willingness to engage in responses to HIV and AIDS and the patterns of care and support that are embedded in family and community relationships (Vincent 2005). Culture can, thus, affect the local dynamics of discrimination or solidarity that may encourage or challenge stigma and discrimination in different settings (UNESCO 2003).

Tackling gender inequity

In parts of Africa and the Caribbean, young women aged 16–24 are up to six times more likely to contract HIV than their male counterparts, while in sub-Saharan Africa 59 per cent of PLWHA are women (UNIFEM 2006). Limited access to resources and institutional power, rooted in wider social norms and institutions as well as the intimacies of everyday life, make women more vulnerable to HIV infection. This socially ubiquitous character of gender makes it difficult to address through specific 'interventions' however:

> …Any young man in Jamaica is constantly being told that he must have more than one woman, take risks and be adventurous to be a man, this is the essence of who he is as a man. This is far more powerful than a message about wearing a condom… There is no point talking to a young man about safe sex, when to be a man is to do the very things that lead him into unsafe behaviour…. [7]

The socially embedded nature of gender in a wide range of social practices (Moore 1994) means that gender inequality also demands concerted action at a range of levels: addressing legal and structural constraints in institutional contexts; community norms and practices; and interpersonal communication (Panos 2006a). It is also important to support women's efforts to gain greater control of their environment — not least the efforts of marginalized women such as sex-workers, and networks of HIV-positive women.[8]

Gender-sensitive participatory communication approaches, like Stepping Stones, have proved useful in getting men and women to talk about the usually taboo subjects of sexuality and gender, and to address some of the barriers to social change at the local level (Hadjipateras 2006). Just as with stigma and discrimination, there are limits to what can be achieved in any particular setting, however, when the constraints of gender and poverty are rooted in wider social structures that stretch beyond the locality. A recent UNAIDS review, which looked at national responses in Cambodia, Honduras and Ukraine, found that structural issues underpinning gender inequity such as the social and economic factors limiting equitable access to land, education and political participation were still largely neglected, and there was a lack of political will to address gender in national HIV and AIDS responses. Despite a plethora of more theoretical guidelines, and over 27 existing guidance documents, the review found that it was the practical 'how to' of tackling gender, and the capacity to address it at the range of different levels needed is still largely missing (UNAIDS 2007).

Despite many promising examples of elements of programming in the areas of gender inequity and stigma and discrimination, their integration into programming that can have a sustainable impact remains a challenge. This is not least because challenging social inequities means challenging the very social arrangements that reproduce inequality and imbalances of power in any setting. Legal and policy frameworks that would challenge prevailing power relationships, however, are often resisted by the powerful, the very people who usually have a disproportionate influence over their making. The kind of integrated and multileveled programming that is needed may also require innovations in development programming, funding and evaluation — appropriate to longer-term, integrated, approaches with multiple and synergistic inputs. At the same time there is a need to create an enabling environment for independent social movements and public action, even while this may have different dynamics and challenge the priorities to official development action. This raises the paradox of trying to combine the instrumental action of development, with the more emergent character of the social and cultural dynamics of civil society. It is here that insights from the theory of complex systems for understanding social change, may prove useful.

SOCIAL LIFE AS A COMPLEX SYSTEM — INSIGHTS FROM COMPLEXITY THEORY

A brief review of some recent attempts to apply the theory of complex systems to social change shows that current models of development planning and action may place too much emphasis on controlling linear, planned changes, where it may be important instead to focus on supporting a range of basic capacities and capabilities to promote the independent action of developments so-called beneficiaries. By attending to the characteristics of society, as a whole, such approaches are able to highlight the range of broad factors that influence the distribution of social outcomes overall — in this case, factors that contribute to vulnerability to HIV infection —instead of a focus on particular instances of risk of infection, which is the level at which most current interventions operate.

Contemporary theorists of globalization point to the way in which a range of influences — flows of resources, images, ideas, and people — impact on particular localities in increasingly complex and unpredictable ways (Appadurai 1996, 13). Given that people act in a range of social settings and contexts with many different influences over long time frames, the difficulties of addressing this complexity of social life through linear, short-term development planning are increasingly recognized. The traditional 'command and control' methods of development planning may be obsolete. Instead, development should focus on ensuring local actors' freedom and capacity for action — the rest will emerge, and should not be expected to follow prescribed patterns based on models of western economic development.[9]

Similar conclusions emerge from recent work on organizational learning in development, which promotes reflection on practice and learning from experience for all development actors — not just programme designers or managers — and holds the potential to deepen participatory approaches to development (Vincent and Byrne 2006). Much of the new thinking in systems theory points to driving social innovation by decentralising initiative and control, and the importance of embedding knowledge and information both in technologies and organizations (Castells 2000, 61–9). This not an argument for *laissez-faire* globalization, but rather an attempt to ensure there is effective communication and feedback throughout social and development action. Further than this, such approaches imply the need for a basic infrastructure for health, wellbeing and problem-solving capacities, as the foundation on which people can act creatively for themselves.

The theories and tools of complex systems approaches have developed across a wide range of disciplines over recent decades in the physical and life sciences in tandem with a parallel development of non-linear mathematics and computer modelling (Nicolis and Prigogine 1989). In 'systems' where there are a lot of interactions and feedback between the constituent parts (something that is clearly a defining feature of social life), complexity theory highlights the inadequacy of linear models of causality in predicting outcomes. At the same time it shows that interactions in the system can give rise to emergent properties that are qualitatively different from the character of the constituents of the system. There may be limits to the extrapolation of such approaches to the realms of human social practice, but a number of authors have argued convincingly that social life displays the kind of complex, emergent character of other complex systems (Byrne 1998; Eve et al 1998). Such an emergent character means that the properties of social life as a whole, cannot be reduced to the sum of the parts — that is a simple combination of the actions of individuals. Such a conviction goes back to the birth of social science and the recognition that there is something distinctive about the social world and the products of social action that can not be deduced from knowing the properties of the individuals that make it up.

An approach to social life rooted in complexity theory suggests in addition that the multiple interactions and feedbacks involved in a society mean that it is very difficult to predict in advance the precise effects of particular social inputs and actions. At the same time, when considering the level of properties of the overall 'system' — in this case a particular society — there may be a restricted set of possible overall general states (in the language of complexity an 'attractor' state for the overall system) and these may be triggered by changes in a limited set of key controlling parameters — such as the degree of inequality within a society (Byrne 1998).

The complexity of health

Byrne (1998) develops the example of the relationship between degree of inequality of wealth in societies and distinctive patterns of health outcomes. In the case of tuberculosis (TB), he argues that TB will manifest as an epidemic in societies wherever a certain degree of social inequity exists. This is not to deny the proximate causality of infection, just to argue that it is insufficient cause for an epidemic to occur. For the latter certain broader and encompassing social influences and causes need to be in place, a key one of which is wealth inequality. The overall social pattern of health in any case will depend on a nested hierarchy of influences, from family and community circumstances, to local institutional arrangements, to wider laws and policies, all interacting with each other in complex feedback loops. In this way, a complexity approach retains an interest in the real social causes and influences on social patterns of health, without expecting to be able to predict exact health outcomes in any particular case. Rather, it can point to key parameters which will have a bearing on tipping a society into one of several likely states — in the above example, either an epidemic of TB or a situation where TB manifests at relatively low levels (Byrne 1998).[10]

The implications of such an approach for development action and planning is to emphasize the importance of a number of basic social processes being in place, such as equitable distribution of wealth, and the provision of basic health and welfare infrastructure, rather than focusing too narrowly on particular interventions that attempt to produced controlled and specific changes in isolation. A parallel can be drawn here with Sen's notion of development as being about supporting 'substantive freedoms' and basic functional capabilities as the foundation upon which development can unfold (Sen 2004). Such an approach emphasizes the positive enabling aspects of freedom that are predicated on certain basic social arrangements that ensure, for example, longevity, access to education, and ability to engage and negotiate in economic and political processes, that can promote overall health enhancing effects at the level of society. There are also clear parallels here with Paul Farmer's notion of 'structural violence' — a consistent set of social, economic and political process that underpin differential access to resources and the determinants of well-being, and contribute to sustaining health inequalities (Farmer 2005).[11]

If we explore further, this example of seeing health as a complex social outcome, now turning to HIV and AIDS, we can see that the narrow focus on influencing sexual behaviour change and the particular risks of individuals and groups in contemporary approaches to HIV prevention is unlikely to have an impact on what is the social systemic nature of HIV and AIDS and various social factors that structure patterns of differential vulnerability. In addition, we can see that a control orientation in the response to HIV and AIDS that focuses on manipulating particular behaviours and individual risks may be counterproductive.

HIV AND AIDS AND THE COMPLEX SOCIAL DETERMINANTS OF HEALTH

Recent epidemiologically informed studies of HIV and AIDS provide a strong complementary supporting case for treating AIDS as a complex social phenomenon. In *AIDS and the Ecology of Poverty*, Eileen Stillwaggon (2006) argues that the hold that HIV and AIDS has taken on many parts of Africa is largely attributable to the multiple assaults on the immunity of impoverished Africans due to inadequate nutrition, water and sanitation and a range of co-infections, not least TB, malaria and parasitic infections, in the context of broader patterns of social inequalities of wealth. AIDS has not taken hold in the affluent societies of the North, largely due to the absence of these factors. In Eastern Europe and the transition countries of the former Soviet Union, it is the collapse of health and welfare infrastructure, coupled with rapidly growing poverty and inequalities of wealth that is behind the emerging epidemics there. These conditions of 'social collapse' she argues, are as much responsible for rising HIV infections than any of the particular specific behavioural manifestations of this social distress in sharing needles in injecting drugs or sex work that may involve engaging in unprotected sex.

Focusing on generalized epidemics of HIV and AIDS, she illustrates that the differences in the overall pattern of HIV and AIDS in different societies is not attributable to different patterns of sexual behaviour, and challenges assumptions about Africans having more sexual partners in than in other parts of the world (Stillwaggon 2006). In many countries in sub-Saharan Africa, rather than only attempting to control and direct people's sexual behaviour, which she suggests has become a veritable obsession in current HIV and AIDS interventions,[12] Stillwaggon presents a range of practical, available and actionable remedies for tackling HIV which address a range of broader determinants of health, many of which are relatively cheap to implement. These include: the eradication of helminths, schistosoma infection and intestinal worms which are endemic in many African countries with a high HIV prevalence; nutritional, clean water and sanitation interventions; promoting the education of girls; changing trade policies that tangle trucks and truckers in protracted border delays; and measures to reunite families who are separated by the migrant labour patterns imposed by contemporary industry.

These interventions all have a synergistic effect on improving overall levels of health, not just of HIV infection, even while standard cost-benefit analysis based on short-term, single-input, single output interventions is inadequate to show the value of those that are multi-input, multi-output long term (Stillwaggon 2006, 170–76). In many ways Stillwaggon is arguing that whether the presence of HIV infection will turn into an epidemic, depends on a broad range of wider social determinants of health that affect people's immunity and susceptibility to infections that are present, just as with any other infectious disease.

So, to tackle HIV and AIDS, a range of broader interventions are important that have no immediate relation to what has become the customary focus — on what she calls the 'just in time' intervention at the last possible moment — only around the behaviour surrounding potential transmission of the virus. Recent work on multiple concurrent partnerships in southern and eastern Africa, does in fact suggest that there may be a distinctive pattern of sexual relations that contribute to higher levels of HIV infection in these regions by linking people up in sexual networks (Epstein 2007), even while it acknowledges the mistaken assumptions around African's having more sexual partners. But Stillwaggon's broader argument still stands — that there is a need to look beyond the immediate proximal setting of HIV transmission to the wider social forces that structure vulnerability.

Strengthening health systems and integrating services

This compelling review of the social ecology of the epidemic clearly suggests that the energy and resources that have been galvanized for HIV and AIDS need an accompanying urgency around the improvement of health systems as a whole, and measures to tackle the basic primary health infrastructure of adequate water supply, sanitation and nutrition. The echoes of the Ottawa Charter for health promotion and the call for 'Health for All' are strong.[13] There might be much to learn from the experiences of primary health care, not least the attempt to build on existing community resources and strengths.[14] In fact, the need for a more integrated approach to HIV and AIDS with action around the broader health issues that interact with it has re-emerged in recent years, with the World Health Organisation (WHO) pioneering decentralised, integrated delivery of HIV and AIDS services in some places as part of its integrated management of adult and childhood illness (Gilks et al. 2006).

Adequate health services and access to affordable treatment will ultimately make the difference to poor communities' chances of surviving HIV and AIDS (Barnett and Whiteside 2002). In the absence of action by formal health services in many cases, community-based organizations in Africa, for example, have risen to the challenge of delivering HIV treatment on a significant scale while they await the much-needed public sector response (UNAIDS 2005). The experience of such organizations points to the need for support for community-based responses that are already making progress; including funding for purchasing antiretrovirals; operational costs and support; and policies to support service decentralization. However, it is clear that this must be in the context of fully resourced health systems: the involvement of local communities may be an inspiration, but it must not be an excuse to avoid government responsibility.

In summary, then, a complex systems approach to health highlights the variety of wider health and social determinants which interact in complex ways to frame the rates of transmission of a particular infection such as HIV, and whether it takes on epidemic proportions in a particular social setting. Just as a complex systems approach raises questions about the adequacy of the current narrow focus in HIV prevention on directing and controlling sexual and other 'risk' behaviour, for addressing the complex social character of HIV and AIDS as a health issue, it also raises questions about this narrow focus for HIV and AIDS as a complex political and communication issue. This is important at a time when such an emphasis on sexual behaviour risks providing a licence for ideologically driven moralizing and social control on the part of various governments and agencies involved in current HIV and AIDS responses.

AIDS RESPONSES: STRENGTHENING GOVERNMENT CONTROL, OR PROMOTING DIVERSE ACTION?

Concern has grown in recent years over the vigorous promotion of 'abstinence only' messages and interventions. One-third of all prevention funds available through the US President's Emergency Plan for HIV and AIDS Relief (PEPFAR) were earmarked for this (CHANGE 2002) — an emphasis that it is claimed rests on Uganda's early response to the epidemic. Calls for HIV prevention communication based on evidence, rather than ideology have been an important challenge to this new moralism.[15] In the present case, a review of the evidence suggests that a balanced combination of prevention interventions was effective in Uganda, where the broad mobilization of society was accompanied by open dialogue and communication, and delayed sexual debut and partner reduction — not abstinence — were associated with falling rates of infection. This moralising approach can also be seen in US policies that liken prevention work with sex workers to the promotion of sex trafficking have seriously hampered work with a key vulnerable population, and the rejection of needle exchange interventions — a public health measure of proven success (Gill 2006).

While it may be important to assemble the available evidence derived from specific prevention interventions associated with particular sexual risk behaviours, it may be equally important to broaden the focus to consider the public action needed on the wider social determinants of health as questions of equity and rights. Recognising the need for a broader social response is also less likely to reinforce the stigma that already marginalized and vulnerable groups face due to moral judgements about their behaviour (Sontag 1991).

The tendency for governments to develop a control orientation in their response to HIV and AIDS and use it in their own quest for legitimacy and control have been provocatively reviewed recently by Alex de Waal, although his principal focus is Africa. Reflecting on the many issues of power and governance surrounding the international AIDS response, de Waal notes how the inflows of HIV and AIDS development funds (in particular linked to the scale-up of treatment) and the scope and influence of non-governmental organisations on the patterns of health and social infrastructure of many African nations, is transforming their governance in subtle but far-reaching ways. Two contrasting scenarios of the impact for such changes are that of increasing government coercion, on the one hand, or raising the profile of neglected health issues in a broader frame of equity and social support, on the other. De Waal (2006) argues that the 'international AIDS apparatus' has been at the vanguard of democratising the aid encounter, promoting a voluntary participation and emphasising the human rights of people living with HIV and AIDS, and in this way, it could be a mechanism for raising a range of voices and neglected issues, and addressing neglect of mass poverty and the social causes of vulnerability (De Waal 2006, 121).[16] Equally, however, the monitoring and compliance necessary for effective supervision of ARV treatment, could strengthen a bureaucracy that is increasingly coercive in an 'unparalleled life controlling intrusion into African societies' (De Waal 2006, 115). Relevant to the latter, is the track record of some African governments using food aid, and more recently antiretroviral drugs, as resources to disburse in patrimonial networks, to bolster their control.[17]

COMMUNICATION FOR SOCIAL CHANGE: A COMPLEX SYSTEMS APPROACH?

Organizing the response to HIV and AIDS too exclusively around interventions into particular behaviours and the imperatives of drug treatment, flies in the face of previous learning from successes in national efforts to tackle AIDS and, as was argued above, neglects the complex character of the epidemic, not least the social challenges of gender inequity and stigma and discrimination. Rather than impose a narrow set of interventions, it is important that national responses be developed to suit national context, but equally that a diversity of initiatives and actors combine in a wide-ranging mobilization that is owned by civil society. This lesson from the experiences of HIV and AIDS responses is supported by the insight from complex systems theory that diversity of sources of information and experiences feeding into a system is important for the system's ability to adapt and learn (Wheatley 1999). Real freedom of action and initiative for those most affected by HIV and AIDS is important to ensure effective responses to their contextual realities in each case. In seeing social change as complex and emergent, systems theory highlights the importance of ensuring diversity and independence of local action. Rather than external control, such an approach emphasizes linking existing initiatives in networks of feedback and communication, something confirmed from developments in participatory evaluation and learning as was noted above.

This, in turn, means developing the social, political and communication practices and institutions appropriate to this task of ensuring genuine participation and ownership. We are reminded here of the focus of participatory communication approaches to support self-defined change on the part of the people who are the supposed beneficiaries of development. It is no accident that when Communication for Social Change programming was being developed in Ethiopia and Zambia in 2004/5, the question of 'scale' was approached with an 'association' model — linking existing initiatives and promoting communication and learning between them, drawing on notions of appreciative enquiry, rather than attempting to replicate the same model in many different places (Chetley 2004). In this way, the successes of contextually grounded programming could be learned from and linked together, recognizing that what was appropriate in one setting may not be simply applicable in another. The wide range of experiences and perspectives captured in the recent anthology of communication for social change also reflects an awareness of the diversity of communication approaches and social movements, with their different routes towards inclusive social change process in different contexts (Gumacio-Dagron and Tufte 2004).

The emphasis on local autonomy of action can be seen in recent critiques of participatory approaches in development, which have highlighted the risks of co-opting people into powerful, pre-set development agendas, under the guise of 'authentic' local participation (Mosse 2004). This has led some to explore who sets the terms of different 'spaces of participation', and to assess how much real control is in the hands of different groups in different development encounters (Cornwall 2004). One of the distinctive things about the early response to HIV and AIDS in the US was creative communication and campaigning driven by being close to the issues on the ground for affected communities, and an ownership of the response (Stoller 1998). This is quite different from some of the more instrumental attempts to get participation of people with HIV and AIDS in national responses on the part of governments and development agencies, with the dangers of tokenism and legitimizing plans and priorities that have already been decided by authorities and experts.

In the Nicaraguan NGO, 'Puntos de Encuentro', we see an organization that, recently, has drawn explicitly on insights from complex systems theory to conceptualise its communication for social change programming. The language and concepts of complex systems theory have helped to explain the way it works — networking a diversity of local actors, with emergent volunteer networks and initiatives — to partner organisations and a donor community used to the linear planning of outcomes and the cause and effect of the logical framework (Lacayo 2006). In fact, the challenges of operating in the world structured by the powerful institutions of development and prevailing economic and political culture, means that Puntos, as with many other organizations, is not always able to realise the potential it sees in the insights of complex systems theory, and the 'emergent' ways in which it attempts to work.

The emergent and dynamic nature of social change also demands a different approach to evaluation: being more an ongoing source of learning and feedback, to capture the emerging model of causal relationships, to learn from the unexpected and 'noise' in the system, and to understand the 'differences that make a difference' among the wide range of interrelationships and connections affecting the focus of development work (Eayang and Berkas 1998). There are clear parallels here with debates on the need for learning focused evaluation and the need to adapt to deal with the context and unexpected change in any setting (Vincent and Byrne 2006).

CONCLUSIONS: STRENGTHENING EXISTING RESPONSES

This chapter has reviewed some recent trends in international HIV and AIDS communication towards tackling the social drivers of HIV and AIDS which may support reflection to address patterns of vulnerabilities to HIV in the Caribbean context. Initiatives that aim to tackle gender inequity and stigma and discrimination illustrate the need for multi-levelled approaches to address social complexity, and build on the participation and empowerment of those most affected by HIV and AIDS. There is a need to further develop of communication for social change approaches in the light of a better understanding of the dynamics of existing social movements and cultural responses, if some of the dangers of co-optation identified in participatory approaches are to be avoided. Where local and social cultural dynamics risk reproducing existing power inequalities, there is a need for processes of critical engagement to challenge power and inequality, but this is a process that has to be owned by people working within their local idioms of everyday practice and discourse.

The theory of complex systems provides useful avenues for further enquiry: pointing to ways to combine support for local freedom of action through the strengthening of key broad social foundations, such as universal provision of basic health and education. Equally, there is a need for a basic infrastructure of communication and dialogue processes that support the expression of local experiences and priorities and involvement of those most affected by HIV and AIDS responses. Such an emphasis may be an important counterweight to the current narrow focus on 'behaviour change' targeted at a range of vulnerable groups, which may serve dubious purposes for a range of contemporary governments who are turning to social authoritarian policies and practices in HIV and AIDS policies.

A willingness to explore participatory development approaches that genuinely work with the grain of local need and respect local initiative cannot be an excuse for neglecting the fundamental social factors which structure vulnerability to HIV and AIDS. These demand an investment of energy and resources to strengthen public health systems and social support infrastructure in many developing countries. Our look at health and HIV through the lens of complex systems theory shows that it is time to renew efforts to tackle the wider determinants of health, and revisit the need for comprehensive primary health care, and the strengthening of health systems, if there is to be real progress on HIV and AIDS. Equally, political will is needed to address the inequity and poverty that drive the epidemic, and to work for legal and institutional policy frameworks that will address the social and structural barriers to the response. It is, ultimately, such social foundations that will lay the basis for tackling the complex social character of HIV and AIDS.

Notes

1. See also W Sittitrai, *HIV Prevention Needs and Success: A Tale of Three Countries*, (Geneva: UNAIDS, 2001); Panos, *Missing the Message: 20 years of learning from HIV/AIDS*, (London: Panos. 2003); E. Green, *Rethinking AIDS prevention: learning lessons from successes in Developing Countries*, (Connecticut: Praeger. 2003); A. Singhall and E. M. Rogers, *Combating AIDS: Communication Strategies in Action*, (London: Sage, 2003).

2. See: *www.communicationforsocialchange.org*

3. See: *www.reflect-action.org*

4. See N. Ford, D. Odallo and R. Chorlton.. 'Communication from a Human Rights Perspective: Responding to the HIV/AIDS Pandemic in Eastern and Southern Africa'. *Journal of Health Communication* 8 no. 6 (2003).

5. See *UNDP Upscaling Community Conversations*: *http://www.et.undp.org/hiv/CC.htm* (accessed June 30, 2006) .

6. This process, which aims to focus on the social drivers of the epidemic in each national setting, is still being developed in early 2008, and the author is part of the UNAIDS technical consultation on social change.

7. Interview by author with Hilary Nicholson of Women's Media Watch, Kingston, Jamaica, April, 2006, cited in Panos. *Breaking Barriers*, (2006a).

8. The Sonagachi collective in Kolkata, India, provides an inspiring example of such organising, see Singhall and Rogers *Combating AIDS*. (London: Sage, 2003).

9. See S. Rihani, *Complex Systems Theory and Development Practice: Understanding Non-linear Realities*, (London: Zed Books, 2002).

10. Malcom Gladwell's *The Tipping Point* gives a popular and resonant account of one of the insights of complexity theory — namely that small changes in some key characteristics of a system when it is at a critical point, can tip the system into much larger changes in their overall configuration: otherwise popularized as 'the butterfly effect' in accounts of 'chaos theory'.

11. Thanks to Sarah Cardey for drawing my attention to this parallel.

12. Not unrelated to the history of assumptions about African sexuality — see chapter 7, E. Stillwaggon, *AIDS and the Ecology of Poverty*.

13. For the Ottawa Charter see: *http://www.who.int/hpr/NPH/docs/ottawa_charter _hp.pdf* (accessed July 10, 2007).

14. Another of which is culture and traditional medicine — see Panos. *Breaking Barriers*.

15. In fact, following a mid term evaluation of PEPFAR by the Institute of Medicine, it seems much more focus will be on the social drivers of HIV when PEPFAR funding is renewed, see: Institute of Medicine (eds). *PEPFAR implementation, progress and promise*, Presidents Emergency Plan for AIDS Relief PEPFAR, 2007.

16. De Waal points to the changing focus of the Treatment Action Campaign in South Africa to look beyond HIV treatment to broader social assistance.

17. Of course African governments are not alone in using resources at their disposal to support patrimonial networks, but Africa is the focus of De Waal's critique here.

REFERENCES

Airhihenbuwa, C. O. and R. Obregon. 2000. 'A Critical Assessment of Theories/Models used in Health Communication for HIV/AIDS', *Journal of Health communication* 5, Supplement: 5–15.

Appadurai, A. 1996. *Modernity at Large: Cultural Dimensions of Globalisation*. Minneapolis, University of Minnesota Press.

Barnett, T. and A. Whiteside. 2002. *AIDS in the Twenty-first Century: Disease and Globalization*. Basingstoke: Palgrave Macmillan, 342.

Byrne, A., and J. Hunt. 2005. *To Change the Dance you must Change the Music: Youth Programmes in Ethiopia aimed at HIV and AIDS*, New Jersey: CFSC consortium: *http://www.communicationforsocialchange.org/mazi-articles.php?id=287*

Byrne, D. 1998. *Complexity Theory and the Social Sciences: An Introduction*. London: Routledge.

Castells, M. 2000. *Network Society*. Oxford: Blackwell.

Centre for Health and Gender Equity. 2004. *Debunking the myths in the U.S. Global AIDS Strategy: An Evidence-Based Analysis*. Takoma Park, MD: CHANGE.

Chetley, A. 2004. *Opportunities to scale up participatory approaches with youth and media: Strengthening Youth Participation in Ethiopia*, March 3–4 . *http://www.healthcomms.org/pdf/ethiopia-UNICEF.pdf*, accessed July 10, 2007.

Cornwall, A. 2004. 'Spaces for Transformation? Reflections on Issues of Power and Difference in Participation in Development'. In *Participation: from tyranny to transformation: exploring new approaches to participation in development*, ed., S. Hickey, and G. Mohan, London: Zed Books.

De Waal, A. 2006. *AIDS and Power: Why there is no Political Crisis – Yet*. London: Zed Books.

DFID. 2005. *AIDS Communication*. London: UK Department for International Development.

Eoyang, G. and T. Berkas. 1998. *Evaluation in a complex adaptive system*: *http://www.winternet.com/~eoyang/EvalinCAS.pdf*. Accessed July 7, 2007.

Epstein, H. 2007. *The Invisible Cure: Africa, the West and the fight against AIDS*. London: Pelican/Viking.

Eve, R., et al. 1998. *Chaos, complexity and sociology: myths, models and theories*. London: Sage.

Farmer, P. 2005. *Pathologies of Power: Health Human Rights and the New War on the Poor*. California: University of California Press.

Ford, N., D. Odallo and R. Chorlton. 2003. 'Communication from a Human Rights Perspective: Responding to the HIV/AIDS Pandemic in Eastern and Southern Africa'. *Journal of Health Communication* 8, no. 6.

Gilks, C.F., S. Crawley and R. Ekpini. 2006. 'WHO public health approach to antiretroviral treatment against HIV in resource-limited settings'. *The Lancet* 368, August 5.

Gill, P. 2006. *Body Count: How They turned AIDS into a Catastrophe*. London: Profile Books.

Green, E. 2003. *Rethinking AIDS Prevention: Learning Lessons from Successes in Developing Countries*. Connecticut: Praeger.

Gumacio-Dragon, A and T. Tufte. 2006. *Communication for Social Change Anthology: Historical and Contemporary readings*. New York: Communication for social Change Consortium.

Hadjipateras, A. 2006. *Joining hands: Integrating Gender and HIV/AIDS*. London: ACCORD, HASAP.

ICRW. 2007. *Towards a Stronger Response to HIV and AIDS: Challenging Stigma*. internal paper for DFID. Washington DC: International Centre for Research on Women.

Lacayo, V. 2006. *Approaching social change as a complex problem in a world that treats it as a complicated one: the case of Puntos de Encuentro, Nicaragua*. *http://www.ohio.edu/commdev/upload/Approaching_social_change_as_a_complex_problem.pdf*. Accessed July 10, 2007.

Moore, H. 1994. *A Passion for Difference: Essays in Anthropology and Gender*. London: Polity Press.

Mosse, D. 2001. 'People's Knowledge, Participation and Patronage: Operations and Representation in Rural Development'. In *Participation: the new tyranny?*, eds. B. Cooke and U. Kothari. London: Zed Books.

Nicolis, G. and I. Prigogine. 1989. *Exploring Complexity: An Introduction*. New York: W. H. Freeman.

Obregon, R. 2004. *The UNAIDS' HIV/AIDS Communication Framework Six Years Later: Is there a future?* Paper submitted to the Working Group on Communication and HIV/AIDS International Association for Mass Communication Research, July 24, 2004, Porto Alegre, Brazil.

Panos Institute. 2003. *Missing the Message: 20 years of Learning from HIV/AIDS*. London: Panos.

———. 2006. *Keeping the Promise? A study of progress made in implementing the UNGASS*.

———. *Declaration of Commitment on HIV/AIDS in seven countries*. London: Panos.

———. 2006a. *Breaking Barriers: Effective Communication for HIV Prevention, Treatment Care and Support by 2010*. London: Panos Institute.

Parker, Richard and Peter Aggleton. 2002. *HIV/AIDS related Stigma and Discrimination: A Conceptual Framework and an Agenda for Action*. Horizons programme, New York: Population Council.

Rihani, S. 2002. *Complex Systems Theory and Development Practice: Understanding Non-Linear Realities*. London: Zed Books.

Sen, A. 2004. *Development as Freedom*. Oxford: Oxford University Press.

Singhall, A. and E. M. Rogers. 2003. *Combating AIDS: communication strategies in action*. London: Sage.

Sittitrai, W. 2001. *HIV Prevention Needs and Success: A Tale of Three Countries*. Geneva: UNAIDS.

Sontag, S. 1991. *AIDS and its Metaphors*. London: Penguin.

Stillwaggon, E. 2006. *AIDS and the Ecology of Poverty*. Oxford: Oxford University Press.

Stoller, N. 1998. *Lessons from the Damned: Queers, Whores and Junkies respond to AIDS*. New York: Routledge.

Tufte, T. 2005. 'Entertainment-education in development communication: between marketing behaviours and empowering people'. In *Media and Global Change: rethinking Communication for Development*, eds. O. Hemer and T. Tufte. Buenos Aires: CLASCO.

UNAIDS. 1999. *New Communicaiton framework for HIV/AIDS*. *http://www.unaids.org/html/pub/publications/ircpub01/jc335-commframew_en_pdf.pdf*

———. 2005. 'HIV-related Stigma, Discrimination and Human Rights Violations: Case studies of successful programmes'. *UNAIDS Best Practice Collection*. Geneva: UNAIDS.

———. 2005. 'Expanding access to HIV treatment through community based organisations'. *UNAIDS best practice collection*. Joint United Nations Programme on AIDS.

———. 2006. *Scaling up access to HIV prevention, treatment, care and support: The next steps*. Geneva: UNAIDS.

———. 2007. *Assessing gender equality and equity as critical elements in National responses to HIV: Cambodia, Honduras and Ukraine*. Geneva: UNAIDS/PCB/.20. CRP1.

UNESCO. 2003. *HIV/AIDS Stigma and Discrimination: An Anthropological Approach*. Proceedings of the roundtable held on November 29, 2002, Paris: United Nations Educational, Scientific and Cultural Organisation.

UNIFEM. 2006. *Transforming the national AIDS response: mainstreaming gender equality and women's human rights into the three ones*. New York: United Nations Development Fund for Women.

Wheatley, M. 1999. *Leadership and the New Science: Discovering Order in a Chaotic World*. San Francisco: Berrett-Koehler.

Vincent, R. 2005. *What do we do with Culture? Engaging Culture in Development*, London: Exchange: *http://www.healthlink.org.uk/PDFs/findings_culture.pdf*

Vincent, R. and A. Byrne. 2006. 'Enhancing Learning in Development Partnerships'. *Development in Practice* 16 no. 5.

RECONCEPTUALIZING SEX

CHAPTER 9

CENTERING PRAXIS IN POLICIES AND STUDIES OF CARIBBEAN SEXUALITY

Kamala Kempadoo

A number of recent studies and debates assume that it is critical for researchers, policymakers and programmers to problematize gendered power and inequalities in order to adequately address HIV and AIDS epidemics. Indeed, everything points to a need for 'gender-mainstreaming' or a 'gender-based approach' in HIV and AIDS work for the interventions and policies to be effective (Gupta and Weiss 2007; Raimondo 2005). Yet, is a gendered approach the miracle cure?

Here, I seek not to dispute the significance of gender and gendered relations of power in the transmission and prevention of HIV. Patriarchy, social constructions of gender and masculine anxieties about female sexuality and homosexuality I agree, must be addressed in HIV policies and programming. However, I also propose that while a focus on gender is critical, unless we turn adequate attention to sexual praxis we may not make much headway in stemming the epidemics. In the following, I offer some thoughts for centering sex in the Caribbean debates, and in so doing, argue for the delineation of a specific field of inquiry in Caribbean studies.

This chapter is part of the outcome of a 2006 study that aimed to assist UNIFEM and its partners to 'better understand and therefore address how gender and sexuality are related to risk and vulnerability' in the Caribbean.[1] It draws from a review of approximately 150 documents (reports, unpublished papers, journal articles, media reports, book chapters, and books) that were identified on the basis of the likelihood of their providing insights into Caribbean sexuality.[2] It also intersects with many other ideas that were presented at the colloquium held by

University of the West Indies HIV and AIDS Response Programme (UWI HARP) in Jamaica in September 2007 as part of the effort to reconceptualise responses to AIDS in the region.

SEXUAL PRAXIS

While we do not have, at this time, a single body of work that can be designated 'Caribbean sexuality studies' we do have multiple sources from which to draw and to gather insights into the subject. Caribbean sexuality is most visible as sedimented social practice rather than social identity, and most commonly appears in studies since the 1980s about violence against women, sexual-economic exchange, same-sex relations, adolescent sexual activity, migration and tourism, and in studies of family and 'mating' patterns (Kempadoo and Taitt 2006). Through such studies, sexuality appears to be configured by heteropatriarchy — and its corollary homophobia — and to be profoundly shaped by an abuse of power and physical violence. Studies also point to its saturation with material interests and needs, as well as to the operation of multiple partnering arrangements. Sexual praxis is, moreover, mediated by age, race, ethnicity and class and, throughout the region, is overshadowed by obfuscating discourses. An active male heterosexual desire is assumed, in many instances, to be a natural condition and, while the significance of notions of virility, fertility, sexual prowess, and violence to manhood are widely acknowledged in popular culture and social studies, male sexual praxis is too often left uncritically problematized. Incest, female sexual agency and expressions of sexual desire, and bisexual behaviour are, likewise, repeatedly signalled in the studies, yet are not well-researched themes.[3]

In hegemonic discourse, Caribbean sexuality is defined by a gender binary where the biological is firmly attached to the social, and in which masculinity and femininity are believed to be lodged in procreative functions and immutable 'facts' of the body. Heterosexuality is most commonly taken 'as the only legitimate sexuality . . . it is sex with the opposite sex that makes a man a man and a woman a woman' (Peake and Trotz 1999). The collapse of sex and gender in everyday, and often academic, discourse elides the existence of persons whose social identities, sexual practices or physical bodies do not adhere or conform to these categories. Caribbean sexuality then regularly appears as rigidly heterosexual and intolerant of sexual difference. Sex folds into gender, and masculinity and femininity are viewed as complements to each other: two parts of a whole. Moreover, sex/gender identities are rigidly defined. What makes a man a man and a woman a woman, other than biology, is commonly represented in stable identity categories that seem to change little over time.

The dominant, almost unquestioned, links between sexuality and gender are lodged in a norm of heterosexuality as 'natural' in African as well as Indian Caribbean communities (Alexander 1997; Chevannes 2001; Lokaisingh-Meighoo 2000), which are reinforced by religion, education, social studies, and the media. Heterosexual behaviour, as the Anglican Bishop of Barbados succinctly puts it, 'is treated as the norm as ordained by God' (Holder 2003; see also Genrich and Braithwaite 2005). Within this discourse 'normal' heterosexual masculinity is not defined or viewed as a problem or as a site that requires particular attention. Rather, 'men-who-have-sex-with-men' (MSM), women-who-love-women, adolescents, 'commercial sex workers' (CSWs), labour migrants, bisexuals, and sex tourists become social groups whose very existences are defined in hegemonic discourse as social problems. The groups are perceived as pools of 'nastiness' and disease, and ultimately as the harbingers of national and regional decline and shame.

Taking sexuality as derivative of, or interchangeable with, gender is, however, problematic. Richard Parker argues that 'whom one is permitted to have sex with, in what ways, under what circumstances and with what specific outcomes are never random: such possibilities are defined through explicit and implicit rules imposed by the sexual cultures of specific communities and the underlying power relations,' where gender is one set of power relations (Parker et al. 2000, 7–8). Sexuality is not conceived as synonymous with gender and gender is one of several factors that shape sexuality. Taking sexuality and gender as overlapping, yet distinct and semi-autonomous terrains, we allow for an examination of 'the articulation between specific features of each system, namely how the configurations bear on the experience of being female [and male] and conversely, how the definitions of gender resonate with and are reflected in sexuality' (Vance 1988).

Yet, even with this distinction and semi-autonomy between sexuality and gender, and the proliferation of studies of sexuality through GLBT and Queer Studies, within gender and women's studies the categories are often collapsed into each other, leading authors such as Gupta and Weiss to argue for a gender-based approach to address sexual matters (2007). Nevertheless, the distinction lurks in the margins, and I propose here that rather then pushing it further into marginality or subsuming it completely by gender, we must recuperate the distinction. It is furthermore my argument that privileging sexuality in analyses of social interactions and identities may be a necessary strategy at this time for addressing HIV and AIDS in the Caribbean due to the centrality of sexual behaviour to the epidemics. A heightened focus on sexuality could then serve the purposes of critiquing, challenging and changing contemporary discourses and practices, while also aiding in the establishment of a specific field of study.

SEXUALITY IN BIOMEDICAL APPROACHES

HIV in the Caribbean is primarily transmitted through heterosexual intercourse and, according to the most recent UNAIDS statistics, the epidemic is not abating in the region. Sexual intercourse, thus, appears resistant to information about how HIV is contracted, transmitted, or may be prevented, and there is concern that although 'HIV and AIDS awareness is close to 100%', this awareness has not translated into 'safer sex' practices (Pargass 2005). There is a 'disconnect', as Marjan de Bruin pointed out several years ago, between knowledge about sexually transmitted infections and sexual behaviour, which continues to interfere with HIV prevention and AIDS treatment activities (de Bruin 2001). Gendered imbalances of power and hegemonic constructions of gender that place great significance, on the one hand, on male sexual prowess, and virility, on the other, female fertility, might well provide many answers.

However, we need to be mindful of other factors that influence the epidemics.

In the first instance, it cannot be overlooked that the biomedical approach that informs many of the current HIV-prevention polices and programmes rests upon certain assumptions about human nature that ignore social relations of power, identity, and desire. As the editors of a recent collection of studies about sexuality and development note:

> At the epidemiological research end, there is an assumption that there exists an objective, socially neutral standpoint from which behaviours can be identified, named and classified; at the intervention end there is an assumption that those addressed by programs will recognize certain desires and actions as sexual behaviours that can be the object of reflexive fashioning (Pigg and Adams 2005, 20).

Sexual passions or desires are believed to be susceptible to rational decision-making processes and individual will power. However, the specific logic or 'intelligence' that informs sexual praxis is overlooked, with the consequence that sexuality remains largely untouched by HIV prevention interventions. Moreover, biomedical approaches often ignore important aspects of the culture within which HIV circulates, including unequal sexual relations of power and sexual agency. As researchers in Africa conclude:

> Biomedical and epidemiological research ... is largely inattentive to socio-cultural contexts and political economies of sexuality, not to mention the agency and interests of people whose sexual practices are now targeted for study. The fact that we have such limited academic and analytical knowledge about sexuality, a pivotal aspect of social organisation at all levels, provides a powerful motivation for future research to be carried out by African scholars, and to be carried out in new ways that are both transformed and transformative (Mama, Pereira et al. 2005, 1).

The significance of sexuality to development policies and strategies is also of importance to this discussion, for while :

[d]evelopment work has tended to focus on sexuality only in relation to disease and violence, on the risks and dangers rather than the pleasures and fulfillments... new possibilities are opening up with the urgency of responding to the HIV and AIDS crisis, and with increasing activism around sexuality worldwide... policymakers must now engage with sexuality' (IDS 2006, 4; see also Adams and Pigg 2005; Gosine 2005).

Sexuality is a new terrain for development experts, and intersections between sexuality and the global economy are only recently recognised.[4] It is then perhaps not surprising that policies and programmes aimed at sexual behaviour change in developing countries do not yet fully address the problem.

Where social, cultural and political dimensions of sexuality have not been ignored, biomedical approaches tend to (re)produce categories of 'at risk' groups. 'MSM', sex workers, adolescents and migrants are commonly identified with deviant sexual practices and as groups that present a health risk to the rest of the population. These groups quickly become, in dominant discourse, 'pools of disease' and 'bridges' through which disease is transmitted to an otherwise 'healthy' national body (Padilla 2007). In other words, biomedical approaches to HIV take up sexuality in such a way that certain social groups are defined as pathological, deviants or social problems. In turn, such pathologization or problematization in terms of disease, risk and ill-health supports legislation that criminalizes same-sex relations and sex work, and feeds stigmas and discriminations against persons involved in sexual commerce, same-sex relations, and sexually active adolescents and migrants (Carr 2003; Kempadoo 2004).

In short, the biomedical approaches that often inform HIV programmes have barely addressed sexuality or its embeddedness in economic relations and global development processes. The inability of such approaches to deal with sexuality as it is lived and practised in social and cultural contexts, or to adequately capture the logic that informs sexual relations, leads to short-sighted and biased policies, programmes and interventions. Taking a gender-based approach may or may not address this problem.

COMPLICATING SEXUALITY

While HIV transmission in the Caribbean appears as straightforwardly heterosexual, a number of other arrangements intervene to make the epidemic difficult to map or influence. Bisexual, same-sex and multiple-partnering arrangements are implicated, as are prostitution and other forms of sex work, 'romance' tourism, and transactional sex. All appear to be common-place scenarios that criss-cross nationality, ethnicity, gender and class. And it is this range of sexual practices, which occur mainly under the social radar and are secretly desired yet publicly frowned upon, that help to sustain the HIV and AIDS epidemics. Cultural secrecy and shame surrounding sexual matters and desires maintain the silences, stigmas and distortions, while laws against prostitution, same-sex intercourse, sex with a minor, and sex tourism push certain practices even further underground. Approaching sexuality as derivative of a gendered binary and a hetero norm elides these very complex sexual interactions and relations, and obscures, rather than illuminates Caribbean sexuality.

Important to any interrogation of sexual praxis is also racial and ethnic relations and identities that may, at times, trump gender relations. One clear illustration of this can be found in the tourism industry. In that site, the exotic appeal of the racial other is fully structured and operational, bringing to the fore a complex interplay between a desire for, and exploitation of, the racial other (O'Connell Davidson and Sanchez Taylor 1999). Traditional heteropatriarchal relations of power are distorted or overturned when female and male tourists seek sexual services from Caribbean men, providing an association with whiteness, or access to 'development' that is otherwise unobtainable by the young men (Phillips 1999). Such arrangements do not fit neatly into classic heteropatriarchal gendered arrangements and, indeed, cannot be fully captured through a gendered lens. In order to properly account for, or address, such relations, we need to grapple with what it conceptually and theoretically means for poor, young black men to be providing sexual services to economically privileged (white) north American or European women, and possibly to be living with HIV themselves and thus able to transmit it to others.

Vulnerability here has a racialised face, which cannot be completely analysed or even comprehended with a traditional gender-based approach.

The extent of transactional sexual arrangements, outside of tourist and sex industries, underscores the significance of economic considerations to sexual relations. Sexuality as a resource that can be deliberately traded for favours, goods, money, housing, education, fashionable clothes, hairdos, travel, etc., plays a fundamental role in the shaping of meanings of sexuality (Ahmed 2003). Giving sex in exchange for a tangible benefit is not an uncommon gesture for women and young men, and can be taken as a profound expression of the way in which sexuality is experienced in everyday life as an embodied resource for 'getting by' or for 'betterment'. Prostitution, too, while most commonly organized through traditional heteropatriarchal arrangements, cannot be captured or explained exclusively through a gendered lens. The significance of 'gigolos', 'rentals' transgenders, and men-who-have-sex-with-men for money, alongside women who service men in the region's sex industries, points to intricate relations of power, identity and desire that inform sexual praxis.

A reading of Caribbean sexuality merely through a gender analysis obfuscates race relations and racialised desires that are deeply embedded in Caribbean prostitution through histories of colonialism, slavery and indentureship, and which continue under postcolonial conditions (Kempadoo 1999, 2004). It also denies the salience of economic inequalities between and within nations, that impel young Caribbean men and women to take up sex work, and overlooks the transgression of traditional gender categories through sexual praxis that occurs in a variety of ways in the sex trade (see also Wekker 2006; de Moya and Garcia 1996; Padilla 2007). It behoves us, then, to ask how the economy is woven together with constructions of race, same-sex desire, and sexuality, and to recognize the multiplicity of sexual expressions in contemporary Caribbean societies. Without an eye for the intricacies of sexual-economic praxis and the ways in which these exceed hegemonic definitions of gender, we lose sight of the multiple ways in which a sexually transmitted infection can spread.

SEXUALITY IN LAW

M. Jacqui Alexander pointed out in the early nineties that a distinction between sexuality and gender is embedded in Caribbean state discourses and laws, evidenced by the criminalization of particular types of sexual praxis (Alexander 1991). People who engage in same-sex relations and those who sell sex are two categories that are defined and treated differently in Caribbean laws, on the basis of sexual practice. National governments regulate sexual behaviour and expressions of erotic desire, differently than they do gender. Indeed, as studies of same-sex relations in Cuba and the Dominican Republic demonstrate, while many men who have sex with men socially identify as masculine, it is their sexual activities and desires, not their gender identification that sets them apart from other men in state policies, laws, and everyday practices (Lumsden 1996; de Moya 1996; Padilla 2007). Moreover, discrimination on the basis of gender is codified in most national laws as unjust and a violation of civil or human rights, yet discrimination on the basis of sexual expression is still possible in many countries due to laws that criminalize anal sex, sodomy, and prostitution. Sexual practice is, thus, firmly etched into Caribbean society as semi-autonomous and distinct from gender identity. The legal distinction forces recognition of the specificity of sexuality and asks for close attention to strategies to bring sexuality out of its abject status.

TOWARD A FIELD OF CARIBBEAN SEXUALITY STUDIES

In the absence of an established field of sexuality studies in the region, yet with many sources to draw on and the urgency required to adequately address the HIV epidemics, it becomes important to focus on sexual praxis, sexual intelligence, and sexualising discourses in research, policy work, and programming. And, if sexuality does not simply derive from gender but constitutes a distinct culture and set of social relations and identities that interact with, yet can be studied separately from, gender, race and the economy, we can use this lens to capture the specificities and variety of Caribbean sexual praxis. However, it is equally important to keep in mind that the conceptual and legal distinction between sexuality and gender is overshadowed by everyday discourse that locks sex and gender together in one body. It is this powerful bind that also serves as a reminder that any examination of Caribbean sexuality cannot be completely separated from gender.

A focus on sexuality as semi-autonomous from gender allows for an examination of the ways in which sexuality is attached to gender as well as to other axes of power. It enables us to analyse 'race' as an important mediating principle, in those instances where constructions of race and ethnicity structure the sexual labour and possibilities for young people, and transform traditional gender relations of power. It helps to inform studies of the production of (new) identities and expressions that may or may not be attached to a gendered binary. The focus also supports continuing explorations into meanings of transactional sex and the ongoing commodification and exploitation of Caribbean sexual energies within local and global economies, and raises questions about ways in which the economic infuses specific meaning into racialised constructions of sexuality. It assists us to see how laws structure sexual inequality and enable discriminatory state regulations and policies. But, perhaps most importantly, it brings sexual intercourse and desires, as well as meanings of sexuality to the forefront of the discussion — those subjects that are still quite widely shrouded by double-entendre, secrecy and shame, and which are subsumed by concerns about gender relations. Sexuality, if accorded its own space and place in academic, political, and everyday discourses, could engender a reformulation of HIV and AIDS policies and programmes and allow us to get to the heart of the epidemic. In such efforts, sexuality — in all its glory and messiness — needs our full consideration.

NOTES

1. Three agencies originally commissioned the study - UNIFEM-Caribbean Office, the Barbados National HIV/AIDS Commission, and the Canadian International Development Research Centre (IDRC) – and it was conducted by this author in collaboration with Andy Taitt. The report was first presented to UNIFEM as 'Gender,

Sexuality and Implications for HIV/AIDS in the Caribbean: A Review of Literature and Programmes' (Barbados, July 2006).

2. For the collection of documents a variety of sources were consulted, including two annotated bibliographies on gender-based violence and gender and HIV/AIDS compiled by the Centre for Gender and Development Studies at the Mona and St. Augustine campuses of the University of the West Indies. Collections housed at the Centre for Gender and Development Studies at the Cave Hill campus, the Women and Development Unit (WAND), and UNIFEM in Barbados were particularly useful for collecting grey material that is often never made public. We also searched online databases through York University Library in Toronto and the UWI Cave Hill Library in Barbados, where we found many recently published journal articles. By email we solicited papers from specific authors, and several people volunteered their work and that of others once they became aware of the study. Because the review was initiated by the UNIFEM Caribbean office whose mandate covers CARICOM countries, the emphasis throughout the collection and analysis of the documents was on those particular territories of the Caribbean, with a bias towards publications written in English due to our own language limitations. Moreover, in attempting to gather information about social practices, an emphasis was on materials that rest on empirical research. Representations of sexuality in novels, art, poetry, songs, television shows, films, and other cultural productions as well analyses of these representations were not a consistent part of the review.

3. For an elaboration of these trends in Caribbean sexual praxis see Kempadoo (2008) 'Caribbean Sexuality: Mapping the Field', *Oso: Journal of Surinamese Studies*.

4. An important breakthrough in debates about gender and development is the emergence of the 'Women, Culture and Development' paradigm (see Bhavnani et al. 2003). Of particular significance are essays in Part One of the collection 'Sexuality and the Gendered Body', which address aspects of queering development and women's heterosexual empowerment in various third world contexts.

REFERENCES

Adams, Vincanne and Stacy Leigh Pigg, eds. 2005. *Sex in Development: Science, Sexuality and Morality in Global Perspective.* Durham: Duke University Press.

Ahmed, Aziza. 2003. 'Children and Transactional Sex in Jamaica: Addressing Increased Vulnerability to HIV/AIDS'. MA Thesis in Population and International Health. Harvard School of Public Health.

Alexander, M. Jacqui. 1991. 'Redrafting Morality: The Postcolonial State and the Sexual Offences Bill of Trinidad and Tobago.' In *Third World Women and the Politics of Feminism*, eds. Chandra Talpade Mohanty, Ann Russo and Lourdes Torres, 133–52. Bloomington and Indianapolis: Indiana University Press.

———. 1997. 'Erotic Autonomy as a Politics of Decolonization: An Anatomy of Feminist and State Practice in the Bahamas Tourist Economy.' In *Feminist Genealogies, Colonial*

Legacies, Democratic Futures, eds. M. Jacqui Alexander and Chandra Talpade Mohanty, 63–100. New York: Routledge.

Barrow, Christine. 2005. 'HIV/AIDS, Sexuality and Adolescent Girls in Barbados: The Case for Reconfiguring Research and Policy'. University of the West Indies, Cave Hill.

Bhavnani, Kum-Kum, John Foran, and Priya Kurian. 2003. *Feminist Futures: Re-imagining Women, Culture and Development*. London/New York: Zed Books.

Bruin de, Marjan. 2001. *Teenagers at Risk: High-risk Behaviour of Adolescents in the Context of Reproductive Health*. Kingston: CARIMAC, University of the West Indies.

Carr, Robert. 2003. 'On "Judgements": Poverty, Sexuality-based Violence and Human Rights in 21st Century Jamaica'. *Caribbean Journal of Social Work* 2: 71–87.

Chevannes, Barry. 2001. *Learning to Be a Man: Culture, Socialization and Gender Identity in Five Caribbean Communities*. Kingston: The University of the West Indies Press.

Genrich, Gillian L. and Brader Braithewaite. 2005. Response of Religious Groups to HIV/AIDS as a Sexually Transmitted Infection in Trinidad. *BMC Public Health*: 1–12

Gosine, Andil. 2005. 'Stumbling Into Sexualities: International Development Encounters Dissident Desire'. *Canadian Women Studies* 24: 59–63.

Gupta, Geeta Rao, and Ellen Weiss. 2007. "Creating an Enabling Context to Prevent HIV infection Among Women and Girls". Washington D.C.: International Center for Research on Women.

Holder, Rev. John. 2003. 'The Bible in The Anglican Tradition.' Anglican Bishop of Barbados.

IDS. 2006. 'Sexuality and Development.' *IDS Policy Briefing* April.

Kempadoo, Kamala. 2008. 'Caribbean Sexuality: Mapping the field', Oso: *Journal of Surinamese and Caribbean Studies 27, 1.*

———. 2004. *Sexing the Caribbean: Gender, Race and Sexual Labor*. New York: Routledge.

———. ed. 1999. *Sun, Sex and Gold: Tourism and Sex Work in the Caribbean*. Lanham: Rowman and Littlefield.

Kempadoo, Kamala and Andy Taitt. 2006. 'Gender, Sexuality and Implications for HIV/AIDS in the Caribbean. A Review of Literature and Programmes'. Barbados: UNIFEM and IDRC.

Lokaisingh-Meighoo, Sean. 2000. '*Jahaji Bhai*: Notes on the Masculine Subject and Homoerotic Subtext of Indo-Caribbean Identity'. *Small Axe: Journal of Criticism* 7: 77–92.

Lumsden, Ian. 1996. *Machos, Maricones, and Gays: Cuba and Homosexuality*. Philadelphia: Temple University Press.

Mama, Amina, Charmaine Pereira, and Takyiwaa Manuh. 2005. 'Editorial: Sexual Cultures'. *Feminist Africa*.

Moya de, Antonio E., and Rafael Garcia. 1996. 'AIDS and the Enigma of Bisexuality in the Dominican Republic'. In *Bisexuality and AIDS in International Perspective*, ed. Peter Aggleton, 21–35. London: Taylor and Francis.

O'Connell Davidson, Julia, and Jacqueline Sanchez Taylor. 1999. 'Fantasy Islands: Exploring the Demand for Sex Tourism'. In *Sun, Sex, and Gold: Tourism and Sex Work in the Caribbean*, ed. Kamala Kempadoo, 37–54. Lanham: Rowman and Littlefield.

Padilla, Mark. 2007. *Caribbean Pleasure Industry: Tourism, Sexuality, and AIDS in the Dominican Republic*. Chicago: University of Chicago Press.

Pargass, Gaietry. 2005. *Gender Review and Assessment of HIV/AIDS Programming of Selected National AIDS Programmes in the Caribbean*. ECLAC Subregional Headquarters for the Caribbean and UNIFEM-Caribbean Office.

Parker, Andrew, Regina Maria Barbosa, and Peter Aggleton, eds. 2000. *Framing the Sexual Subject: The Politics of Gender, Sexuality, and Power*. Berkeley: University of California Press.

Peake, Linda, and Alissa D. Trotz. 1999. *Gender, Ethnicity and Place: Women and Identities in Guyana*. New York: Routledge.

Phillips, Joan L. 1999. 'Tourism-oriented Prostitution in Barbados: The Case of the Beach Boy and the White Female Tourist'. In *Sun, Sex, and Gold: Tourism and Sex Work in the Caribbean*, ed. Kamala Kempadoo, 183–200. Lanham: Rowman and Littlefield.

Pigg, Stacy Leigh and Vincanne Adams. 2005. 'Introduction: The Moral Object of Sex'. In *Sex in Development: Science, Sexuality, and Morality in Global Perpective*, eds. Vincanne Adams and Stacy Leigh Pigg. 1–38. Durham: Duke University Press.

Raimondo, Meredith. 2005. 'Intensifications: Representing Gender and Sexuality at the UN General Assembly Special Session on HIV/AIDS'. In *Just Advocacy? Women's Human Rights, Transnational Feminism, and the Politics of Representation*, eds. Wendy S. Hesford and Wendy Kozol, 195–221. New Brunswick: Rutgers University Press.

Vance, Carole S. 1988. 'Pleasure and Danger: Towards a Politics of Sexuality'. In *Pleasure and Danger: Exploring Female Sexuality*, eds. Carole S. Vance, 1–27. London: Pandora Press.

Wekker, Gloria. 2006. *The Politics of Passion: Women's Sexual Culture in the Afro-Surinamese Diaspora*. New York: Columbia University Press.

Chapter 10

Afro-Surinamese Women's Sexual Culture and the Long Shadows of the Past

Gloria Wekker

Introduction

Since the AIDS epidemic struck at the heart of many global communities, commentators have reflected on the irony of this particular, late twentieth-century meeting of Eros and Thanatos. The metaphorical death that individuals, engaged in the pursuit of Eros, encounter may very well metamorphose into a very real, material death. Yet, it has also become clear that this scourge does not attack communities and individuals at random; systematic sets of socio-economic circumstances appear to be operative that make some groups more vulnerable to this particular disease than others: poverty, gender inequality, low educational and high unemployment levels of women, high risk sexual patterns, repressed alternative sexualities, labour mobility and migration have been named as some of those factors. Yet, what that systematicity consists of exactly in particular settings, still needs to be determined. The most general claim of this article is that while a biomedical approach may be of service in detecting on the ground, epidemiological patterns of sexual risk, a more informed, sociohistorical understanding of sexual configurations is necessary in order to successfully respond to HIV and AIDS.

In this chapter, I will zoom in on Afro-Surinamese or Creole sexual cultures, the cultures of the descendants of the enslaved, especially as they manifest in Paramaribo, Suriname. I understand sexuality as a cultural construction. Sexuality is not God-given, nor biologically programmed into our genes, nor, moreover, is it frozen or transhistorically and transculturally given. We construct it together, with some of us having more power to steer its manifestations and its outcomes. According to Foucault (1978), sexuality is a thick terrain, where different power nodes come together, pertaining to other institutions in society, e.g. kinship, marriage, mating, relationships, property, economics and gender; it is expressive of such power relations.

Even with such a small multi-ethnic, transnational population as Suriname's, with 440,000 people living in Suriname and about 330,000 in its Trans-Atlantic counterpart and former colonial metropole, the Netherlands, there is lot of variation in sexual cultures and, one supposes, in vulnerabilities. I will demonstrate that there is a firm historical embeddedness of some sexual behaviours, which are nowadays regarded as 'high risk'. I am referring specifically to an old and widespread phenomenon, called the *mati work* by those who engage in it, which is found in working-class Afro-Suriname. The mati work entails both men and women having sexual and erotic relations with partners of the same and of the opposite sex, either simultaneously or consecutively. Mati, both male and female, typically, have children. These behaviours carry long shadows from the past, having first been documented in colonial literature in 1912. While most accounts of the female variant of the phenomenon place it in the context of turn-of-the-nineteenth century, when many men were absent from Paramaribo, due to migrant labour in the forest and the interior, this does not account for the male variant, which has not been studied yet.[1] I have argued that these behaviours may very well have much longer and thicker roots than has generally been assumed (van Lier 1986, Janssens en van Wetering 1985). The mati work, in my understanding, forms part of a complex conglomerate of West African derived configurations of sexual subjecthood (Wekker 2006). These behaviours, I furthermore argue, are more widespread than just Afro-Suriname and elements of the configuration may be observed in Africa, in parts of the Afro-Caribbean and the African American Diaspora. Because of a particular combination of colonial-political and demographical factors, Afro-Suriname forms a site where this configuration was enabled to develop relatively unhampered.

In this chapter, I want to propose a more historically and socially grounded approach to the understanding of HIV and AIDS in the Caribbean, on the basis of research that I have conducted over the past two decades on constructions of Afro-Surinamese female sexual subjectivity. First, I will foreground our general lack of knowledge concerning black Diasporic sexuality, its genealogies and local understandings. The 'sex negativity' (Rubin 1984) which was so characteristic of the US academic landscape in the '80s, when it was first remarked upon, continues to plague the study of sexuality in a variety of ways. I will also sketch a key finding of my research, which forms a cornerstone to the exercise I undertake later in the article. That is, I will offer an informed image of the contours of historical, nineteenth century, Afro-Surinamese folk sexual culture. I arrived at this hypothetical model by way of a close reading of pertinent historical sources and by extrapolating my findings back into the past. I am centrally interested in the question how the enslaved were able to reconcile two opposed cultural and ideological systems, a Western and a West African system, in the context of which they had to realize their sexual subjecthood. To a significant extent, current Afro-Surinamese sexual culture still possesses the same ten characteristics which I hypothesise for the more distant past. Finally, I will indicate why the socio-historical approach that I propagate offers more depth than a biomedical approach, with its search for culprits and victims, and which, by its typical rapid assessment procedures can only offer limited and superficial understandings of complex sexual cultures.

I AM A GOLD COIN

Over the past two decades, I have been engaged in a project (Wekker 1992, 1993, 1994, 1997, 1999, 2001, 2004 and 2006), which explores the ways in which 25 working-class, Afro-Surinamese women make sense of their sexual subjectivities, whether they are now located in Suriname, in the Netherlands or in the US. At the outset of this project, which started with my dissertation research, it seemed remarkable to me that, in African Diaspora Studies, we gradually and painstakingly have come to know about the music, songs and family patterns of the enslaved, about their religious belief systems and their food intake, their aesthetic preferences with regard to verbal and material arts, the bodily stresses and diseases that they suffered from, about birth and death rates, about their motor behaviours, but that we know so little about how the enslaved and their descendants saw themselves as sexual subjects in the world. It seemed to me that it had taken African Diaspora studies an inordinately long time to engage with sexuality, whether during or after slavery. As literary critic Hortense Spillers remarked in the early '80s:

> [...] In my attempt to lay hold of non-fictional texts — of any discursively rendered experience concerning the sexuality of black women in the United States, authored by themselves, for themselves — I encountered a disturbing silence [...]. Black women are the beached whales of the sexual universe, unvoiced, misseen, not doing, awaiting *their* verb (1984, 74).

To this day, we lack a theory or a set of theories about black sexual lives. It is a worthwhile epistemological exercise to contemplate the questions that we have asked about the past, but more important even to think about those that we have *not* asked and why; whose interests has this deafening silence been serving? This exercise may also illuminate why dominant discourses within current research on HIV and AIDS seem so strongly invested in apportioning blame and why it is so infinitely more difficult to get funding for research that is fundamentally interested in genealogies and constructions of sexual configurations than for — more or less applied — projects that aim to tackle the AIDS pandemic. I cannot escape the impression that in all these different domains we are confronted with one of the legacies of the fact that the US is the dominant global academic power. Sexuality has for a long time been shunned as a legitimate area of research, not only within History, but also in Anthropology, in African Diaspora Studies and other disciplines. It was only in 1961 that AAA (American Anthropological Association), passed a motion that made sexuality a legitimate area of research. Ten more years passed before the Association was prepared to deal with research on homosexual behaviour (Carrier 1986). Anthropologist Gayle Rubin, at the time, spoke about a broad canvas of 'sex negativity' in Western cultures, embedded in a history which has seen sex as sin, as disease, as excess, as danger, as losing control. Rubin notes:

> ...Western cultures generally consider sex to be a dangerous, destructive, negative force. Most Christian tradition, following Paul, holds that sex is inherently sinful... This culture (i.e. US culture) always treats sex with suspicion. It construes and judges almost any sexual practice in terms of its worst possible expression. Sex is presumed guilty until proven innocent. Virtually all erotic behavior is considered bad unless a specific reason to exempt it has been established. The most acceptable excuses are marriage, reproduction and love....*But the exercise of erotic capacity, intelligence, curiosity, or creativity all require pretexts* that are unnecessary for other pleasures, such as the enjoyment of food, fiction, or astronomy (Rubin 1984, 278, author's emphasis).

This general sex negativity is still evident in the academy; for a long time those who did sex studies were professionally punished, quaranteened, finding no avenues to get ahead, tenure-track positions withheld, being accused of being too narrow and too specific (Newton 2000; Lewin 2002).

The result is a fundamental lack of knowledge about the sexuality of US enslaved or enslaved in any other 'New World' territory and their descendants. Coupled with the understandable reluctance, after Abolition, on the part of working-class and middle-class African American women (Clark Hine 1989), to be known as sexual beings to researchers, the fundamental study of black sexuality has suffered appreciably.

My dissertation research was entitled *I Am a Gold Coin* (1992), after the proverb working-class Afro-Surinamese women mentioned most often when asked to name a proverb that said something meaningful about their own sense of (sexual) self. 'I am a gold coin/ I pass through many hands/ but I do not loose my value', speaks to the working-class value system, whereby a woman may have had many — either male or female — partners, but that does not diminish her value, as would be in the case in a middle-class setting. The proverb, which, like so many others in rich African-Surinamese oral culture, is coined by women themselves, compares working-class women to gold coins that pass from hand to hand, but they do not diminish in value.[2] It is not monogamy, having one man be the biological as well as the social father of one's children, nor being legally married that encapsulates one's value, it is how women carry themselves through life, being capable of taking care of those entrusted to them, economically, psychologically and spiritually.

My dissertation has resulted in several findings and I will now introduce the most central building block of women's sexual subjectivity. The genealogies and the content of sexual subjectivity in this African Diasporic context are radically different from those constructed in Western contexts. We encounter a plural, multiplicitous self, which is not the highly singularized self of the Enlightenment nor is it the fragmented self which has been brought to light under the contemporary transformations of postmodernity. Central to the understanding of this self is the fact that African-Surinamese women (and men) have a plethora of terms at their command to make statements about the self. In contradistinction to Indo-European languages, which have only one self-referential term available ('I'), creating an illusion of stasis, trans-situational continuity, boundedness and indivisibility, the Afro-Surinamese self-lexicon is multiplicitous, malleable and dynamic. The lexicon can be divided into three categories: first, regardless of gender, a person can make statements about the self, in masculine and feminine terms, meaning that a person is understood to be made up out of male and female instantiations. Second, one can speak about 'I' in singular and in plural terms, indicating the multiplicity and the contextual saliency of the self. Third, third person constructions are used. In the last case, the Winti, the gods and spirits within the Afro-Surinamese Pantheon that carry a person, are invoked to make a statement about 'I'; as a man with drinking problems stated: '*Mi winti no wan' m'e dring' moro*', my winti do not want me to drink anymore/ 'I' do not want to drink anymore (Wekker 1992, 2006).[3]

This conceptualization of self as a plurality journeyed with Fante-Akan people of the Gold Coast (Ghana) who became Surinamese in the context of slavery and who developed a creole grammar in the form of Sranan Tongo (Wooding 1988). The plural 'I' brings together the secular and the sacred, in that a person draws characteristics from her/his biological parents, but also from spiritual parents, from his/her winti. This self, then, should not be assumed to draw an inheritance from Western cosmological systems, but rather from those based in West Africa.

There are various sexual repertoires present in the working class, among which is an institutionalized form of sex among both men and women, called the mati work, in which people have opposite and same-sex sexual relationships, either consecutively or simultaneously. The local understanding of this institution does not make use of foreign categories like homo- or bisexuality, but is correlated with the sexual/spiritual multiplicitous self. In the case of women, one important instantiation of the self, is a strong male winti, the god Apuku, who is fiercely jealous and who loves to lie down with real-life women. Thus it is believed that a woman who is carried by Apuku loves to lie down with women, as well. Men, who are carried by Aisa, the most important female deity, will display comparable behaviour, they love to lie down with men (Wekker 1992, 2006).

There is compelling evidence to suggest that such multiple constructions of sexual subjecthood are present in working-class women's cultures elsewhere in the African American and the Caribbean Diaspora: titillating bits and pieces of evidence come from Haiti (Herskovits 1937) Cariacou and Grenada (Smith 1962; Lorde 1982), Jamaica (Kerr 1952; Silvera 1992), Curaçao (Clemencia 1995), Trinidad (Herskovits 1947), St Vincent (Rubenstein 1987) and St Kitts, Dominica, Saint Lucia (Elwin 1997). Comparable evidence exists for West Africa, Dahomey and Ghana. Ashanti women, who had same-sex relationships were embedded in a similar sexual/spiritual complex as Afro-Surinamese women and were described as *obaa banyins*, women who have a 'heavy soul' (Herskovits 1938). The comparable idea of being carried by the male god Apuku and having a 'heavy soul' seems suggestive of the continuity of sexual-cultural constructions in the black Diaspora which need to be more fully probed. Interestingly, this same conceptualization is used in Zimbabwe. Epprecht (1998) notes:

Women who had strong homo-erotic feelings, it should be noted, also had means to express them in ways that were not perceived as sexual. Principally this involved claiming possession by a male spirit such as *svikiro* or *tokoloshi*. A woman so possessed could take multiple female 'wives', or refuse to be married, without challenging the dogma of heterosexual appearances.[4]

Using sexuality as a privileged point of entry, I want to further explore the gendered, historical characteristics of this sexual culture. Central to my endeavour has been the question of how we can reconcile and think simultaneously the two systems that the enslaved had to deal with in building and ordering their world, in the domain of sexual subjecthood. According to Gilroy:

> the system of plantation slavery was nothing if not the confrontation between two opposed yet interdependent cultural and ideological systems and their attendant conceptions of reason, history, property and kinship. One is the diluted product of Africa, the other is an antinomian expression of western modernity (1993, 219).

In the next section, I will explore the organization of sexual subjecthood in Surinamese slave society, privileging the view from below/ from within, with an emphasis on the worldview and agency of enslaved women and men. This entails deciphering how the enslaved managed to reconcile the opposed principles mentioned above. It importantly includes knowledge relating to gender: the enslaved's ways of being men and women (Morrissey 1989; Beckles 1989, 1999; Shepherd et al. 1995; Brereton 1995). It has by now become commonplace to note that slavery was lived differently by men and women, and so, we need to ask, how was sexuality lived? The closest we have come to Surinamese sexuality, is that we have learned about marriage and mating patterns from plantation and church archives (Lamur 1985; Everaert 1999), but I am more interested in the living human beings underneath those patterns and statistics and there we are still a long way away from being enlightened. Some of the questions that are of interest to me include: How did the enslaved conceive of themselves as sexual beings? What did they do? What gave them pleasure? How were relationships between men and women, ideally, conceived? And, were opposite-sex dyads the only meaningful and conceivable relationships? Weren't same-sex relationships part of the sexual repertoires of the enslaved? About such intimate, experience-near, phenomena like how they looked at themselves and what they found attractive in each other, we are still very much at a loss. According to a well-known metaphor used by Clifford Geertz (1984), I am concerned here with the inner layers of an onion, the formations of the self and the institutions upholding it. However, these questions also and inevitably involve the outer layers of the 'onion', for example, ideas and practices regarding family and its formation, religion, economics and power.

SEXUALITY DURING SLAVERY

Suriname during colonial times lends itself exceptionally well to the study of sexuality. Due to a particular combination of demographical and culture-political factors, the enslaved lived in an environment that enabled them to elaborate rather freely on their West African cultural heritage. The ratio of whites to blacks, during most of the eighteenth and nineteenth centuries, was one to 25 in general and in many plantation districts it was one to 65 (van Lier 1977). Out of fear for this multitude of slaves, the Dutch plantocracy had as a general policy to remove the slaves from themselves, that is, the plantocracy, as far as possible, spatially, culturally, linguistically and psychologically. The enslaved in Suriname were, contrary to their North American counterparts, for example, forbidden to speak Dutch, the master's language. Until well after 1830, moreover, the African element in the Surinamese slave body was continually replenished, because it was cheaper for the planter class to import new slaves than to create conditions in which they would reproduce themselves (van Stipriaan 1993; Lamur 1985). Obviously, as in all slave societies, interracial sexuality was formally forbidden, but widely practiced. Most important for my argument is that the real and metaphorical distance between the plantocracy and the enslaved enabled the latter to elaborate rather freely on their own cultural complexes. Because the enslaved were left to their own devices, as long as they performed the labour that was expected of them, they could develop their languages and (sexual) culture.

The task before us is to discern the contours of the two opposed yet interdependent cultural and ideological systems that were operative in the domain of sexual subjectivity. In the first instance, there was the dual marriage structure, which has been called the basic building block of Caribbean societies and whose principles were laid like a template over these societies (Smith 1996). Like in Jamaica, Trinidad and Tobago, elsewhere in the Caribbean and the Southern United States, upper-class white men, who could afford to maintain two families, were formally married to a white wife, had a white family, and also had an informal wife of colour and family. Raymond Smith argues, convincingly, that this Creole kinship structure was established in the formative stage of West Indian society. In Suriname, absenteeism of the white planter class had always been high during slavery and there were few white families, until the beginning of the twentieth century. Here, as elsewhere, the operative rule was the same: men marry status equals and have non-legal unions with status inferiors. One of Smith's illuminating insights is that

> ...it (the dual marriage system) wove a complex tapestry of genetic and social relations among the various segments of Creole society. Once established (—) it was capable of ordering conjugal relations outside the simple black-white conjunction; it could generate the forms of sexual and conjugal behavior appropriate to equals and unequals of all kinds. (—) The West Indian system of kinship and marriage was an extension in cultural logic and social action of the dominant structural element in Creole society, the racial hierarchy — an element that pervaded every aspect of social life: economic, political, religious and domestic (1996, 70).

As I have noted elsewhere (Wekker 2001, 2006), to the central position Smith gives to racial hierarchy, we immediately have to add the simultaneously operating element of gender hierarchy. Being white was not enough; it was the combination of whiteness and maleness which determined one's sexual possibilities in this asymmetrical system. For the few white, Jewish and light-skinned Creole women in Suriname, it was unthinkable that they would be allowed to have a sexual relationship with a coloured or black man. During the days of slavery, this possibility represented a serious transgression of racialised sexual boundaries. White women — and in their train Jewish and light-skinned Creole women — were seen as sexually innocent. Put on a pedestal of being non-sexual, they had to embody the Surinamese version of 'the cult of true womanhood'. Since they were identified with the nation and its continuation, it was essential that their sexual activities were policed and that they should be protected: their offspring should be (as) white (as possible). An unmarried women having 'carnal conversation' with a black man would be tortured severely and banished from the colony, while a married woman would undergo the same fate in addition to being branded (Schiltkamp en de Smidt red. 1973). The black man would be killed. Black men certainly did not have the same sexual prerogatives as white men, so being male was not enough either. This point bears repeating in other terms: it was (and is, to an extent) the *combination* of one's gendered and racialised (and classed) positions that determined one's prerogatives and limitations in the dual marriage system. A dominant racist gender ideology and a gendered racial ideology both pointed to the obvious: various actors in the system were differentially empowered, that is, having different sexual positions and possibilities.

Thus the Western system in the domain of sexual subjectivity prescribed that the structural positions available to enslaved women were those of concubine to a white or an enslaved man and the lighter her skin color was, the more likely the chances that she would be enlisted to render sexual services to white men (Sharpe 2002). Formal marriage to a white man was not possible in this inegalitarian system; only so-called 'Surinamese marriage', that is, concubinage, was an option. In fact, inequality on the basis of 'race', gender and class was the *sine qua non* of this sexual template, while this inequality was also expressive of power differentials.

In the shadows of the dual marriage structure, the Surinamese enslaved were able to develop their own cultural complexes, including cultural notions and practices in the sexual domain that were based on West African 'cognitive and behavioural grammatical principles' (Mintz and Price 1992) governing sexual personhood. Mintz and Price argue that the aim of the discipline of African American Studies should be to identify underlying principles, common basic assumptions (which will often be unconscious) about, for instance, social relations or, as in this case, sexual relations. Such principles can define the perceived similarities in African, African-American and African-Caribbean cultural patterns. Mintz and Price propose:

> An African cultural heritage, widely shared by the people imported into any new colony, will have to be defined in less concrete terms, by focusing more on values, and less on sociocultural forms, and even by attempting to identify unconscious "grammatical" principles, which may underlie and shape behavioral response (1992, 9–10).

It is the cognitive orientations of Surinamese blacks in the domain of sexuality that I submit to further research. My project, fundamentally, references the shaping and the content of what it meant to be human, with a specific focus on conceptions about subjectivity, about gender, and about — something we now call — sexuality, which circulated among the slaves who lived in Suriname in the eighteenth and nineteenth centuries.

WEST AFRICAN PRINCIPLES IN THE DOMAIN OF SEXUALITY

We can now enquire what the ingredients were of the other, West African, ideological system that was present during slavery in Suriname. I imagine the cognitive and behavioural grammatical principles governing sexual personhood, which the enslaved elaborated upon in Suriname like jazz: improvising upon certain basic themes, musicians (m/f) in various parts of the Diaspora have produced riffs, that are remarkably similar. On the basis of extensive interviews with 25 working-class women and reading existing historical sources against the grain, I have concluded that these principles included (and still include) a conglomerate of interrelated notions. I see these notions as anchor points of a yet to be fully determined sexual configuration. While the existing historical record cannot conclusively 'prove' the presence of this configuration, I propose its ten ingredients as hypotheses to be tested in future research.

1. As I noted earlier, the basic building block of this system is a notion of personhood in which the secular and the spiritual were/are intertwined. The anthropomorphic gods and spirits which carry a person, the winti, form an inextricable part of one's personhood and are especially powerful in determining one's sexual practices.

2. Same-sex as well as opposite-sex dyads formed part of the sexual configuration. Female same-sex behaviour was conceptualized as governed by the women being carried by a strong masculine spirit, called Apuku. This same conceptualization is found for female same-sex behaviour in various parts of the Caribbean (Elwin 1998) and in different parts of Africa, for example, in Zimbabwe (Epprecht 1998). Likewise, same-sex behaviour among men was understood as the men being carried by a strong female spirit, Mama Aisa. This understanding had as a corollary that sexuality was seen as activity; one did not need, as in the West, to claim a particular (exclusive) sexual identity (Wekker 1999).

3. This sexual system was undergirded by a flexible gender system in which gender did not act as a constraint on the basis of biological sex. As has been described for gender systems in Nigeria, the social relations between men and women were mediated through a flexible gender ideology and a linguistic system with certain gender-free aspects (Amadiume 1987). That ideology and the linguistic system made it possible for both genders to possess the same roles and status. The flexible gender system encouraged that women, like men, could occupy positions of power and authority. The correlation between sex and gender was not emphasized, but rather the relationship between gender and power was emphatically asserted. Men as well as women could acquire power and authority.

4. This, again, had connections with an understanding that women were (and very much are) full sexual subjects. This entails the understanding that, like men, women are sexual beings and that

they can act on their desires, without being stigmatised as less worthy. In Sranan Tongo, this notion is expressed by several proverbs, for example 'Mi na gowt' moni', I am a gold coin, as we have seen. Another preferred proverb is '*Uma na lep' bana, a no man pori*', woman is like a ripe banana, she cannot spoil' (Wekker 2006). This is quite contrary to Western conceptions of women's sexuality, in dominant versions of which women are constructed as passive and in need of being resuscitated by stronger, male passion and, as everyone knows, 'nice girls don't like sex'.

5. People regard(-ed) sex, including in its same-sex modality, as an extraordinarily pleasant part of life, in which one could (and can) engage to a quite advanced age. Regular sex was seen as a necessity for one's inner well-being, for mental and physical balance and health.

6. The sex of one's object of passion was less important than sexual activity and sexual fulfilment per se. This, again, runs counter to a modern Western conceptualisation of sexual identity, in which, remarkably, one's own sexual categorizing is determined by the sex of one' s object of passion. One's categorization into hetero- or homosexuality is, in other words, ascertained on the basis of the sex of those one is attracted to. Paraphrasing Geertz' pronouncement on Western notions of personhood (1984), one might certainly say that this is a rather peculiar phenomenon, in the context of the world's sexualities. Arguably in its starkest manifestation, Suriname has been home to the working-class sexual configuration that has been *central in the mati work*.

7. The importance of fertility and parenthood for both men and women. In realizing mature and successful personhood, reproduction was central for both sexes.

8. Conjugal relations were brittle and less prominent than the relations with consanguineal, uterine, kin. The bafflement of anthropologists in encountering a family system in which women were prominent in both economic and emotional terms, has led to the concept of matrifocality. Dominant readings of this family system, have rendered men, by and large, as sexual entrepreneurs and women as

sexual dupes and dopes.

9. My research has pointed to a different interpretation in which women had a preference, evident already during slavery, of a relational arrangement with a man, in which they had autonomy and in which they perceived an exchange relationship between sex and money.

10. In this system, quite large age differences between sex partners, both in opposite-sex and same-sex modalities, were possible and acceptable.

Generally, a cultural mood and mode of possibility and additivity, a both/ and attitude, instead of exclusivity, expressed in an either/or worldview, was characteristic. In the framework of this article, I cannot possibly go into all these ingredients at length, but let me elaborate on another anchor point of this configuration; women's preference for a relational arrangement with a man, in which they have autonomy.

Women's Agency and Preference for autonomy

From historical sources it can be established that enslaved women and their parents did not easily consent to marriage. In a famous quote, dating from Suriname in the middle of the nineteenth century, the undesirability of marriage and the connection between sex and money for women is illustrated.

Some colored people consider marriage as very oppressive, through which crushing links they do not want their daughters tied. One even has examples that colored parents who, living together for better and worse in unmarried state (like most colored people) and having produced children, absolutely refused their daughters to enter into a marriage contract. A certain colored father answered a white man, who asked for his daughter's hand: "Get married, get married immediately? No! It does not go like that; should you want to live together first with Louisa, you can do that, then one can see how things go, but my daughter has to be free and will not permanently engage herself blindly" (Teenstra 1842, 48–49; transl. mine).

206

There is another source on Afro-Suriname, which has received relatively little attention. It is a rich, oral source, which alerts us to the attitude of a prosperous female slave regarding relationships between men and women. Master storyteller, Aleks de Drie bases his oral knowledge on the stories of his *uma afo/* mother's mother's mother, born around 1837 (de Drie en Guda 1985, 16). In one of his fascinating stories, *Prensés Apîaba/* Princess Apîaba, de Drie introduces us to an African princess, who had been sold into slavery. The story should be situated in the second half of the nineteenth century. The governor, probably van Sypensteyn 1873–1882, treated her with special attention, because of her status and gave her a house and a yard. She loved to dance winti, on top of a sheep; she would cut its head off and drink its blood. Apîaba had a well in her yard, from which she not only got water, but also money. A light-skinned man, watching the princess dance, fell in love with her. He proposed to her, but Apîaba who liked the man well enough, had little use for him:

Well look, for you to set up life with me, that is not nothing, it is a sweet thing. But I do not need anything from a man. Because look, did you not see that I lowered a bucket into the well and when I hauled it up, the bucket was full of money. A woman, well, she needs money. And that I already have. So I do not need you anymore. And my winti, when they come on top of me, I cannot be with a man. When you come here, I can make my servants put something nice for you to eat, but nothing else (de Drie en Guda 1985, 129, author's transl.).

From this oral source several important themes emerge. First, there is Apîaba's relationship with her winti, her 'spirits' and the money they provide her with, in return for her honouring them. In the juxtaposition of those relationships and one with a real life man, she makes the greater significance of the first type of relationship to her very clear. Second, the story shows that women made a firm connection between being in a relationship with a man and money. Having money of one's own made a relationship with a man highly improbable. Third, the desire for an independent position points to the agency of enslaved women. It was the preferred mode by women, facilitated by the equal work burdens men and women carried and the independent food provision. Everaert (1999), in his study of plantation records, illuminated a gendered pattern among the slave population: enslaved men with high status had multiple wives, if they could afford it, while high status enslaved women were more typically single or had younger, male partners.

Enslaved women's desire for independence was equally operative in relationships with white men as in those with enslaved or free men. Enslaved women had their own reasons, based on the West African archive, to reject marriage and to want an independent status from men and this wish dovetailed with the structural position offered to them in the dual marriage system, the other, Western system that was operative in slave societies. As we have seen, the dual marriage system *did not structurally offer marriage to slave women in their relationships* with white men, but it did produce some mobility in terms of status for themselves and their children and a varying measure of freedom.[4] This constraint coincided for slave women with their own negative feelings towards marriage. I read the longevity and tenacity of the rejection of marriage as a testament to this coincidence.

Thus, it is not surprising that only nine per cent of present-day working-class Creole women with a steady relationship are married (Jagdeo 1992). Terborg found that Creole men and women preferred, for different reasons, to live in concubinage or in a visiting relationship (Terborg 2002). One of my respondents, Nana, a 60-year-old cook, indicated that she never really thought about marriage and she referred to some of the impediments for women, which by the 1990s had been repealed, but were still very much part of women's consciousness around marriage:

> I don't see the point of getting married. All married men have their outside-women, anyway. You don't profit from marriage. You have more obligations, you have to bring him into everything you do, whether it is taking out a loan, buying a refrigerator, or going to a government office. They will tell you: your husband has to sign. Suppose I want to leave him, then maybe he does not want to separate: it's going to be one headache. Some men are so *pertinent/* insolent, even when you are separated, and you are with another

man, they will still come to you and demand all kinds of things. No let me stay by myself, it is better that way!!! (Wekker 2006, 137).

Mis' Juliette, my main 84-year-old informant, also had quite distinct ideas about the undesirability of marriage:

I never wanted to marry, or make *verbontu*/union[5] with a man. Even when a man is beautiful, I cannot put beautiful in my pot to cook. *Mi kan or' nanga man, ma dan a mu' gi mi sensi. Mi no law*/ I can have a sexual relationship with a man, but then he must give me money. I am not crazy. When I am with a man, I do not tell him all of my business, for example that I am playing *kasmoni*. I always rented my own house, the contract was in my name. *No wan mannengre*[6] *sa kis' mi oso na tap' en nen*/ not one man-negro will get my house to his name. Then he is going to send me away and start living there with another woman.

Thus, a system that was inherently saturated with inequalities, the dual marriage system, could in practice be reconciled with a subjugated, but relatively egalitarian system that fueled enslaved women's own understandings of their position in relationships with men.

While from the worldview of the dual marriage structure, the voidness of the category of marriage with a status unequal was a way of *creating and expressing* racial, gender and class inequality, from a West African perspective, the point to be grasped is that enslaved women preferred to be in a relational arrangement that granted them as much freedom as possible and that they considered conjugal relations as less prominent than the relations with consanguineous, uterine kin. It was and is not wife-hood that is paramount in African household and family organizations, but motherhood (Oyewumi 2001; Amadiume 1987). I propose that the centrality of motherhood, a reliance on uterine kin as opposed to consanguineous relations and forms of femininity which stressed independence from men and full sexual subjectivity, which various enslaved took with them to the 'New' World, different though their provenience and cultural archives were, became part of the organising principles upon which their lives were based.

Concluding Remarks

I have been arguing, on the basis of longitudinal interviews with contemporary working-class Afro-Surinamese women and a critical reading of existing historical sources, that it is worthwhile to take an in depth view of their sexual understandings, practices and relations, in order to accomplish a twofold goal. In the first place, to ascertain the historical depth of these sexual configurations and to look for their presence in other parts of the black Diaspora. Since the historical record does not give a voice to the subjugated, this project might allow us to open windows unto the consciousness of the enslaved and to see patterns that do not belong merely to Afro-Suriname, but that can be considered part of the 'cognitive and behavioral grammatical principles' in the domain of sexual subjecthood in the black Diaspora. Secondly, my aim was to show that a grounded, socio-historical perspective in the response to HIV and AIDS yields more insights and openings for intervention than a statistical, biomedical approach. In particular, I wanted to warn against a flattening move, which automatically and myopically conceives of *all* working-class women, who have difficulty making ends meet, as monolithically vulnerable to the contraction of HIV. My tracing of different sexual repertoires among Afro-Surinamese women points to the necessity for more sensitivity to on-the-ground realities, including attention to their sources of empowerment, but also to differences between women. Women who engage in the mati work are not the proverbial victims or, necessarily, transmitters of risky sexual practices, but they are embedded in a culture which empowers them sexually, at least in their relationships with women. Such empowerment is manifest, for instance, in the active exchange of sexual knowledge between women, inter- and intragenerational. Moreover, all women, whether they are active in opposite-sex sexual relations only, involved in opposite-sex dyads or in both same-sex and opposite-sex relations, have an historically embedded desire for sexual agency and autonomy. This cultural archive should be acknowledged and built upon.

Structural inequities between men and women are certainly present and, against a background of unequal pay for the same labour and the differential responsibilities that men and women frequently carry for the maintenance of their families, some women depend on men for financial sustenance in exchange for sexual activities. The different socio-economic situations, notably including whether women have access to foreign currencies, all need to be acknowledged in a multi-faceted model. These insights should offer possibilities for a more nuanced approach to the trope of the categorically oppressed, vulnerable working-class woman (Dworkin 2005).

Along complementary lines, I want to caution against another seemingly Pavlovian reaction: in many Caribbean and North American spaces, a punitive discourse circulates in which multiple partnering, involving same-sex practices — MSM — especially among men who have a steady female partner, is inevitably dismissed as inherently undesirable and dangerous, being on the 'down low'. Here again, I argue that it is necessary to acknowledge and understand these behaviours as historically embedded.

NOTES

1. The male mati work, so far, has not been studied. In the latest incarnation of my work, I have started to record the life history of a 56-year-old male mati.
2. For a more elaborate analysis of this proverb, see Wekker 2006.
3. I am not familiar with comparable research about linguistic complexes in the domain of self in other black Diasporic contexts.
4. Wadzanai, recalling the experiences of an elderly female relative, interviewed by Marc Epprecht, Harare, 25 March 1997 (1998).
5. The advantages in terms of mobility or obtaining freedom, to enslaved women who had a relationship with a white man should not be overestimated (cf Beckles 1989, Barrow 1996).
6. The *verbontu*, which is meant here, was introduced among the slaves by the Moravian Brethren (EBG) as a substitute for marriage. It acquired another content among Creoles, certainly not meant by the Brethren, as the oath that lovers take to be sexually faithful to each other, all their lives.
7. *Mannengre/* lit. man-negro, means men, generically. To my delight, Juliette also called my white male colleagues mannengre.

REFERENCES

Amadiume, I. 1987. *Male Daughters, Female Husbands. Gender and Sex in an African Society*. London: Zed Books.

Barrow, C. 1996. *Family in the Caribbean: Themes and Perspectives*. Kingston: Ian Randle Publishers.

Beckles, H. McD. 1989. *Natural Rebels. A Social History of Enslaved Black Women in Barbados*. London: Zed Books .

———. 1999. *Centering Woman: Gender Discourses in Caribbean Slave Society*. Kingston: Ian Randle Publishers.

Brereton, B. 1995. 'Text, Testimony, and Gender: An Examination of some Texts by Women on the English-speaking Caribbean, from the 1770's to the 1920's'. In *Engendering History: Caribbean Women in Historical Perspective*, eds. Verene Shepherd, Bridget Brereton, and Babara Bailey, 63–94. London: James Currey Publishers; Kingston: Ian Randle Publishers.

Carrier, Joseph, Foreword. Blackwood, Evelyn. ed. 1986. *The Many Faces of Homosexuality: Anthropological Approaches to Homosexual Behavior*, xi–xiii. New York: Harrington Park Press, Originally published as *Journal of Homosexuality* 11 no, 3/4.

Clark Hine, D. 1989. 'Rape and the Inner Lives of Black Women in the Middle West. Some Preliminary Thoughts on the Culture of Dissemblance'. *Signs: Journal of Women in Culture and Society* 14, no. 4: 912–20.

Clemencia, J., 1995. 'Women Who Love Men. A Whole Perspective From Kapuchera to Open Throats.' Paper deliverd at the Caribbean Studies Association conference. Curaçao. May 23–26.

De Drie, A. and Trudy Guda, eds. 1985. Sye! Arki Tori! Paramaribo: Ministerie van Onderwijs, Wetenschappen en Cultuur.

Dworkin, Shari L. 2005. 'Who is epidemiologically fathomable in the HIV/AIDS epidemic? Gender, Sexuality, and Intersectionality in Public Health'. *Culture, Health & Sexuality*, November-December; 7 no. 6: 615–23.

Elwin, R., ed. 1997. *Tongues on Fire: Caribbean Lesbian Lives and Stories*. Toronto: Canadian Scholars' Press (Women's Press).

Epprecht, M. 1998. 'The "Unsaying" of Homosexuality Among Indigenous Black Zimbabweans: Mapping a Blindspot in an African Masculinity'. *Journal of Southern African Studies* 24, no. 4.

Everaert, H. A. M. 1999. *Een zoektocht naar de aard van man-vrouw relaties onder Surinaamse slaven: De suikerplantages Fairfield, Breukelerwaard, Cannewapibo en La Jalousie in de periode voorafgaand aan de emancipatie*. Amsterdam: Universiteit van Amsterdam.

Foucault, M. 1978. *The History of Sexuality. Volume I. An Introduction*. Harmondsworth: Pelican.

Geertz, C. 1984. '"From the Native's Point of View": On the Nature of Anthropological Understanding'. In *Culture Theory: Essays on Mind, Self, and Emotion*, eds. R. Shweder and R. LeVine. Cambridge: Cambridge University Press.

Gilroy, Paul. 1993. *The Black Atlantic: Modernity and Double Consciousness*. Cambridge: Harvard University Press.

Herskovits, M. 1937. *Life in a Haitian Village*. New York: Knopf.

Herskovits, M. and F. Herskovits. 1947. *Trinidad Village*. New York: Knopf.

Herskovits, M. Dahomey. 1967. *An Ancient West African Kingdom*, Vols. I and II. Evanston: Northwestern University Press, 1938.

Jagdeo, T. and C. Survey. 1992. *Stichting Lobi*. Paramaribo: Drukkerij Boschman.

Janssens, M. and W. van Wetering. 1985. 'Mati en lesbiennes. Homoseksualiteit en etnische identiteit bij Creools-Surinaamse vrouwen in Nederland.' *Sociologische Gids* 32 no. 5/6: 394–415.

Kerr, M. 1952. *Personality and Conflict in Jamaica*. Liverpool: University Press.

Lamur, H. 1985. *De Kerstening van de Slaven van de Surinaamse Plantage Vossenburg, 1847–1887*. Amsterdam: Universiteit van Amsterdam, Antropologisch – Sociologisch Centrum.

Lewin, E. and W. Leap, eds. 2002. *Out in Theory: The Emergence of lesbian and gay Anthropology*. Urbana, Chicago: University of Illinois Press.

Lier, R.A.J. van. 1977. *Samenleving in een grensgebied. Een sociaal-historische studie van Suriname*. Amsterdam: Emmering.

———.1986. *Tropische tribaden. Een verhandeling over homoseksualiteit en homoseksuele vrouwen in Suriname*. Dordrecht: Foris Publications.

Lorde, A. 1982. *Zami. A New Spelling of my Name*. New York: The Crossing Press.

Morrissey, M. 1989. *Slave Women in the new World. Gender Stratification in the Caribbean*. Lawrence: University Press of Kansas.

Mintz, S. and R. Price. 1976. *An Anthropological Approach to the Afro-American Past: A Caribbean Perspective*. Philadelphia: Institute for the Study of Human Issues Publications. 1992.

Newton, E. 2000. *Margaret Mead Made Me Gay: Personal Essays, Public Ideas*. Durham: Duke University Press.

Oyewumi, O. 2001. 'Ties That (Un)bind: Feminism, Sisterhood and Other Foreign Relations'. *Jenda: A Journal of Culture and African Women Studies* 1, no. 1.

Rubin, G. 1984. 'Thinking Sex. Notes for a Radical Theory of the Politics of Sexuality.' In *Pleasure and Danger. Exploring Female Sexuality*, ed. C. Vance, 267–319. Boston/ London: Routledge/ Kegan Paul.

Rubenstein, H. 1987. *Coping with Poverty*. Adaptive Strategies in a Caribbean Village. Boulder/ London: Westview Press.

Schiltkamp, J. and J. de Smidt. eds. 1973. *Westindisch Plakkaatboek. Plakkaten, Ordonnantieen en andere Wetten Uitgevaardigd in Suriname*. Amsterdam: Emmering.

Sharpe. J. 2003. *Ghosts of Slavery: A literary Archeology of Slave Women's Lives*. Minneapolis: University of Minnesota Press.

Shepherd, V., B. Brereton and B. Bailey eds. 1995. *Engendering History: Caribbean Women in Historical Perspective*. New York: St. Martin's; Kingston: Ian Randle Publishers.

Silvera, M. 1992. 'Man Royals and Sodomites: Some Thoughts on the Invisibility of Afro-Caribbean Lesbians.' *Feminist Studies* 18. no. 3.

Smith, M.G. 1962. *Kinship and Communit in Carriacou.* Hew Haven: Yale University Press.

Smith, R. 1996. *The Matrifocal Family. Power, Pluralism and Politics.* New York: Routledge.

Spillers, H. 1984. 'Interstices. A Small Drama of Words.' In: *Pleasure and Danger. Exploring Female Sexuality*, ed. C. Vance, 73–100. Boston/London: Routledge/ Kegan Paul.

Van Stipriaan, A. 1993. *Surinaams contrast: roofbouw en overleven in een Caraïbische Plantagekolonie 1750–1863.* Leiden: KITLV Uitgeverij.

Teenstra, M.D. 1842. *De Negerslaven in de Kolonie Suriname en de uitbreiding van het Christendom onder de Heidensche Bevolking.* Dordrecht: Lagerweij. 1842.

Terborg, J.R.H. 2002. *Liefde en conflict: seksualiteit en gender in de Afro-Surinaamse familie.* Proefschrift Universiteit van Amsterdam.

Wekker, G. 1992. 'I Am Gold Money (I Pass Through All Hands, But I Do Not Lose My Value). The Construction of Selves, Gender and Sexualities in a Female, Working-Class, Afro- Surinamese Setting'. (Unpublished PhD dissertation, Los Angeles: UCLA).

———. 1993. 'Mati-ism and Black Lesbianism. Two Idealtypical Expressions of Female Homosexuality in Black Communities of the Diaspora.' In *If you Seduce a Straight Person, Can You make them Gay? Issues in Biological Essentialism versus Social Constructionism in Gay and Lesbian Identities*, eds. J. P. De Cecco and J.P. Elia, 145–158. New York: The Haworth Press.

———. 1994. *Ik ben een gouden munt, ik ga door vele handen, maar verlies mijn waarde niet. Subjectiviteit en seksualiteit van Creoolse volksklasse vrouwen in Paramaribo.* Amsterdam: Vita.

———. 1997. 'One Finger Does Not Drink Okra Soup. Afro-Surinamese Women and Critical Agency'. In *Feminist Genealogies, Colonial Legacies, Democratic Futures.* eds. M.J. Alexander and C.T. Mohanty. New York and London: Routledge.

———. 1999. 'What's Identity Got To Do With It? Rethinking Identity in light of the Mati Work in Paramaribo, Suriname'. In *Female Desires: Same-sex Relations and Transgender Practices Across Cultures.* eds. E. Blackwood and S.E. Wieringa. New York: Columbia University Press.

———. 2001. 'Of Mimic Men and Unruly Women. Social Relations in Twentieth Century Suriname.' In *Twentieth-Century Suriname. Continuities and Discontinuities in a New World Society.* eds. R. Hoefte and P. Meel, 174–97. Kingston/Leiden: Ian Randle Publishers/KITLV Press.

———. 2004.'Sranan, Swit' Sranan. Populaire beeldvorming over etnische en genderongelijkheid in Suriname.' In: *Wandelaar onder de palmen. Opstellen over koloniale en postkoloniale literatuur. Opgedragen aan Bert Paasman. Eds.* M. van Kempen, P. Verkruijsse & A. Zuiderweg red., 539–50. Leiden: KITLV Uitgeverij.

———. 2006. *The Politics of Passion. Women's Sexual Culture in the Afro-Surinamese Diaspora.* New York: Columbia University Press.

Wooding, C. 1988. Winti: een Afro-Amerikaanse Godsdienst. Een cultureel-historische Analyse van de Cosmologie en het Etnomedische Systeem van de Para. Rijswijk: Eigen Beheer. 1972.

CHAPTER 11

CONTRADICTORY SEXUALITIES

From Vulnerability to Empowerment for Adolescent Girls in Barbados

CHRISTINE BARROW

A deeper understanding of sexual identities and the role of gender inequality in sexual decision-making and performance is critical to the development of effective prevention strategies to curtail the spread of HIV. The key to understanding vulnerability to infection lies in the socially embedded realities of sexuality, gender and power. Drawing on the findings of ongoing qualitative research with adolescent girls in Barbados,[1] we focus on the discourses and contradictions of young feminine sexual identity and, from this perspective, challenge prevailing models of *risk* behaviour that have underpinned the response to HIV. We argue that both normative femininity that privileges virginity followed by monogamy, and the Caribbean counter-discourse of *bashment* that promotes an active, assertive sexuality represent unsafe sexual identities for teenage girls and that their empowerment is a critical precondition for sexual protection and HIV prevention. The process of renegotiating the politics of safer sex against hegemonic masculinity and the unequal relations of gender and generation must be relocated from the private to the public domain as an issue of social justice and human rights.

We set the stage by reporting on the official response to HIV and AIDS in Barbados, on the spread of infection to women and youth, and on research evidence of risky sexual behaviours among adolescents. We then present the case for qualitative research on sexuality, gender and power, and introduce sexual identities in the lives of adolescent girls. This provides the contextual framework for their narratives on sexual choices and the process by which they construct their sexual selves. The conclusion suggests how the HIV and AIDS policy response might be reframed through the lens of vulnerability and sexual health rights.

HIV, GENDER AND YOUTH

Barbados, a small island developing state in the Caribbean, has a commendable record of social development and response to HIV and AIDS. Presently ranked at 31 on the UNDP Human Development Index (HDI), the highest in the Caribbean region, successive governments have devoted priority attention, political will and resources to combating the twin epidemics. The success of treatment and care is evident in the 50 per cent reduction in mortality from AIDS-related infections, and a reduction in vertical HIV transmission from mother to child by 82 per cent. But the dependence on the bio-medical response model, supplemented by care and support, education and information campaigns, has failed to stem the spread of infection (Barrow 2006). The response continues to rely on traditional Information, Education and Communication (IEC) approaches, notably as Health and Family Life Education (HFLE) in secondary schools, though perhaps with less enthusiasm from officialdom and a greater awareness of the limitations of their ABC message, with emphasis on the 'A' for the younger generation.[2] The most problematic question in the context of HIV, remains unanswered as it has in other lifestyle epidemics, that is how to induce the behavioural changes necessary for self-protection and to stem the tide of infection.

The feminization of AIDS is a world-wide phenomenon (Anderson et al. 2002; Inciardi et al. 2005, S19; UNAIDS/WHO 2007). In Barbados during 2006, for the first time, equal numbers of women and men were diagnosed as HIV-positive. Of serious concern also is the spread of HIV to the younger female population. Infection rates for adolescent girls reveal an alarming trend throughout the Caribbean region. For Barbados, using the cumulative total between 1984, when the first case was identified, and December 2005, girls outnumber boys in the 10 to 19 year age group by 2.3 to 1 for HIV infection and by 2.5 to 1 for AIDS cases.[3]

With the spotlight turned on *teenagers at risk*, we have learnt much about youthful sexual behaviour. In Barbados, the results of a series of knowledge, attitudes, beliefs and practices (KABP) surveys among young people provide disturbing evidence, albeit among a minority, of unsafe practices including: early sexual initiation, short-term relationships and multiple partnering — both serial and concurrent — and casual one-night stands (Blades 2002, 10; Carter 2001, 29; Dann 1987; Ellis et al. 1990, 7–8; PAHO 1999, 15–16). Early sexual debut correlates with high-risk practices and multiple partnering and is, therefore, perceived as a key predictor of risk (UNICEF/UNAIDS/WHO 2002, 11). There is also evidence that adolescent girls: are the victims of *forced* sexual initiation[4] (PAHO 1999, 17); are under pressure from male partners to become pregnant and bear a child (Blades 2002, 13); are engaged in transactional sex for material gain (Stuart 2000, 129); and are twice as likely as their male contemporaries not to use condoms (Carter 2001, 25, 30).[5]

Official statistics on the sexual abuse of girls, gender violence and relatively high abortion rates add further cause for concern. Even as we acknowledge the under-reporting of sexual abuse and inaccuracy of official figures, the record shows fluctuations, but no decline in the incidence and reveals girls as the victims in over 90 per cent of reported cases.[6] Researchers describe the disturbing cultural 'normalcy' of sexual abuse and gender-based violence (Barrow 2003; Clarke 1998; Le Franc and Rock 2001; Le Franc 2002; Rock 2002). No accurate figures are available on gender violence in Barbados, but the global discourse on HIV and AIDS has turned attention to violence against women as a primary driver of the epidemics. From a policy perspective, where sexual coercion and violence are commonplace, abstinence or the insistence on condom use is unrealistic. Furthermore, partner violence is still officially viewed as an intimate, private matter in many countries and is missing on the HIV-response agenda (Piot 1999, Wood et al. 1998).

In Barbados, adolescent motherhood has continued to decline, reaching 15.4 per cent of all births in 2006, but teenage abortions in the public hospital during that year accounted for 16.5 per cent of the total.[7] Early motherhood may no longer constitute the social problem it did in previous generations, but adolescents clearly continue to engage in unprotected sex, and are exposed to pregnancy and now to HIV. Although, as mentioned, only a small proportion of adolescent girls in Barbados is reported to be 'at risk', perhaps no more than 15 per cent or so, it was this accumulation of evidence that prompted this study of their sexual vulnerability.

FROM QUANTITATIVE INDICATORS TO QUALITATIVE RESEARCH

KAPB questionnaire surveys have provided a substantial statistical data-base on youthful sexuality, though somewhat overwhelming in detail and replication. Most significantly, they have opened our eyes to the disconnect between sexual knowledge and behaviour — the 'KAP gap' — thereby challenging the premise on which the official HIV-education response has been based. Emerging clearly from these studies is the message that knowledge and information are essential, but not sufficient to change risky sexual practices. However, the limitations of these quantitative indicators and macro-level analyses are well documented. An understanding of sexual behaviours cannot be reduced to attitudes, beliefs and other psychological ingredients, and HIV infection must no longer be interpreted as personal irresponsibility and misfortune. While sexuality cannot be separated from the body and mind, it is also socially constructed and driven (MacPhail and Campbell 2001, 1,614; Wood et al. 1998, 234).

It follows that research methodologies must shift to qualitative approaches that are contextual and relational, and investigate the *Why?* of unsafe sexual behaviours. The absence of incentive and agency for behaviour change among young people is a function of multiple differentials including ethnicity and poverty, but also gender and age. Contradictory messages confuse social and gender identities and performances. Thus, peer group and male sexual pressures conflict with the values and norms of formal social institutions, including families, schools and churches. Mass media and advertising messages increasingly target youth and promote male and female identities centred on sexuality, while mothers, teachers and other adults suppress any evidence of sex.

In this research, we seek to understand how social identities of femininity and youth are acted out within unequal power relationships, so reinforcing vulnerability and the spread of HIV to adolescent girls, as well as exposing them to unwanted pregnancy, abuse and exploitation. In other words, we are less concerned with sophisticated statistical correlations, such as the goodness-of-fit index (GFI), between specific predictors — such as personality, peer group pressure or family poverty — and risky sexual practice or early sexual debut. We take a different approach by listening to how adolescent girls explain sexual choices and shape sexual identities against the backdrops of normative and subaltern sexualities and cultures. To unpack the key drivers of HIV, we must interrogate sexuality, gender, generation and power; hence the rethink from individual *risk* to social *vulnerability*, and the concern to understand how the interplay between gendered identities and power relations shapes sexual decision-making and undermines the capacity for self-protection.

For this study, we conducted focus group discussions and individual one-on-one interviews with young adolescent girls (aged 11–16 years) in four selected secondary schools in Barbados. The sampling was purposive. The girls were selected as volunteers from among those identified by teachers and guidance counselors as most vulnerable, sexually and socially. Sessions were conducted in an informal manner with open-ended questions and were designed to privilege their voices — to provide the space for them to air their opinions, concerns and anxieties. As they expressed their views and spoke of their experiences, it became clear that their narratives drew on two contradictory discourses of feminine sexuality to shape their own sexual and social identities and codes for living. Both discourses are strongly heterosexual: one, a normative femininity that for young adolescent girls denies sexuality and condemns any evidence of sex as dangerous and immoral; the other, a counter discourse of *bashment* that promotes an active and assertive sexuality. As our participants centred romantic love, trust and fidelity, they also celebrated *bashment*, thereby simultaneously accommodating and resisting the dominant meanings of hetero-normative femininity.

NORMATIVE FEMININITY

Mainstream heterosexuality is dimorphic, double standard and deeply contradictory. Men want sex, much of it and with many partners; women want love and commitment. Male sexuality is free, active and dominant; female sexuality is constrained, passive and vulnerable. The sexual behaviour that makes him a *real man*, sullies her reputation. Male sexual practice is perceived to be driven by unrestrained biological urges and is promoted, celebrated and enjoyed. In the Caribbean, where male homosexuality is heavily stigmatized, the sexual initiation of boys is encouraged by parents and brings great relief as evidence of heterosexual normality (Chevannes 2001, 144; Dann 1987, 59–64). But girls' sexuality is a source of anxiety and their mothers are constantly on the lookout for signs. The discourse of desire and pleasure is forbidden and missing (Fine 1988), their sexuality is denied and controlled, and any evidence condemned and covered up. Hetero-normativity also connects sexuality with violence against women and girls. They are victims, not sexual agents.

Normative femininity defines and regulates the sexuality of women and girls by tying it in with a conservative family orthodoxy of love and fidelity with the promise of marriage, motherhood and social respectability (Holland et al. 1998, 108-113; LaFont 2001; Wilson 1969). The church adds a moral layer of purity, virginity and abstinence. This discourse is powerful — entrenched and legitimated as it is by the legal system and major social institutions of society. In the lives of children and adolescents, it is strongly promoted by the family, education and religion. However, a recent review of Caribbean youth development reports on the failures of these institutions, as well as government and society in general, to support young people as they mature into adulthood (World Bank 2003).

Illustrating this scenario, the adolescent girls participating in this research reported that communication about sex with adults, including family members, teachers, guidance counselors, nurses and clergy, is poor and confined to a restrictive and protective conversation centred on abstinence (see also Jejeebhoy and Bott 2005, 32–35). They also perceive these professionals in health and education to be judgmental and *'dangerous'*— meaning that they leak confidential information to others, including parents. While most spoke very positively about relationships with their mothers in terms of love, care and support, they avoided communication on sexual matters: 'Yuh can't tell she everything 'cause she is yuh mummy'; 'My mudda ask me, "if you having sex you could tell me, you know". Who? Not me'.

According to the girls, mothers suppress sexuality in their daughters, urging them to wait and stay away from boys. Mothers believe that discussions on sex will lead to premature sexual debut. They warn their daughters not to make the same mistakes they did, and turn a blind eye to evidence of sexual activity until it becomes glaringly obvious, when they 'take dramastic (dramatic/drastic) measures'. One girl claimed that her mother would 'thrash me, publicly at that', and another stated: 'My mother would tell my father and he would find him (the boy), and then find me and lock me up, so I can't go anywhere.' Mothers are themselves steeped in a culture of masculine hegemony. Their relative lack of education, and sex education in particular, also points to their incapacity to empower their daughters and to encourage a reshaping of their sexual identities.

Normative femininity is centred on the twin pillars of abstinence for girls and monogamy for women, and is widely perceived and promoted as a *safe* feminine code. But within this discourse, female sexuality is controlled by men and defined in terms of servicing the male sex drive. Women and girls are disempowered, their sexual safety compromised. In their study of young women's sexuality and sexual practice in England, Janet Holland and her colleagues concluded that 'the conventions of heterosexual masculinity and femininity powerfully contribute to sexual risk-taking and the instability of safer sexual practices' (Holland et al. 1998, 3. See also Weiss et al. 2000, 237–239).

Bashment

Bashment, on the other hand, represents a subversive female sexual subjectivity and behavioural code, a popular peer-group performance of

Afro-Caribbean youth sexuality and conspicuous consumption for girls as well as boys. It is promoted by mass media images, music, dance and entertainment.[8] Appearance, and looks, is important — girls are large-bodied, big-bottomed and full breasted. A *bashy* girl and her counterparts, the *ghetto* or *block* girl, is admired for her display of *bling*, brand-name clothing and accessories that accentuate her sexuality — expensive gold jewellery, elaborate hairstyle and make up, flashy finger nail extensions, and the latest model cellular phone or I-pod. Hers is a loud and self-confident public style. She demands to be the centre of attention and is out to have a good time — to *mek sport* and enjoy life. She has *attitude*, meaning that she is a mature, no-nonsense woman, who knows what she wants and meets life head on. She is streetwise, her life experiences have toughened her up and 'nuhbody caan' mess with she'. She flaunts her sexual prowess, attracts men and knows how to handle them, and manages relationships without falling in love and becoming vulnerable.

Her mirror opposite is the normative good 'li'l girl' or 'church girl', who is quiet and modest, leading a 'dull and boring' life according to the mores of home, school and church. She is the virgin who is timid and 'scared of sex', 'saving sheself for somebody'. Expressly challenging this restrictive femininity encoded in the denial of sexuality, maturity and fun, *bashment* celebrates risk. In so doing, it fuels moral panic and a language of control reflected in the pejorative public labeling of non-conformist girls as sexually 'force-ripe' and socially deviant. A Juvenile Court magistrate recently added her voice, commenting on those who seemed to be 'virtual sex addicts'.

> The drug lords have a lot of money and they get the girls involved. It's become very fashionable among the girls 14 to 15 years old to have a drug lord boyfriend. So they go and sometimes they disappear for months. Two, three months and you can't find them and they are holed up somewhere with one of these drug lords who are usually in their mid- to late 20s. (*Saturday Sun* July 28, 2007)

Paradoxically, the outrage of mainstream moral authorities appears to enhance the very behaviour it is designed to suppress.

Bashment disrupts the discourse of normative femininity by celebrating the agency and empowerment of young women. There are parallels here with those who 'inhabit marginal social spaces' and who 'resist, and sometimes rebel, against gendered and sexual regimes that privilege masculine heterosexual needs and desires, and actively work against dominant ideologies and practices that seek to deny their existence' (Kempadoo 2004, 4), their existence as sexual beings, we might add for adolescent girls in Barbados. For them, this subversive counter-identity provides a compelling alternative, an escape from the dullness and submission imposed by a social order that suppresses their emerging sexuality and maturity. Celebrated as freedom, affluence and sexual agency, in reality however, this too is operationalized and enacted in the context of a dominant male heterosexuality, putting young girls at great risk.

Adolescent sexual realities

We turn now to the narratives of the girls as they presented their own sexual choices and experiences, navigating against, between or within these contradictory feminine identities. Highlighted here are four dimensions of decision-making, namely: love or sex; postponement or sexual debut; fidelity or multiple-partnering; safety or risk? Their responses, as they shaped meanings about their sexual selves, revealed that life is not a simple choice between normative femininity and *bashment*, but 'a complex process of becoming' (Allen 2003, 216. See also Butler 1990).

Love or Sex?

The girls all endorse the conventional ideal of heterosexual relationship development through defined stages — from friendship, to boy/girlfriend or 'talking' one-to-one, to falling in love, to sex, and ultimately, to marriage for life. Love is pivotal to the process and encompasses 'trust', 'honesty', 'commitment', 'faithfulness' and 'respect': 'No matter what happens, he'll be there for you'. Fourteen years is considered an appropriate age for a girl to have a boyfriend and be in love. They denied quite vehemently that they were too young: 'I do not believe that because you older you know more about love than somebody our age. I don't buy that!' When asked if persons of their age fall in love, they responded with 'How yuh mean? Yuh en got nuh feelings?' For them, love is a prerequisite and prime motivator for sex, later on in the relationship. Several also claimed that they would be proactive and express interest directly, rather than wait for a male to do so or approaching discretely through an intermediary: 'Well, tuh be honest, I like to be straightforward. So I go and tell he, "my friend, I like you." Dat is true, very, very true, "my sexy friend, I like you."'

But they were also well aware of the gulf between the ideal and the real. In their words, the distinction between sex and love has become unclear and confused: 'Once it was mekkin' love, but now sex, is just sex. Yuh ain't got tuh love de body (the person) tuh do it, is just plain sex now.' While girls fall in love, boys proclaim love for ulterior motives: 'Fellas does use "I love you" tuh get sex, yeah. "I love you" don't mean nuttin.'

They pointed to the dangers of intimacy. Relationships are short-lived — 'a month, a week, a day!' Young, immature girls fall in love too quickly, get involved for the wrong reasons, and end up suffering emotional pain: 'Yuh does get hurt.' Loving, enduring relationships were cynically perceived as an ideal, virtually impossible to achieve.

'Love, wuh (what) is love? Love ain' nuh word. Love is when you mother and father loves yuh. Nuh man wuh never love yuh … I ain' know wuh love is, dah is de trute (truth);' 'My mother say, "love is a contract between two fools."'

The majority also claimed that sex was not important in their lives: 'Tuh me dah is like a hobby, for de sport', though some pointed to the physical benefits: 'relaxing,' 'it mek yuh feel good,' 'it does get yuh hormones high.' They also spoke of girls for whom persistent sexual activity had become a norm and a need: 'People can't control demself cause dem hormones does be kicking.' But their own sexual pleasure was hardly mentioned.

Postponement or sexual debut?

Between 15 and 16 years was considered to be the earliest age appropriate for sexual initiation, though some participants were in favour of postponement to late teens:

'Dah does be part of a relationship right, but further on in life.'

'It (sex) is not important now cause yuh got yuh school work and yuh don't want a b.a.b.y (spelt out).' They were adamant that, for young girls, sex should not be rushed or forced: 'Yuh have to know when yuh ready.' Too many, they argued, become sexually active at too young an age.

On the other hand, girls achieve a reputation among their friends by boasting about sexual encounters while others with no such experience are left out of the conversation. Peer pressure fuels curiosity and sexual debut: 'Dah was experimenting. I did just wan' know wuh it dih feel like.' Most significant, is the heavy and continuous pressure from boys and men: 'Well, this generation boys just look for sex and dah is all.' Initially they use persuasive techniques and 'bribe with sweet talk.' Failing that, insistence intensifies as they taunt, undermine a girl's reputation and threaten physical assault, so that resistance becomes futile:

'And den de man might say, might say, "You is a bare lil girl, you don't trust me, and I love you" and all uh dah foolishness. And dem (the girls) gine feel now, "Oh shoot, he gine go and tell my friends" so and so, and so and so. So it is more, sometimes it is more that they don't want people to talk about it, and say that they are that kindah li'l girl, can't tek it, and stuff like dat.'

Looking back, the girls revealed that they were caught off guard and were unprepared for their first sexual experience. Several expressed regret: 'Tuh me I would say, sex is not all important 'cause tuh me I would say I regret de day I did dat. I say so all de time. I regret the day, de hour.' Male deception and harassment are clearly evident in the narratives of Sheena and Kamisha, but in general, the girls denied that they were forced to have sex.[9] Kamisha's experience also illustrates the pressure on girls to have a child.

Sheena had her first sexual relationship at age 13 with Mark, aged 18, in a storeroom at school: 'Because he was just confusing me all de time. And every time he see me, he telling me junk like "little girl, come along little girl" and ting. And I just get fed up and say dat I wuh gih he a little piece to make he happy and stop confusing me.' She says that there was no relationship between them and that she was 'kinda' pressured into having sex.

Kamisha describes her first sexual experience at age 13 with her 18 year old boyfriend of about 4 months: 'Well it was like this. I knew the fella, was seeing him and stuff. He was one o' my family friends. And we just start talking, start dealing with one another and every time dat we come onto the phone, we talk. He was always talking about he want children, he want children. So I would be like listening tuh what happen tuh him in the past and stuff like dat. And outside one night he just like, he was by me, we was outside talking, he about he want ... he want tuh have sex. I say "No", because I ain't ready fuh it, nor I ain't want to do it. And he keep forcing me and pressuring me, and pressuring me all de time. And I just get fed up and I say, "Alright, yeah right". And after we finish we was going through town because it was two days after my birthday, and we was going through town and like I had a glush, a big glush, like something hitting through my body and I just drop everything 'cause it hurt me real bad. And when we got home de night, he told me dat he had ahhmmm, come inside of me. And I was pretty vex 'cause I say I trust he and everyt'ing and he come and do something dat I wouldn't expect he tuh do'.

An economic exchange equation underpins these sexual liaisons. Tempted by gifts of *bling*, girls are under pressure to '*give sex*' in return when boys and men spend money on them.[10] Girls must also '*give sex*' in order to maintain a relationship. Otherwise, boys and men move on. And yet, paradoxically: 'He like a girl 'til he get it. Den he tell she "Nope, can't work out. You gimme it (sex) too quick". He gone, just left de girl'.

The girls agreed that, in the final analysis, boys choose girlfriends who are quiet, respectable and church-going, who 'don't overplay dem sexuality' and keep themselves to themselves — 'a personal girl', one that 'he can carry home'. The 'personal girl' resonates with the image of the 'lil' girl', scorned by the participants, but also admired. Ultimately, it is these girls, who concentrate on school work and postpone sex, that are seen to be 'strong,' 'tekking them time and choosing wuh dem got tuh choose.' Free from sexual pressure, they are able to secure a successful future: 'When yuh ain' got nuh boyfriend, yuh able to keep yuh life pun track.'

Fidelity or multiple partnering?

Fidelity was perceived by the girls as an impossible ideal, since male concurrent multiple partnering is commonplace and culturally condoned. Though they hope things will work out otherwise, they expect their boyfriends to 'cheat'. Their response is to propose 'back up' relationships for themselves: 'When yuh boyfriend horning yuh, yuh does doan know, so you should got a flam.' A 'flam' is a standby ready to step in and become your boyfriend should your main relationship break up: 'a man to fall back on. You aint' gotta wait. If de man done wid yuh, you don' got to care.' Experience and variety was also seen as an advantage:

'You can't be so clingy. If you are with this one person for a long time, by the time you get old you would have no experience. I'm not saying that you have to be with a lot of men, but as in you won't know what you would be missing. But you would never know. If from the first you are with one person, you would never know. What I am saying is that if you are there all the time with vanilla, you would never know if chocolate taste better.'

Fun was also mentioned as a positive quality in young people's relationship experience: 'You can't have one relationship that is too serious all the time. You are only going to be 15 for one year. We have the rest of our life to be dull.'

One girl implied that one man cannot satisfy all your needs: 'Yuh like one ting 'bout he and den yuh like another ting from another fella.' But most disagreed, fully aware of the implications for a girl's reputation within the context of a gender double standard of morality. Girls who are sexually involved with more than one partner simultaneously run the risk of being labeled 'sluts', 'rats' or 'skanks'. They are condemned as 'nasty', loose and promiscuous: 'dem don't care nuttin' 'bout demself' and 'would just do anything, anywhere, wid anybody.'

For girls, then, serial multiple partnering was proposed as an acceptable strategy enabling them to contest the restrictions of feminine sexual normativity and also to resist being positioned as 'sluts'. Alarmingly, they did not question the sexual history of their partners or undergo HIV testing together, and considered themselves to be safe. In their minds, HIV infection happens to others who are sexually promiscuous. Thus, they objectify HIV, maintain their own moral propriety, distance themselves from high risk groups, leave their own risky sexual behaviour unchallenged, and live for the here and now.

Safety or risk?

During the focus group sessions, the girls acted out an assertive femininity with encouragement from their peers, emphasising a no-nonsense attitude in dealing with male pressure for sex and unsafe sex (without a condom) and their boyfriends' multiple partnering: 'Dem ain't got no pressure on me. A'right den. Not me. No is no and if you doan like dat, lump it. Simple.' But their accounts of translating these intentions into action revealed ambivalence and a lack of agency.

The girls were well educated on HIV transmission and condom use. They also spoke of the persistence of unsafe sex due to pressure from men and boys who 'like it rough and bareback'. Nevertheless, they insisted that they were not at risk (see also de Bruin 2002, 6). The onus is on them to put restraints on sexual activity and to set safe standards by insisting on condoms, but they claimed to be too embarrassed to purchase condoms and also expressed doubts about their efficacy — they break and 'some fellas does put a hole in de back of it.' Also putting limits on precautions is the unpredictability of sexual activity. Sex is unplanned and 'just happens', 'anywhere, any time.' Adolescent spontaneity and risk, linked directly to the influence of drugs and alcohol, often override knowledge and caution:

'Yu high, you just think, well I want something now. You just want it, hit it, quick so. And when you done wid da dey, you remember you din' had no condom. Couple months later you got bumps coming up 'pon you skin. You got some disease … AIDS'.

Far from being a straightforward, practical issue, condom use is loaded with symbolic meaning and circumscribed by gendered power dynamics (Holland et al. 1998, 39, 52; Lear 1995, 1,314–15). Even raising the issue is interpreted as an insult and the male response is:

'"You don' trust me. If you love me you gine do it (sex without a condom)." Da's de sorta guilt trip dem does put yuh pun.'

'Some boys does tell you, "I love you so you ain't gotta use a condom, 'cause I love you."'

'Dem (men and boys) does be like "man, I ain't got nutting, I ain't got nutting (no disease). Man, you ain't trust me, I thought you did trust me."'

When a girl produces a condom, 'she's a rat,' and if he voluntarily wears one, she may conclude that 'he feel dat she dirty.'

Lisa (age 16) explains her dilemma. She has been involved in a relationship with Deon (age 18) for the past 11 months:

'Sometimes if, like if we stop talking and like say we stop talking and then we start talking back, I wuh be like, you got tuh use a condom, know wuh I mean? And he wuh look at me like, hard. He know that I know that if he was supposed tuh go out there and do something (have sex) that he wuh use protection. It is only with me that he don't use protection. But he was like, "You serious?" And I was like, "Alright."'

Lisa thus preserves the relationship and presents a less than convincing argument for her safety based on her assumption that Deon uses a condom *outside* his main relationship with her. Her statement also illustrates the lack of sexual communication between partners: 'He know that I know ....' In general, what talk there is relates to the physical act of sex and male pleasure: 'wha's he favourite position.' Ironically, the ideal of trust and love, defined according to a masculine script, is incompatible with condom use. Girls give in to please men: 'If yuh like he real bad, yuh would gi he unprotected sex.' It is her responsibility to say 'No' to unsafe sex, but his decision to purchase and use a condom.

For *bashment* girls, the key signifier of maturity and popularity is a sexual relationship with an older man of style and reputation — a 'bad boy', 'gangster', 'thug', 'money man' or 'ghetto man' (See also Kempadoo 2004, 49). These liaisons are defined as transactional; in this context love was not mentioned. For the men, referred to today as *sugar-daddies*, the motivation is sex: 'yuh know he only looking fuh what yuh got between yuh legs.' For girls the attraction is economic — money, clothing and jewelry — as well as notoriety and protection:

'Money, drive 'bout in big cars, bling bling, all o' dat.'

'Look at she. She is a boss. Look she man is a pure, pure thug. Nobody can't mess 'round she. Girls get a level of respect when they deal with certain fellas. Alright, if he supposed tuh be a bad man and she got he pun lock, she got tuh got someting.'

'If somebody interfere wid you, dem wuh protect yuh, right. And yuh family too.'

However, it is within these mixed-age relationships that the girls 'go missing,'[11] and are at their most vulnerable. They have no agency to refuse sex or to negotiate condom use, or to protect themselves from pregnancy, HIV, violence and sexual abuse, or to end the relationship.[12]

'If somebody force yuh to have sex, yuh don' have nuh choice if dey don' wanna use a condom you can't tell them wuh to do.'

'De men does threaten. Dem girls frighten. De men is tell dem dey can't leave... I know girls that get beat from their men and don't leave.'

The gender disparity in HIV-infection rates among adolescents has been attributed, not only to higher female physiological susceptibility but also to the involvement of girls with older men who control the sexual process and are more likely to be sexually experienced and HIV-positive (Allen et al. 2002, 198; Inciardi et al. 2005, S16–17).

FROM VULNERABILITY TO EMPOWERMENT

The politics of heterosexuality and gendered power relations is extremely complex involving a mix of contradictory discourses and multiple practices. There is no single adolescent sexual sub-culture in Barbados. Adolescent sexual worlds are dynamic and complex, and research on HIV and AIDS must avoid the premature closure, over-simplification and recourse to stereotyping that has become all too common in the search for predictors of risk behaviours (Wood 1998, 240). Although the sexuality of the adolescent girls participating in this research cannot be summed up and understood by recourse to either *bashment* or normative femininity, these scripts provide socializing backdrops, shaping their identities and their choices. For them, *bashment* promotes and celebrates sexual style and prosperity, and offers fun and freedom within a live-for-now ethos, while the normative feminine message promoted by mothers, teachers and priests promises respectability, safety and the realization of personal goals in the future to those who restrain sexuality and postpone sexual debut.

But both constitute unsafe identities for adolescent girls, contextualised as they are within a hegemonic masculine heterosexuality esteemed as biologically natural, socially normal and morally proper. To be conventionally feminine requires a girl to have a boyfriend and be in a relationship, to trust and fall in love, to resist sexual pressure, to appear innocent about sexual matters and concerned to preserve her reputation. As a virgin, she may be safe for now, but even she is under strong peer pressure and demands from boys and men to initiate sex. And her older sister, who is often powerless to resist her partner's predatory sexual posturing, to initiate condom use, to question his sexual history, or do anything about his multiple partnering, gives her body for his sexual pleasure while denying her own. On the other hand, disrupting the passive feminine code, *bashment* is positioned against the trap and emotional pain of romantic love, sexual self-denial, the boredom and restrictions of home and school, the social and moral pressure to remain a *good little girl*, and passive conformity to adult moral authority. But the *bashment* girl's performance represents a mere illusion of female empowerment, realized as it is in relationships with older men that also expose her to unprotected sex, pregnancy and HIV, and to sexual and physical violence. Her performance also constitutes social deviance, fuels moral panic and exposes her to heavy condemnation by family, school, community and society.

The vulnerability of the girls who participated in this research is revealed as their choices accommodate normative feminine codes and also as they resist by taking up a *bashment* posture. There is a wide gulf between knowledge and practice. They are well informed, but have not personalized HIV and AIDS. It is pregnancy they fear; HIV infection happens to others, those in risk groups. They take the risk of 'quick' unprotected sex in the belief that they will 'get away with it', and assume their norm of serial monogamy to be a safe option. Their narratives also revealed a disconnect between intention and action.[13] Girls insist that 'No means no', but give in under male pressure, occasionally coercive. Their accounts provided the occasional glimpse of an alternative pattern of female empowerment, gender equity, and safer sex as they contested the double standard of sexual morality, insisted that condom use should be a joint responsibility and warned against giving in to male and peer pressure and following the crowd. But they lack the agency to put these changes into practice in sexual encounters with boys and men, shaped as these are by male definitions of love, trust and sexual entitlement, and by male material and ideological power. As they seek to construct their own sexualities and navigate through the hazards of sex and relationships in the context of HIV, their questions and concerns posed across the generations are met with silences, contradictory messages and the reinforcement of a repressive hetero-normativity. While they may have taken the first step by challenging the virgin ideal and restrictive femininity, this has led them to a *bashment* sexual identity, rather than to the formulation of a model of youthful female sexuality that promotes safety, well-being and resilience, and also represents emergent maturity with fun, freedom and desire.

Safer sex has been written into the HIV response as an issue of individual responsibility and private morality. But decisions about risk are governed not by rationality, but by the multiple and often contradictory pressures of relationships and daily life. The extent to which girls are empowered to control their sexual lives and ensure their own safety in relationships is clearly a critical question for the design of HIV-prevention strategies. It is not just a question of bridging the gap between knowledge and practice and either abstaining or using condoms. Sexual activity is interactive, contextualized and shaped by power dynamics, most importantly the inequalities of gender and generation that reinforce vulnerability.

There is a clear need to rewrite the politics of safer sex against the idea of a natural and normative dominant masculine heterosexuality and social pressure to deny and suppress youthful female sexuality, and according to a social identity script, yet to be written, for adolescent girls on the verge of sexual debut and falling in love — a script that centres female sexual pleasure with safety, gender equity and the empowerment of women and girls. Safer sex practice is based on a complex process of communication about sex, but this is not yet widely practised in Barbadian culture, either between sexual partners, among friends, or between mothers and daughters, teachers and pupils. The peer groups of young girls in this research are not a source of advice and agency, but rather, pressure girls to engage in risky behaviours in the belief that they are immune to the consequences. Those that play safe are marginalized and ostracized (Fisher et al. 1992; Wood et al. 1998, 236).

The process requires the provision of discursive social space in peer education and informal social settings for young girls, with and without their boyfriends, male contemporaries and adult facilitators, to consider alternative sexual choices and life styles. These conversations should facilitate the development of a critical consciousness about their sexual health and sexual rights, and the construction of identities that challenge normative relations of gender and generation. They should also build confidence and the collective capacity to negotiate the boundaries of pleasure and risk in relationships and to safeguard their own sexual well-being (Campbell and McPhail 2002; Weiss et al. 2000, 242). The process of reshaping relations of gender and generation must also work with men — who already have the power to refuse sex or use a condom — to change male predatory and risky sexual behaviours and to promote zero tolerance for sexual exploitation and violence against women and girls. The transformation from hegemonic masculinity to gender equality and female empowerment cannot be realized within the domain of the personal and private. It requires a systemic approach involving key social institutions and social policy. Finally, the discourse of sexual identities and cultures must be inserted into public debates about gender, youth, patriarchy and citizenship rights, and placed on the national agenda alongside other issues of social justice, such as child abuse and gender-based violence.

NOTES

1. The author gratefully acknowledges funding and support from UNICEF, Caribbean Area Office in Barbados for this research.
2. HFLE messages tend to be objective and remote, rather than personalized and internalized, and the programme has not lived up to expectations (de Bruin 2002, 27; Campbell and MacPhail 2002, UNICEF 1995). In common with their counterparts in a Trinidad and Tobago study (Baird et al. 2007, 246–47), the girls in this research said that real-life stories and interaction with persons living with HIV would have more impact on their attitudes and behaviour.
3. In Trinidad and Tobago and in African countries where the epidemic is more advanced, the adolescent gender imbalance is between 5 and 6 females to 1 male (Anderson et al. 2002,1; UNICEF/UNAIDS/WHO 2002,17).
4. In a study that spanned nine countries of the Caribbean, of the one-third of adolescents who had been sexually active, almost half of the girls (49 per cent) reported that their first sexual experience had been forced (PAHO 2000).
5. Similar gender disparities have been reported for other countries of the Caribbean (Allen et al. 2002, de Bruin 2002, Kurtz et al. 2005, PAHO 2000, Rivers and Aggleton 1999, World Bank 2003,15).
6. Statistical information from the Child Care Board (CCB) of Barbados.
7. Abortion was legalized in Barbados with the passage of the Medical Termination of Pregnancy Act, 1983.
8. *Bashment* in Barbados is fed by a global entertainment culture of youth and has roots in Jamaica dancehall, a liberating space for the expression of black female sexuality from the restrictions of middle class respectable norms (Cooper 2004). The link has been explored elsewhere (Barrow, 2008).

9. Unlike their counterparts in Jamaica (de Bruin 2002, 13), the girls in this study avoided the language of abuse and rape to describe their experiences. This may be related to the normalcy of gender violence, but is possibly also because they considered the labels of *'abuse'*, *'rape'* and *'rapist'* to be inappropriate to their relationships and the boys and men with whom they are involved. Research from elsewhere also reports that girls believe that sexual coercion is normal and that sexual action on the part of their peers or boyfriends that is non-consensual is not seen in this way, only that with strangers (Jejeebhoy and Bott 2005, 6, 11; Wood et al. 1998, 238).

10. Not mentioned in this research but noted, for example in Jamaica, is sexual exchange and economic dependence on men for everyday needs such as food, school expenses and family subsistence (de Bruin 2002, 21; Kempadoo and Dunn 2001,14, 51).

11. At regular intervals, police reports appear in the local press indicating that teenage girls are *missing* from home, the assumption being that they are living with men as alluded to in the earlier quotation from the Juvenile Court magistrate. It appears that most turn up after a short period of absence.

12. Research findings from Jamaica, taking a male perspective into account, report that *'women deserve to be beaten'* if they fail to perform domestic and sexual services and to demonstrate respect for their partners. Male violence is expected and condoned in cases of female infidelity, real or suspected (de Bruin 2002, 13; Bailey et al. 1998, 30–31, 8–85). Violence against women is a symbol of manhood. Barry Chevannes reports on 'the ability, if not the right, of man physically to discipline woman, without social sanction. Boys do not have this right. When they do, it is a sign of having made the transition to men' (Chevannes 2001, 56).

13. In similar vein, Janet Holland and her colleagues also report that young women may be empowered at the *intellectual* level, but not at an *experiential* level, in that they are unable to act on their ideas and intentions in practice to reduce risk in sexual encounters (Holland et al. 1998,9).

REFERENCES

Allen, C., D. DaCosta Martinez, U. Wagner, K. McLetchie, A. DeGazon Washington, T. Chapman-Smith and M. Wright. 2002. 'The Sexual Behaviour of Youth in Tobago: A Report on the Development of a Health Promotion Project', *West Indian Medical Journal*, 51, no. 3: 197–99.

Allen, L. 2003. 'Girls Want Sex, Boys Want Love: Resisting Dominant Discourses of (Hetero) sexuality' *Sexualities* 6, no. 2: 215–36.

Anderson, H., K. Marcovici and K. Taylor. 2002. *The UNGASS, Gender and Women's Vulnerability to HIV/AIDS in Latin America and the Caribbean*. Washington, D.C.: Pan-American Health Organisation, Women, Health and Development Programme.

Baird, D., E. Yearwood and C. Perrino. 2007. 'Small Islands, Big Problem: HIV/AIDS and Youth in Trinidad and Tobago', *Journal of Child and Adolescent Psychiatric Nursing*, 20, no. 4: 243–51.

Bailey, W., C. Branche, G. McGarity, and S. Stuart. 1998. *Family and the Quality of Gender Relations in the Caribbean.* Jamaica: University of the West Indies, Institute of Social and Economic Research.

Barrow, C. 2003. 'Children and Social Policy in Barbados: The Unfinished Agenda of Child Abuse,' *The Caribbean Journal of Social Work* 2: 36–51.

_____. 2006. 'Adolescent Girls, Sexuality and HIV/AIDS in Barbados: The Case for Reconfiguring Research and Policy', *Caribbean Journal of Social Work,* 5: 62–80.

_____. 2008. 'Sexual Identity, HIV and Adolescent Girls in Barbados' *Social and Economic Studies.* Special Issue: Crisis, Chaos and Change, Vol, 57, no. 2.

Blades, M. 2002. *A Force to Reckon with: Youth Against AIDS (Focus Groups Report).* Barbados: UNIFEM Caribbean.

Bruin de, M. 2002. *Teenagers at Risk: High-Risk Behavior of Jamaican Adolescents in the Context of Reproductive Health — Observations and Impressions.* Jamaica: The Jamaica Adolescent Reproductive Health Activity.

Butler, J. 1990. *Gender Trouble: Feminism and the Subversion of Identity.* New York: Routledge.

Campbell, C. and C. MacPhail. 2002. 'Peer Education, Gender and the Development of Critical Consciousness: Participatory HIV Prevention by South African Youth', *Social Science and Medicine,* 55 no. 2: 331–45.

Carter, R. 2001. *Report on the National KABP Survey on HIV/AIDS.* Barbados: Ministry of Education, Youth Affairs and Sport.

Chevannes, B. 2001. *Learning to be a Man: Culture, Socialisation and Gender Identity in Five Caribbean Communities.* Jamaica: University of the West Indies Press.

Clarke, R. 1998. *Violence Against Women in the Caribbean: State and Non-state Responses.* New York: UNIFEM.

Cooper, C. 2004. *Sound Clash: Jamaican Dancehall at Large.* New York and Basingstoke: Palgrave Macmillan.

Dann, G. 1987. *The Barbadian Male: Sexual Attitudes and Practices.* London: Macmillan.

Ellis, H., M. Hoyos, F. Jones, T. Roach, M. Sounder, and E. Walrond. 1990. 'A Knowledge, Attitude, Belief and Practices Survey in Relation to AIDS amongst Children ages 11-16 Years Old in Barbados', *Bulletin of Eastern Caribbean Affairs* 16 nos. 4&5: 1–12.

Fine, M. 1988. 'Sexuality, Schooling and Adolescent Females: The Missing Discourse of Desire', *Harvard Educational Review,* 58 no. 29.

Fisher, J., S. Miscovich and W. Fisher. 1992. 'Impact of Perceived Social Norms on Adolescents' AIDS-Risk Behaviour and Prevention'. In *Adolescents and AIDS: A Generation in Jeopardy,* ed. R. Clemente, 117–35. London: Sage Publications.

Holland, J., C. Ramazanoglu, S. Sharpe and R. Thomson. 1998. *The Male in the Head: Young People, Heterosexuality and Power.* London: The Tufnell Press.

Inciardi, J., J. Syversten and H. Surratt. 2005. 'HIV/AIDS in the Caribbean Basin', *AIDS Care,* 17 (Supplement), S9–S25.

Jejeebhoy, S. and S. Bott. 2005. 'Non-consensual Sexual Experiences of Young People in Developing Countries: An Overview'. In *Sex without Consent: Young People in Developing*

Countries, eds. S. Jejeebhoy, I. Shah and S. Thapa, 3–45. London and New York: Zed Books.

Kempadoo, K. 2004. *Sexing the Caribbean: Gender, Race and Sexual Labor.* New York and London: Routledge.

Kempadoo, K. and L. Dunn. 2001. *Factors that Shape the Initiation of Early Sexual Activity among Adolescent Boys and Girls: A Study in Three Communities in Jamaica.* Jamaica: University of the West Indies, Centre for Gender and Development Studies.

Kurtz, S., K. Douglas, and Y. Lugo. 2005. 'Sexual Risks and Concerns about AIDS among Adolescents in Anguilla', *AIDS Care,* 17 (Supplement), S36–S44.

LaFont, S. 2001. 'Very Straight Sex: The Development of Sexual Mores in Jamaica', *Journal of Colonialism and Colonial History,* 2, no. 3.

Lear, D. 1995. 'Sexual Communication in the Age of AIDS: The Construction of Risk and Trust among Young Adults', *Social Science and Medicine,* 41, no.9: 311–23.

Le Franc, E. 2002. 'Child Abuse in the Caribbean: Addressing the Rights of the Child'. In *Children's Rights: Caribbean Realities,* ed. C. Barrow, 285–304. Jamaica: Ian Randle Publishers.

Le Franc, E. and L. Rock. 2001. 'Commentary: The Commonality of Gender-based Violence', *Journal of Eastern Caribbean Studies* 26, no.1: 74–82.

MacPhail, C. and C. Campbell. 2001. '"I think condoms are good but, aai, I hate those things": Condom use among Adolescents and Young People in a Southern African Township', *Social Science and Medicine* 52: 613–27.

PAHO. 1999. *Report: Barbados Adolescent Health Survey.* Prepared for the Ministry of Health, Barbados.

_____. 2000. *A Portrait of Adolescent Health in the Caribbean, 2000.* Minneapolis: University of Minnesota, WHO Collaborating Centre on Adolescent Health.

Piot, P. 1999. *HIV/AIDS and Violence against Women.* UNAIDS Panel on Women and Health.

Rivers, K. and P. Aggleton. 1999. *Adolescent Sexuality, Gender and the HIV Epidemic.* UNDP, HIV and Development Programme. University of London, Institute of Education, Thomas Coram Research Unit.

Rock, L. 2002. 'Child Abuse in Barbados'. In *Children's Rights: Caribbean Realities,* ed. C. Barrow, 305–29. Jamaica: Ian Randle Publishers.

Stuart, S. 2000. The Reproductive Health Challenge: Women and AIDS in the Caribbean'. In *The Caribbean AIDS Epidemic,* eds. G. Howe and A. Cobley, 122–38. Jamaica: University of the West Indies Press.

UNAIDS/WHO. 2007. *AIDS Epidemic Update.* Geneva, UNAIDS and WHO.

UNICEF. 1995. A Strategy for Strengthening Health and Family Life Education in CARICOM Member States.

UNICEF/UNAIDS/WHO. 2002. *Young People and HIV/AIDS: Opportunity in Crisis.*

Weiss, E., D. Whelan and G.R. Gupta. 2000. 'Gender, Sexuality and HIV: Making a Difference in the Lives of Young Women in Developing Countries', *Sexual and Relationship Therapy,* 15, no. 3: 233–45.

Wilson, P. 1969. 'Reputation and Respectability: A Suggestion for Caribbean Ethnology', *Man* 4, no. 1: 70-84.

Wood, K., F. Maforah and R. Jewkes. 1998. '"He Forced Me to Love Him": Putting Violence on Adolescent Sexual Health Agendas', *Social Science and Medicine* 47, no. 2: 233-242.

World Bank. 2003. *Caribbean Youth Development: Issues and Policy Directions*. Washington, D.C.

NEWSPAPERS

Saturday Sun, Barbados.

Chapter 12

How risk and vulnerability become 'socially embedded'
Insights into the Resilient Gap Between Awareness and Safety in HIV

David Plummer

Introduction: The 'KAP gap'

People engaged in HIV-related work have long been concerned about a persistent gap between awareness, knowledge and safe practice. It appears that being aware and knowledgeable about HIV does not have a simple correlation with being safe. This gap — between knowledge, attitudes and practice — is sometimes referred to as the 'KAP gap'.

The existence of the 'KAP gap' in the Caribbean was recently confirmed in a survey of HIV-related knowledge, attitudes and beliefs conducted in six Eastern Caribbean states: Antigua and Barbuda, Dominica, Grenada, St Kitts and Nevis, Saint Lucia and St Vincent and the Grenadines. The survey was a joint initiative of the Pan American Health Organisation (PAHO), Family Health International (FHI) and the US Agency for International Development (USAID) (Ogunnaike-Cooke et. al. 2007). A total of 5,897 young people between the ages of 15 and 24 was recruited, consisting of just under 1,000 participants from each participating country. Key results can be found in table 12.1.

The survey demonstrated that awareness of HIV and AIDS is universal: nearly 100 per cent of the sample of young adults had heard of HIV and AIDS in all countries. The study also documented high levels of knowledge about HIV prevention: knowing about sexual abstinence as a prevention strategy ranged from 86 per cent to 94 per cent; knowing about being faithful to a single uninfected partner as a prevention strategy ranged from 80 per cent to 92 per cent; and knowing about consistent condom use as a prevention strategy ranged from 75 per cent to 88 per cent.

In contrast, the evidence relating to sexual practice revealed a substantial gap between knowledge and safety (the 'KAP gap'). Between 60 and 74 per cent of young people between 15 and 24 years of age reported having been sexually active and of them, between 87 per cent and 99 per cent had had sex with at least one non-marital, non-cohabiting partner in the last 12 months. Only between 16 per cent and 44 per cent of the sample used condoms with non-marital, non-cohabiting sexual partners consistently.

The survey also found that between 22 per cent and 26 per cent of participants experienced their first sexual intercourse before the age of 15 and that between 31 per cent and 46 per cent of the sample had *multiple* non-marital, non-cohabiting partners in the last 12 months. In other words, despite near universal awareness of HIV and high levels of knowledge about prevention, the adoption of the 'ABCs' (abstinence, being faithful and using condoms) of HIV prevention is far from universal: only a minority of 15 to 24 year olds have not had sex, the overwhelming majority of those who had had sex reported at least one casual (non-marital, non-cohabiting) partner in the past year, many had multiple partners, and condom use was low to moderate, at best. The gap between awareness and practice is illustrated in table 12.1.

UNPACKING THE 'KAP GAP' AND THE SUSTAINABILITY OF PROTECTIVE BEHAVIOURS: METHOD

The above findings raise key questions for HIV control: (i) what factors contribute to maintaining the gap between HIV awareness and safe practice? (ii) how can that gap be reduced? and (iii) how do we ensure that safe behaviours are sustainable? These complicated issues almost certainly are multi-factorial. However, further inroads into the HIV epidemic will depend on elucidating factors that militate against safety and entrench risk.

To investigate these militating factors we took a dual approach: (i) we revisited the work of other Caribbean researchers to search for clues; and (ii) we undertook our own qualitative investigations. A qualitative

Table 12.1
Key indicators for HIV-related awareness, knowledge and practice among 15-24 years olds in 6 eastern Caribbean countries.

Respondents aged 15 to 24	Antigua & Barbuda	Dominica	Grenada	St Kitts & Nevis	Saint Lucia	St Vincent & the Grenadines
Number of respondents per country	989	988	971	982	988	979
AWARENESS						
Ever heard of HIV/AIDS *	100%	100%	100%	99%	100%	100%
KNOWLEDGE						
Knew of abstinence as an HIV prevention strategy *	93%	87%	91%	88%	86%	94%
Knew of faithfulness to one infected partner as an HIV prevention strategy *	85%	87%	90%	80%	83%	92%
Knew of consistent condom use as an HIV prevention strategy *	86%	80%	75%	88%	81%	77%
ACTIVITY						
Sex before the age of 15 *	25%	23%	25%	22%	26%	22%
Ever had sex *	62%	71%	67%	60%	74%	72%
Sex in the last 12 months **	74%	77%	80%	82%	85%	79%
PRACTICE						
Sex with a non-marital, non-cohabiting partner in the last 12 months ***	98%	99%	97%	98%	90%	87%
Sex with multiple non-marital, non-cohabiting partner in the last 12 months ***	41%	31%	43%	46%	40%	38%
Consistent condom use with non-marital, non-cohabiting sexual partner ****	39%	44%	31%	16%	21%	19%

Denominators: * = all persons in sample surveyed; ** = all persons in sample who had ever had sex; *** = all persons in sample who had sex in past 12 months; **** = all persons in sample who had non-regular, non-commercial partners in past 12 months;
Source: based on Ogunnaike-Cooke S, Kabore I, Bombereau G, Espeut D, O'Neil C, Hirnschall G (2007) *Behavioural surveillance surveys (BSS) in six countries of the Organisation of Eastern Caribbean States (OESC) 2005-2006.* Washington: Pan American Health Organisation (PAHO)

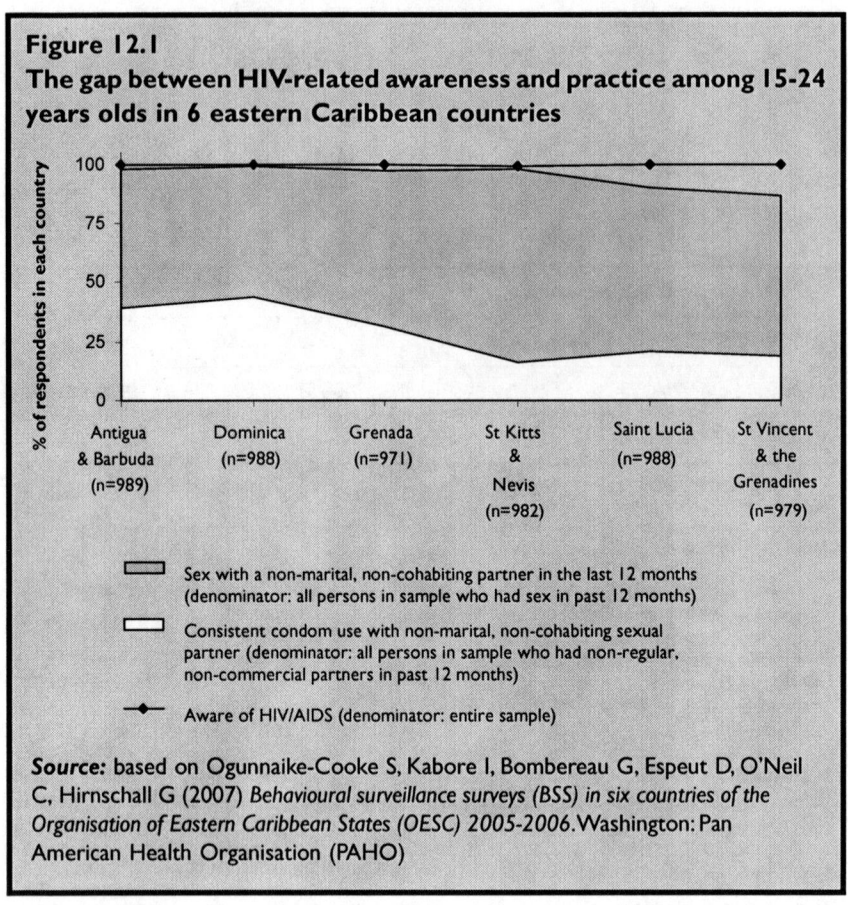

Figure 12.1

The gap between HIV-related awareness and practice among 15-24 years olds in 6 eastern Caribbean countries

Sex with a non-marital, non-cohabiting partner in the last 12 months (denominator: all persons in sample who had sex in past 12 months)

Consistent condom use with non-marital, non-cohabiting sexual partner (denominator: all persons in sample who had non-regular, non-commercial partners in past 12 months)

Aware of HIV/AIDS (denominator: entire sample)

Source: based on Ogunnaike-Cooke S, Kabore I, Bombereau G, Espeut D, O'Neil C, Hirnschall G (2007) *Behavioural surveillance surveys (BSS) in six countries of the Organisation of Eastern Caribbean States (OESC) 2005-2006.* Washington: Pan American Health Organisation (PAHO)

approach is ideally suited to the tasks of exploring poorly understood phenomena and interpreting the quantitative data (which, as we have seen, have already documented the KAP gap), to decipher social trends in relation to prevention, for unearthing explanations (for the KAP gap, and protective behaviour change reversal) and for developing more useful theory to explain our observations.

From the outset, we theorised that gender roles are playing a role in restraining HIV prevention. For this reason, we decided to approach the study primarily from a gender perspective. Interview data based on 140 interviews in eight countries, from a larger project of ours on Caribbean masculinities, were used. This project involved interviewing young men over the age of 18 years about their experiences of gender and risk while they were growing up, particularly in peer groups, family, community and school. Purposive sampling was undertaken to identify participants who were well placed to shed light on the existing data. As such, participants did more than simply give an account of their own experiences — they were also used as field observers of complex social systems and the data, therefore, captures observations of many additional participants and social systems (including villages, communities, schools and peer groups). To date interviews have been conducted in eight Caribbean countries — Anguilla, Grenada, Guyana, Jamaica, St Kitts and Nevis, Saint Lucia, St Vincent and the Grenadines, and Trinidad and Tobago. Only young Caribbean men have been interviewed for this research. The findings reported here are preliminary and further interviews in additional countries are planned for the coming year along with more detailed analyses.

WHEN VULNERABILITY AND RISK ARE 'SOCIALLY EMBEDDED' – RESULTS

The central outcome of the present study is the proposition that risk and vulnerability are deeply 'socially embedded' and that this sustains a range of unsafe practices and restrains the adoption of safer alternatives. Despite high levels of awareness and knowledge of HIV, there are complex countervailing social and cultural codes that are 'woven into the social fabric' that work against sustained protective behaviour change. The present research identified five key areas in which socially embedded codes, roles and practices reinforce risk, they are: gender roles, peer group pressures, stigma and taboo, economic power and as a paradoxical effect of religion.

Male gender roles I: risky obligations

The data from our research and that of other Caribbean researchers confirm that enacting masculinity involves internalising a wide range of expectations concerning how males should act in order to be considered appropriately gendered and sufficiently masculine. For example, Bailey and colleagues found that from an early age: 'there is the expectation that the boys will take risks while girls are encouraged to be passive (Bailey et al. 1998, 17).

This idea — the expectation that boys will take risks — is one of the key findings of the present research and applies in all countries studied to date.

The expectation that boys ought to be risk-takers has important implications for activities where risk taking has health consequences. In particular, risk-taking is directly relevant to the spread of HIV providing the expectation that males should take risks applies to sexual practice. Perhaps unsurprisingly, the link between risk taking and sexual practice has been confirmed by other researchers. In the following excerpt, Bailey and colleagues note the connection between gender role expectations and sexuality: 'By the age of 10... boys began to realise that toughness, physical strength and sexual dominance, all features of traditional masculinity, were expected of them' (Bailey et al. 1998, 53).

The linkage between social expectations of males and sexual dominance lays the foundations for HIV patterns. It also raises the possibility that the need to stop the spread of HIV might come into direct conflict with male gender expectations and therefore HIV interventions will require more than awareness and information to be effective — to be effective, the interventions will need to reshape gender roles.

Research by Chevannes and his colleagues elaborate on this point. Chevannes's work demonstrates strong links between the successful enactment of masculinity and sexual practice, and he points out that these involve more than simply adopting a heterosexual identity, it is public image that counts: 'Manhood is demonstrated by sexual prowess... it is usually measured... by the number of female sexual partners' (Brown and Chevannes 1998, 23).

Of course, the existence of 'social expectations' says nothing about how influential they are. It may be that such expectations exert little or no influence over men and/or that they are able to exercise their free will and agency to reject them. This latter possibility seems to be the premise behind many communications and prevention campaigns, which generally take a rationalist approach where information is assumed to produce change. While in some cases this may be so, we have already seen that information alone often does not correlate neatly with practice. Moreover, even though social obligations can be overridden and conformity need not be universal, the presence of widely held social expectations can nevertheless exert sufficient influence over sexual practice to shape the epidemiology of sexually transmissible diseases, including HIV.

It is also worth noting that all societies attach paramount importance to their young people achieving an appropriately gendered identity and the penalties for failing to conform can be heavy (including violence and murder). Our conclusion, therefore, is that social expectations of men as risk-takers are highly influential. In Barry Chevannes's words: 'For many men, meeting the demands of a male identity is a far greater moral imperative than the virtues of honesty and respect for property *and even life*'. [our emphasis] (Chevannes 1999, 11).

Male gender roles II: taboos on safety

The existence of expectations of how masculinity ought to be enacted implies a complementary set of expectations of what failed masculinity is. Our research found extensive evidence of these expectations which, because of their binary relationship with dominant masculinity, take the form of taboos.

In the following quote, Bailey and colleagues illustrate these expectations and the consequences of not meeting them: here toughness is considered to be definitive of 'real men', while departing from accepted standards is taboo and results in name calling and other sanctions. 'The culture demanded physical responses from boys and made toughness the hallmark of the real male. Young boys knew that if they performed outside the expected, traditional roles they would be ridiculed and labelled 'sissy' by boys and girls' (Bailey, et al. 2002, 8).

Similar observations are reported in the research of Parry (2004). First there is the expectation of how boys should behave (the obligation to be macho); second there is the expectation of how boys should not behave (the taboo of effeminacy) and third there are the sanctions imposed on those who transgress (targeting and teasing). 'Boys have a real macho image to live up to. If a boy acts in an effeminate way he will be targeted and teased by the other students' (Respondent quoted by Parry 2004, 176).

Our research data were rich with examples of how this binary system of obligation and taboo orchestrates and restrains young men's lives.

Not surprisingly, the system of gender obligation and taboo extends to sexual practice too and this has implications for HIV. As we have previously seen, having multiple female partners is a way of enhancing masculine status — something that is highly valued by young men. Conversely, the further a male strays from meeting those expectations, the more 'suspect' he becomes and the deeper the taboos are. This system of expectations works to undermine strategies that rely on abstinence and monogamy — a male is obligated to be heterosexually active and failure to do so comes at considerable social cost. Having more partners is equated with higher status and even being 'faithful' can result in loss of face: 'For males, multiple partnerships could become also a matter of status... (65). The term "one burner" applied to a faithful male in some Jamaican communities was a phrase of derision' (Bailey et al. 1998, 66).

One of the deepest masculine taboos of all is homosexuality and our research revealed that this taboo is highly influential on all men. We found that homophobia exerted a profound influence over male behaviour in a wide variety of settings – both gay and straight. Here is an example from Crichlow: 'Someone who did not have as many women as they did was "sick", "suspected as a buller"[1] or not "the average young black male."' (Crichlow 2004, 206).

The paradox exposed by the research is that homophobia does indeed exert pressure on heterosexual men to take sexual risks (Plummer 2005). Clearly the way to affirm your masculine reputation and to avoid any suggestion that you might be gay is to have multiple female partners. The implications for HIV-prevention programmes are obvious, particularly when there is also an expectation that 'real men' should also be risk-takers!

Who says so? Peer groups that's who!

Earlier it was argued that the successful enactment of masculinity entails conforming to a range of expectations. This finding raises questions about where these expectations emanate from and how they are enforced.

The present research identified a number of sources of gender expectations: parents, teachers, and society at large. However, by far the most significant factor in the lives of modern young men is the peer group. Caribbean research confirms that the peer group is a major source of gender norms and is a key enforcer of masculine codes of conduct. In Parry's take on the issue, despite the rhetoric that men act out their roles to impress women, in fact male gender roles are enacted more often than not for a male audience. The study suggested that the audience for whom 'masculinities' were enacted was primarily male (53) '… If maleness and manhood is primarily demonstrated through the approval and endorsement of other men, then its underlying concern derives from the fear of being exposed or unmasked as a fraud by other males' (Parry 2000, 54).

Notice here that a key to the enactment of masculine roles is not simply to behave like a 'real man', but to be seen to be doing so. The motivating force is the taboo of failing to be a man and being judged adversely by peers as a consequence.

It is common for many of the difficulties that young men experience to be ascribed to 'bad' parenting or schooling, but, according to our research, this view over-simplifies and risks misrepresenting the situation. It certainly is true that parenting can leave boys vulnerable to 'bad influences' (that is, the peer group) or conversely, the family can substantially buffer boys against them. But what has become clear from Caribbean research is that parents and teachers often find themselves locked in a tug-of-war with the powerful influence of the male peer group. Here is Chevannes's (1999) view: 'the peer group or the wider community or society exert influences that are not only greater than the influence of parents, but which contradict those nurtured within the family.'

So deep does the influence of the peer group run that Chevannes concludes that peer group loyalty acquires an almost sacred status and, indeed, competes with religion in the struggle to control boys' lives.

> An adolescent boy's friends exact an affinity and a loyalty as *sacred* as the bond of kinship as strong as the sentiment of *religion*. They socialise one another, the older members of the group acting as the transmitters of what passes as knowledge, invent new values and meanings [Our emphasis] (Chevannes 1999, 30).

Note the references to transmitting knowledge and inventing meanings in this excerpt. These references are an indication that peer groups have an important culture generating function. Our own research confirms that far from being passive 'sponges' of outside influences, peer groups have their own dynamic, semi-autonomous cultures, which exert enormous influence over young men's behaviours and the way the peer group impinges on the wider world.

Peer culture is passed down through generations — it neither emanates from adults nor does it require involvement of the outside adult world. Instead, it passes from older to younger peers in the street and school ground and is actively moulded and remodelled by the groups during the process. This process, which I have previously called 'rolling peer pressure' (Plummer 1999), offers insight into the interaction between commercial exploitation of youth culture and the influence of youth culture on society at large through music, clothing styles, speech patterns and so on. Peer culture generates social trends, and commercial interests 'discover' them and market them back to young people, who buy them precisely because they strike a chord. 'Rolling peer pressure' also provides an explanation for how antisocial units, such as gangs, develop and operate at arms length from adults and the law. For young men the influence of the peer group is immediate and as far as they are concerned, peer group obligations are the law.

As we have seen, males are subjected to gendered obligations and taboos and these affect their sex lives. While it is typically said that speaking about sex in the adult world is taboo, this is certainly not the case among younger peer groups, whose environment is saturated with sexual references.

Sex then was very much in the environment of the young boys and girls… they did pick up a great deal of information from observing their environment and from listening to "people", particularly the age group just older than themselves (Bailey et al. 1998, 29).

This quote too makes reference to 'rolling peer pressure' where the sexual culture is passed from older to younger peers as part of a constant flow of peer culture from generation to generation. Ultimately, it is the peer group that shapes and determines male identity and roles; it is the peer group that polices and enforces those roles, sometimes brutally; and it is the peer group that shapes male sexual practice, although this may be completely out of alignment with the seemingly remote priorities of public health (and can be at loggerheads with it).

It is the peer group that will put the final touches, so to speak, to the construction of his male identity — his anti-homosexual heterosexuality, power and control over women through control over financial and other resources, paternity, and the importance of respect (Chevannes 1999, 30).

Of course, the 'importance of respect' is not intended to imply a respect for life. On the contrary, securing 'respect' for masculine honour sometimes costs lives.

Other cases where risk is 'socially embedded': Economic power, stigma, and religion

While we found that gender roles are central to embedding HIV risk, we also found evidence that other social factors also contributed to entrenching risk: economic power, taboo and religious beliefs. It may be that these effects are secondary to gender, for example the economic effects may well be due to the way men use their wealth both as a way of affirming their gender roles and of exercising masculine power.

Economic power and the economies of risk

Money is equated with power, and money and material assets feature prominently in the gender dynamics identified in our research. As we have seen, a major priority for young men is to establish and defend their masculine reputation and a key way to 'score points' is to have numerous female sexual partners. 'Money was seen as an absolutely vital resource for a male in relationships. Much of his status was given in the equation where money was exchanged for respect, loyalty and sex' (Bailey, Branche, McGarrity and Stuart 1998, 77).

Our data reveal that young males view wealth as an important means of attracting female partners. Of course, the amount of money salted away in the bank is not the most important factor, what matters is that boys are able to display their wealth for all to see — it pays to advertise! As a result a high premium is placed on brand-name items of clothing, cars and other accessories. These *brand name* items serve a number of purposes: they are a statement of financial means because they are known to be expensive; they often consist of items such as well-known sports clothing, which symbolize masculinity; and they attest to the boy's allegiance to peer group gender norms because they conform to certain 'street styles'.

Rebellion and risk-taking are also taken as signs of successful masculinity by peers, and extra status can be gained when wealth symbols are combined with rebelliousness and used to subvert external (adult) authority. Examples from our data include wearing brand name items of clothing which technically conform to school uniform requirements and, therefore, cannot be banned but which successfully elevate the status of the wearer (e.g. black brand name sports shoes). Taboos also come into play in relation to money, and, of course, the big taboo when masculine success is staked on material wealth, is poverty.

Boys often attract rejection and teasing if they are poor, but they can regain some status by being bad (under the gender logic used by the young men in this study bad boys are 'cool' because they are considered to be more like 'real men' while good boys who are thought of as, most likely, gay). The wealth-gender nexus can be transgressed by wearing imitation brand name items that give themselves away because of variant spellings and other details. Wearing short pants is also considered a sign of insufficient masculinity: first, because graduating to long pants is seen as a rite of passage towards manhood; and second, because long pants that are too short or too tight are evidence that the boy's family cannot afford new clothes for him. According to our informants, only 'bullermen' wear tight clothing.

We find the gender binary being projected onto wealth, such that wealth is associated with masculine status and poverty is taboo. The ramifications of this relationship are far-reaching. Using wealth to procure sexual partners has implications for the quality of future relationships. The ostentatious display of costly accessories to attract multiple partners in order to bolster masculine status has implications for HIV.

A further dimension that has emerged from the project is that education is increasingly not seen as manly — on the contrary, the epitome of manhood is the physical, outdoor male. As a result, boys are leaving school early and are not reaching the educational standards they used to (their earning power is compromised). Being less well-educated, being physically oriented but being pressured to possess wealth leaves boys with very limited options: to become a successful musician or sportsman, where only an elite few make it to the top, or to engage in crime, where you can prove your manhood everyday, even if that means getting killed (albeit according to peer-based codes with your masculine honour enhanced).

A conclusion of the present research is that the simplistic notion that poverty drives the AIDS epidemic needs revisiting and unpacking. From our evidence, it appears that it is money and the way it conflates with gender that is driving HIV: men, their power and their money form the basis for risk and vulnerability of others. This evidence has been corroborated by studies elsewhere (for example see Shelton, Cassell and Adetunji, 2005). In the international context, this reformulation also makes sense: HIV prevalence is high at sites where there are concentrations of young men with significant disposable income: trucking routes, mines, logging camps and military bases. Greater wealth has also been associated with increased risk for women in some settings (Shelton, Cassell and Adetunji 2005). HIV has spread rapidly across areas that have opened up their economies (China, Eastern Europe). It is money which funds the sex industry, and buys drugs and alcohol. It is through money that masculinity can be expressed and men's reputations made.

Stigma and taboo

The Caribbean is severely affected by HIV: one in every 38 people in Trinidad and Tobago is estimated to be HIV-positive (UNAIDS 2006). Yet HIV remains largely invisible in everyday life, almost certainly because it is so deeply stigmatised. The effects of stigma are insidious, including that it hides the epidemic and facilitates denial; it disrupts vital support networks and undermines social cohesion; it wounds vulnerable people; it impairs access to care; it licenses antisocial acts against people suspected of being infected or at risk; and it undermines the political leadership needed to act constructively and humanely (Plummer and McLean 2007).

The stigma associated with HIV is more complex than simply stemming from a fear of a serious viral infection. There are two lines of evidence which support this claim: first stigma is not as heavy for other dangerous infections such as antibiotic resistant tuberculosis and certain types of influenza (e.g. avian influenza) which, unlike HIV, are readily transmitted by coughing. Second, stigma is not as heavy when HIV is acquired medically (for example) rather than through homosexual sex. Both of these cases suggest that the fear of a transmissible infection is amplified by other factors, not least of which are associations with the classes of people who are classically infected (gay men, drug users and sex workers) and the taboos associated with them (homophobia). In all of these cases, stigma helps to embed the vulnerabilities and risks that promote HIV into the social fabric to the detriment of public health.

Religion

While religion is a sensitive topic in the Caribbean, it is important for academics to engage with religion and, on occasion, to challenge it. With regard to HIV, a key issue is whether religion in the Caribbean might be helping to alleviate the effects of the HIV epidemic or aggravating it (albeit inadvertently).

In the current study there is evidence that religion does indeed contribute to intensifying HIV risks, at least in some situations. This adverse impact seems to arise in three main areas. First, different religious voices are delivering different (mixed) messages when it comes to sexual safety, some of which are more pragmatic than others; some of which strenuously oppose certain forms of prevention (such as condoms) despite the evidence for their effectiveness. Second, religion can reinforce stereotypes of dominant masculinity, which turn out to have associated sex roles that can work against HIV control as discussed earlier. Third, religion contributes to deepening HIV-related stigma, particularly sexual stigma and homophobia. Deepening HIV-related stigma pushes the epidemic further underground and makes engaging with the epidemic and effective HIV control more difficult.

There is strong preliminary evidence from our research of young gay men who feel obliged to get married for appearances sake, because of social pressure. There is also evidence that many have outside sexual partners but are not consistently taking precautions because of religious taboos about condoms (In this respect, these young men are no different from their heterosexual counterparts who are acting in a similar way, as the above survey shows). Of course, this situation would not arise if they did not feel pressured to enter unsuitable relationships in the first place. Furthermore, as we saw earlier, there is evidence that homophobia puts pressure on the sexual practices of heterosexual men too, including pressures to take multiple partners, which is a standard way of affirming manhood and of avoiding the loss-of-face that results from being labelled as 'less of a man' or as gay. The gay Trinidadian academic, Crichlow captures this double bind when he says of his adolescence:

I found a desperate assurance in my hyper-masculinity through religion, sports, aggressiveness, loudness, having many intimate women friends, and practising occupations or trades constructed as "manly" in my family and the community at large (Crichlow 2004, 190).

A final point needs to be made regarding religion. It would be a misrepresentation to suggest that Caribbean religion speaks with one voice on these issues. On the contrary, there is a wide diversity of religious opinion about HIV, which ranges from pragmatic, progressive approaches through to dogmatic, conservative ones. In my opinion, it is the political divide between conservative and progressive which is impacting on HIV strategies, sometimes adversely so and in the name of religion.

CONCLUSION: WHERE TO FROM HERE?

Gender is the engine that drives HIV, and masculinity emerges from the present study as a key force behind HIV vulnerability. Through a system of gendered obligations and taboos, masculinity entrenches a range of risky roles and behaviours which amplify the epidemic. Thus, while the Caribbean was one of the first regions where the HIV epidemic was recognized and it remains second only to Central Africa in prevalence, Caribbean prevention efforts have had less than ideal results as evidenced by the resilient gap between HIV awareness and safe practice among young Caribbean men and women (the so-called KAP gap).

Although young people are universally aware of HIV and have a high level of knowledge of how to prevent it, safe behaviours do not seem to follow readily. The present research suggests that the KAP gap persists because risk and vulnerability are deeply embedded in the 'social fabric' —— in the roles, behaviours, expectations and taboos that accompany gender, peer groups, economic power, stigma and religion. The obligations and taboos of masculinity undermine safety because society attaches high importance to all members achieving a satisfactory gender identity. Paramount in a boy's priorities is the need to prove his manhood. According to male peer-group culture, this is best achieved through risk-taking and having multiple sexual partners. Deep homophobic taboos and the stigma associated with not measuring up to peer-group expectations undermine the safety of both gay and straight men (and their partners), regardless of whether we are considering condoms, monogamy or abstinence.

The way forward, then, is to revisit the rationalist assumptions that underlie our communication and prevention strategies. Unless we engage with the ways in which risk and vulnerability are 'socially embedded' progress will always be limited. Rather than aiming for individualistic behaviour change with little reference to social context, we should be aiming for broader social change with embedded behavioural outcomes. In the case of gender this includes refashioning dominant masculinities so that sexual prowess and risk-taking are replaced with more positive qualities. In this regard, there is cause for optimism: social and historical research has shown that gender roles are in a constant state of flux and dominant masculinities have changed radically over time and vary widely across cultures.

Acknowledgements

Thanks to the Commonwealth, UNESCO, Joel Simpson and The University of the West Indies for assisting this research.

NOTE

1. 'Buller' and 'bullerman' are words used in parts of the Anglophone Caribbean to refer to male homosexuals and are often extrapolated to be used against men who are 'soft' or who do not act in stereotypical masculine ways.

REFERENCES

Bailey, W., C. Branche, G. McGarrity and S. Stuart. 1998. *Family and the Quality of Gender Relations in the Caribbean.* Mona, Jamaica: Institute of Social and Economic Research.

Bailey, W., C. Branche and A. Henry-Lee. 2002. *Gender, Contest and Conflict in the Caribbean.* Mona, Jamaica: SALISES.

Brown, J. and B. Chevannes. 1998. *Why man stay so – tie the Heifer and loose the bull: An examination of gender socialisation in the Caribbean.* Mona: University of the West Indies.

Chevannes, B. 1999. *What we sow and what we reap – problems in the cultivation of male identity in Jamaica.* Kingston, Jamaica: GraceKennedy Foundation.

Crichlow, W.E.A. 2004. 'History, (Re)Memory, Testimony and Biomythography: charting a Buller Man's Trinidadian Past'. In *Interrogating Caribbean Masculinities,* ed. R. E. Reddock, 185–222. Mona, Jamaica: University of the West Indies Press.

Kirby, D., B.A. Laris and L.Rolleri. 2005. *Impact of Sex and HIV Education Programs on Sexual Behaviors of Youth in Developing and Developed Countries.* North Carolina: Family Health International.

Ogunnaike-Cooke, S., I. Kabore, G. Bombereau, D. Espeut, C. O'Neil, and G. Hirnschall. 2007. *Behavioural Surveillance Surveys (BSS) in six countries of the Organisation of Eastern Caribbean States (OESC) 2005-2006.* Washington: Pan American Health Organisation (PAHO).

Parry, O. 2000. *Male Underachievement in High School Education.* Mona, Jamaica: Canoe Press.

———. 2004. 'Masculinities, Myths and Educational Under-achievement: Jamaica, Barbados and St Vincent & the Grenadines'. In *Interrogating Caribbean Masculinities* ed. R. E. Reddock. Mona, Jamaica: University of the West Indies.

Plummer, D. 1999. *One of the Boys: Masculinity, Homophobia and Modern Manhood.* New York: Haworth Press.

Plummer, D. and A. McLean. 2005. 'Crimes against Manhood: Homophobia as the Penalty for Betraying Hegemonic Masculinity'. In *Perspectives in Human Sexuality, eds.* G. Hawkes and J. Scott Melbourne: Oxford University Press.

———. forthcoming. 'The price of prejudice: the corrosive effect of HIV-related stigma on individuals and society'. In *Challenging HIV & AIDS: A New Role for Caribbean Education*, Kingston, eds. M. Morrissey, D. Plummer and D. Bundy. Kingston: Ian Randle Publishers.

Shelton, J. D., M.M. Cassell and J. Adetunji. 2005. 'Is Poverty or Wealth at the Root of HIV?' *The Lancet* 366:1057–58.

UNAIDS. 2006. *Report on the global AIDS epidemic.* Geneva: UNAIDS.

POLICY AND
MACRO PERSPECTIVES

CHAPTER 13

RISKING EDUCATION

Placing Young Gay, Bisexual and Other MSM in the HIV Prevention Equation

R. ANTHONY LEWIS

SETTING UP

Among the groups especially vulnerable to HIV in Jamaica are men who have sex with men (MSM). Estimates suggest that infection rates in this group are higher than those in the general population (WHO/ PAHO/UNAIDS 2006; Ministry of Health 2005, 2006 and 2008). In response to the situation, Jamaican government policy recommends that 'MSM should have the right of access to prevention knowledge, skills and services and to treatment, care and support within a non-threatening environment' (Ministry of Health 2005, 24). As noble as this goal is, much remains to be done for its achievement, as many gay, bisexual and other MSM, because of the socioeconomic conditions within which they exist, often find themselves outside of the HIV-education loop (Royes 1999). Further compounding their situation is the extreme homophobia of the Jamaican culture, which drives them underground and makes them an invisible population (Human Rights Watch 2004). This invisibility often carries over into HIV-prevention programmes, making it difficult for these men to be reached (Royes 1999). Against this background, it is important to explore how men who have sex with men, particularly the more difficult to reach subgroup of young men who have sex with men (cf. Gunter 2007), might be better integrated into HIV-prevention programming.[1]

Data from the Ministry of Health indicate that at the end of 2006, among reported AIDS cases for whom information on mode of infection was available, more than 90 per cent reported engaging in heterosexual

sexual practices. On the other hand, among the reported male AIDS cases for whom information was available, homosexual or bisexual practices were reported by 14 per cent. Cumulatively, the data also reveal that from 1980 to 2006, 71.5 per cent of reported cases have been heterosexual, with 2 per cent homosexual male and 2.8 per cent bisexual male (Ministry of Health 2006). The data point to the fact that HIV infection in Jamaica, as elsewhere in the Caribbean (CAREC 2003), is overwhelmingly the result of unprotected heterosexual sex. This fact, Royes notes, came to light at the turn of the 1990s, when the Ministry of Health observed that there was 'a growing number of AIDS cases among women and children' (1999, 6).

Muturi (2008), citing Bertrand (2004), Melkote, Muppidi and Goswami (2000) and Parker (2004), points out that over the last several years, in response to the growing HIV and AIDS crisis, many organizations have pumped millions of dollars into prevention programmes, focusing mainly on changing patterns of sexual and drug use behaviour. While some of these programmes have been geared towards marginalized groups (cf. Human Rights Watch 2004), interventions have mainly focused on demographics that reflected the changing nature of the Jamaican and wider Caribbean epidemic, viz. the heterosexual population. Thus, while MSM, the group most affected by the epidemic in the early years, have benefited from targeted HIV services (Royes 1999), responses to the disease have largely centred on the heterosexual community (cf. Ministry of Health 2006 and 2008).

ASKING A FEW QUESTIONS

The primary question that arises in this chapter is whether the heavy emphasis in policy and programming on addressing the heterosexual mode of HIV transmission has contributed to the reinforcement of conditions that fuel the spread of the virus among young gay, bisexual and other MSM. The backdrop to this issue is the view echoed by Muturi (2008), Royes (1999), Human Rights Watch (2004) and WHO/PAHO/ UNAIDS (2006), that Jamaican (and Caribbean) AIDS statistics mask the true nature of the HIV epidemic among particularly vulnerable groups, including gay, bisexual and other MSM. The dramatic rise in infection rates among heterosexuals had triggered the need for increased awareness of heterosexual risk. However, this required that HIV be dissociated from male homosexual activity, since it had led to HIV-positive people — particularly males — becoming social outcasts seen as having contracted the virus through homosexual activity (cf. Carr 2002 and 2003) This perception had the knock-on effect of preventing those most vulnerable to the disease, especially persons not engaging in (male) same-sex practices, from seeking HIV-related information and health care (Human Rights Watch 2004).

The flip side of the attempt to reverse perceptions of HIV as a 'gay disease' has been not only the increased focus on the heterosexual community but unfortunately an underestimation of the significance of data on same-sex exchanges as a mode of HIV transmission. The Ministry of Health statistics cited earlier show, for instance, the sexual practices of over 40 per cent of reported male AIDS cases in 2006 as 'unknown'. The sexual practices of almost a quarter of male AIDS cases between 1980 and 2006 also fall into this category (Ministry of Health 2006). Additionally, WHO/PAHO/UNAIDS (2006) reports for the mid-1990s have suggested that prevalence rates among groups of Jamaican gay, bisexual and other MSM ranged from a low of 30 per cent to a high of 67 per cent. The Ministry of Health's report to the United Nations General Assembly Special Session (UNGASS) (2008), though pointing to somewhat lower prevalence rates of between 25 and 30 per cent for 2006–2007, notes that there is cause for concern as these figures suggest the existence of a concentrated HIV epidemic among gay, bisexual and other MSM. It is probable, however — as Human Rights Watch (2004) points out — that given the high levels of homophobia in Jamaica, the percentage of HIV cases acquired through male-to-male sexual contact is higher than what official statistics suggest. A further question in this chapter, then, is how information about sexual and reproductive health and HIV risk is communicated to young gay, bisexual and other MSM at a point in their lives when it will make a difference.

The chapter explores the issue in three motions. The first is an examination of the conjunction of factors that contribute to masking concerns related to gay, bisexual and other MSM in HIV-prevention education. This includes the manner in which the Jamaican curriculum is policed to exclude any discourse on same-sex behaviour, typified by the ban placed on three texts that address same-sex activity and partnering. Here, the focus is on the implications of the ban on the vulnerability of young gay, bisexual and other MSM to HIV. This leads to the second move in the chapter, which is the analysis of data on MSM sexuality and HIV. The data confirm that the school is one of many social institutions through which same sex discourse is excluded from the lives of young gay, bisexual and other MSM. Finally, the case for advocacy aimed at providing a more holistic conception of sexuality and sexual risk is made following a socio-programmatic analysis of Whitman's (2004) mapping of a set of Caribbean regional initiatives. The essential ingredient of these is the use of health promotion within the education system as a conceptual framework for addressing issues such as youth vulnerability to HIV.

NO GAY VIBES IN SCHOOLS

On Wednesday, October 31, 2007, the Jamaica *Gleaner* newspaper published a story titled 'Same-sex lessons — Ministry-recommended textbook lists homosexual unions as family option'. The controversial textbook was the Caribbean Secondary Education Certificate (CSEC) level home economics text, *Home Economics: C-SEC and Beyond - Management*, by Rita Dyer and Norma Maynard. According to the report, a section of the text reads: 'When two women or two men live together in a relationship as lesbians or gays, they may be considered as a family. They may adopt children or have them through artificial insemination.' Within a day of the story's publication, the paper reported that the Ministry of Education and Youth had distanced itself from the textbook. The newspaper quoted a release from the ministry advising that it did not endorse the text by Dyer and Maynard, which it said was 'neither recommended nor approved by the ministry for use in schools.' Thus, contrary to what the original *Gleaner* headline had suggested, it seemed that the textbook had slipped into use without passing through the ministry's textbook review process.

On November 2, the *Gleaner* ran another news story, stating that the minister of education had ordered that the textbook be removed from the classroom. Following the report, the minister of education ordered an audit of textbooks approved for use in schools. In less than three weeks, another news story appeared, reporting that a second textbook had been pulled from schools. This time it was one that did in fact figure on the ministry's approved booklist. According to the *Gleaner* report on the matter on November 18, 2007, the offending text, Michael Keene's *New Steps in Religious Education for the Caribbean Book 3*, contained the statement 'Many people do find it difficult to accept that same-sex relationships are indeed normal.' The story quoted Dr Charlene Ashley, Director of Communications at the Ministry of Education, as saying that the book would no longer be distributed and that it would be replaced before the start of the next school year.

The reaction to the books mirrored that to Joseph Robinson's teacher's manual *Preparing for the Vibes in the World of Sexuality* (2000) because of its inclusion of anal intercourse in the definition of sex. According to a news report from the online news magazine *Salon.com*, a senior cleric in the Roman Catholic Archdiocese of Kingston, Monsignor Kenneth Mock Yen, expressed outrage at what he claimed was the Robinson's attempt to equate homosexuality with heterosexuality. Mock Yen remarked that such information should never be allowed into schools (*Salon.com* August 23, 2000). Similarly, the Opposition spokesman on education at the time decried the indecency of the manual, forcing the then minister of education to respond. The minister pointed out that his ministry found the presence of the manual with the kind of information it contained unhelpful to students. He withdrew permission for the text to be used in the education system as presented, stating that the Ministry of Education could not 'promote the acceptance as normal of a practice which is contrary to [Jamaica's] laws' (*Gleaner*, August 17, 2000, A3). The content of the book was later modified before being allowed to be used in the education system.

One sees in the concerns about the texts a reflection of Jamaican social and cultural anxieties over homosexuality as both subject and practice (Carr 2003; Chevannes 1993; Human Rights Watch 2004; Royes 1999). Under the former People's National Party (PNP) and the current Jamaica Labour Party (JLP) administrations, the Ministry of Education has seen it fit and necessary to police the curriculum to ensure that discourse on same-sex practices is excluded. Indeed, this is seen as part of its duty of protecting national values. Yet, this approach prevents members of the school population from receiving information that is pertinent to their understanding of HIV. Such an omission is critical since the *National HIV and AIDS Policy* envisages that schools play an important role in addressing HIV education nationally. It states that the education system has a responsibility to help incorporate reproductive and sexual health education into the 'curricula for *all* students and school personnel and [to] ensure that similar reproductive and sexual education is made accessible to youth out of school to protect them from HIV and other STIs (my emphasis)' (Ministry of Health 2005, 21). While this is necessary for young people generally, it is even more so for young gay, bisexual and other MSM, who are among those at greatest risk of HIV infection (USAID 2004). Their greater need provides a rationale for same-sex practices to be identified and named in education as a means by which they can accurately perceive their risk in relation to HIV and other STIs.

The *National HIV and AIDS Policy* laments the ill-preparedness of the education system for addressing HIV. It notes that for school-age children, 'HIV and AIDS issues have not been adequately incorporated into the formal education system' and points to the fact that despite the existence of the Health and Family Life Education curriculum and the Management Policy for HIV and AIDS in Schools, 'policy direction is needed to help educators better prepare young people as sexual beings' (Ministry of Health 2005, 4). Thus, Barrow's concern regarding 'the effectiveness of official HIV and AIDS policies based on the premise that Health and Family

Life Education (HFLE) provides the knowledge-base for behaviour change' (2007, 1) in Barbados may also hold true for Jamaica. This suggests that deliberate omissions and blind spots in relation to risk education in the curriculum need urgently to be interrogated and addressed if HIV-prevention programming is to advance.

CONTEXTUALIZING THE MSM CHALLENGE: UNPACKING HIV AND AIDS DATA AND HIV PREVENTION STRATEGIES

Another reason for the education system to urgently address issues related to gay, bisexual and other MSM has already been alluded to: that is the disproportionate impact of the virus on some groups of gay, bisexual and other MSM. This is borne out by the AIDS statistics for Jamaica. Disaggregated by sex, the data show that girls and young women between the ages of 15 and 19, and 20 and 24 years old are several times more likely to be diagnosed with AIDS than their male counterparts (Ministry of Health 2006). Of the 138 AIDS cases in the 15–19 age group, 28 are males and 110 females. In the 20–24 age group, there are 269 males and 365 females. This suggests that girls in these age groups are up to four times more likely to be HIV-positive than their male counterparts. With estimates of HIV incubation ranging between eight and 10 years (World Bank 2000), it is likely that these girls and young women could have contracted the virus from as early as 10 years of age. Analysis of their sexual networks and practices would undoubtedly reveal, as it has in other parts of the world displaying similar trends, that sex with older men as well as coercive sex are major drivers of the HIV epidemic among females in these age groups (cf. Garvey 2003). Yet, while AIDS in these cohorts predominantly impacts adolescent girls and young women, there is an almost 1:1 ratio of male to female cases in the age cohort immediately above theirs, that of 25 to 29 (704 males to 784 females). This reflects a steep jump in the number of male cases, suggesting that the rate of HIV infection among boys in their late teens and among young men increases much faster than it does among their female counterparts. The next age cohort, 30–35 year olds, reflects an even greater disparity between male and female AIDS cases: 1,108 males to 863 females (Ministry of Health 2006). That male AIDS cases relative to female AIDS cases balloon in the manner reflected in the data suggests not only the possibility but the probability of male-to-male same-sexual activities contributing to the rise in HIV infections. Additionally, the disproportionate number of total male AIDS cases and the high number of those for whom the mode of infection remains unknown are significant and worrying.

Concern for this situation is expressed in the *Caribbean Regional Strategic Framework 2002 – 2006*, which underscores the significant risk that exists for gay, bisexual and other MSM in the context of a homophobic Caribbean. While noting rising infections among women, the document points to strong indications that male-to-male sexual contact remains an important route of transmission in the Caribbean. It sums up the challenge thus:

> Given the strong homophobic culture that pervades much of the region, this mode of HIV transmission is grossly under-reported, particularly as it relates to bisexuality. The strong stigma and potential discrimination attached to homosexual and bisexual behaviour results in a reluctance to report infection through this type of contact. Approximately twenty per cent of AIDS cases among men are reported to be due to sexual contact with other men, whereas 22 per cent of cases among men are reported as "mode of transmission: unknown." Most of such "unknown" cases — 80 per cent of which are male — are probably through male-to-male sex, which would attribute more than 40 per cent of all cases among men to be a result of homo-/bi-sexual transmission. Of all heterosexual AIDS cases, men are still the majority (60%), and it is possible that a certain number of them do not report bisexual activity. In total, approximately 50 per cent of cases among men could be related to male-to-male sexual contact (2002, 4).

The *Framework* indicates clearly that despite the level of risk faced by gay, bisexual and other MSM in the Caribbean, 'very few prevention campaigns have addressed the specific issues related to homosexuality and bisexuality in the region' (6). It further notes that anti-gay stigma has led to a social context 'dominated by lack of trust and open communication, poor dissemination of information and unsafe sex practices' which impacts the wider community 'through the bridge of bisexual practices in which risk of HIV is not openly acknowledged' (6).

It is noteworthy that although all national and regional policy statements on HIV and AIDS point to the importance of addressing the needs of especially vulnerable groups such as gay, bisexual and other MSM, very little has been achieved in practical terms to reach these men. Same-sex issues have not, for instance, been integrated into mainstream HIV prevention initiatives, even if they have been given special treatment and support in outreach programmes by non-governmental organizations. Thus, in Jamaica, for instance, it has essentially been Jamaica AIDS Support for Life (JASL) that has had active outreach programmes to gay, bisexual and other MSM since its inception in 1991 (Royes 1999). Through its Targeted Interventions Department, JASL has designed activities specifically geared towards men who have sex with men, whether they identify as gay or not. The Ministry of Health remains one of the strongest financiers of the programme. Yet, the inadequacy of such efforts in comparison to the need has led the Caribbean Vulnerable Communities Coalition (CVC) to express the hope that Caribbean regional and national strategic plans would pay greater attention to the work necessary to give members of especially vulnerable populations such as the gay, bisexual and other MSM community a more central role in the fight against HIV (CVC 2005).

GAY, BISEXUAL AND OTHER MSM: UNPACKING THE DATA

In making the argument for the mainstreaming of education on same-sex risk, it is important to establish that a gap exists in the prevention information circuit. Gunter (2007) began mapping that gap through his study of the risk perception of 89 young gay, bisexual and other MSM (mean age: 21 years old). He collected data on a range of issues, including information on personal risk assessment in relation to HIV, actual and preferred sources of HIV information, as well as on sexual behaviours generally. When asked what they thought their risk of becoming infected with HIV was, 42 per cent of respondents saw themselves as being at little or no risk. Forty six per cent had rarely or never learnt about sex at school and 57 per cent had never or rarely been told about sex by their parents or guardians. More significantly, 72 per cent of respondents said they had rarely or never learnt about homosexuality in sex education at school. Of the sample, only 17 per cent reported learning about homosexuality at school sometimes or all the time. On the other hand, only 20 per cent indicated that their parents or guardians sometimes or always spoke to them about homosexuality, with 46 per cent reporting never or rarely receiving such information from parents or guardians. When asked if they would prefer to receive information on sexuality from the school, an overwhelming majority of 80 per cent said 'no' but, interestingly, 28 per cent of respondents cited guidance studies (a subject or mix of subjects involving vocational, personal development and family life issues) as a preferred source of information on life skills for young gay, bisexual and other MSM. A slight majority of 57 per cent said they would prefer to receive such information from their peers (age mates). Most respondents (63%) preferred to receive information from friends and 30 per cent expressed preference for receiving information from the media.

It is important to assess these data as responses to and indicators of the exclusion of homosexuality from public and domestic discourses on sex and sexuality. This means that the preference expressed by the subjects in the study for receiving life skills information from particular sources may reflect their views of what has been safest for them in an intolerant and hostile society. It is, therefore, noteworthy that the most strongly favoured sources of information are peers, followed by JASL (62%). On the flip side, schools (20%) and churches (14%) are least favoured. This would indicate that the young men's responses derived from and reflected the manner in which schools and churches have traditionally treated them and the issue of same-sex sexuality.

One of the conclusions that may be drawn from Gunter's research is that it studied young gay, bisexual and other MSM who were members of an existing network of friends that could support and promote HIV-prevention education. They were also familiar with and comfortable with JASL. This echoes information gleaned from Royes's study (1999), which concluded that there was a high level of knowledge of HIV and AIDS, particularly regarding protection against HIV, among young gay, bisexual and other MSM. In fact, the substantive concern of the men interviewed by Royes was how social structures such as institutional homophobia constrained their ability to act against HIV. On the other hand, the group for whom there was greatest concern was that comprising men not found in the traditional underground networks of gay, bisexual and other MSM. It is this group, 'the larger number of hidden or bisexual men spread throughout the island' (Royes 1999, 3), that are most at risk as a result of an information deficit. She argues for sensitivity and diversity training as a means of addressing the concerns of these men. She proposes that this address issues of sexuality and sexual identities and involve a number of sectors, including health care, entertainment and tourism. She suggests further that this be done as part of tertiary and in-service training to create a more empathetic and human rights aware cadre of professionals for the future (Royes 1999 and 2003).

As can be gleaned from Gunter's study (2007), the prevention information communicated to gay, bisexual and other MSM in public spaces often does not include discussions of same-sex sexual practices. The controversy over the textbooks and the safer sex manual emblematizes the structural constraints that govern the actions of young gay, bisexual and other MSM: information regarding sexual and reproductive health is oriented towards heternormativity. Thus, alternative sexual practices and identities are not only excluded from the discourse on sexuality but also from that on sexual risks. It is therefore important to assess the long-term consequences on youth of the insistence that sex serves no other appropriate function than procreation and that it belongs only within the confines of marriage. Even if this affirms the idealized value system of the existing socio-religious environment, the realities of youth suggest the need for an alternative approach that leaves room for sensitively and sensibly (re)presenting all their concerns as sexual beings (cf. Royes 1999 and 2003). It is for this reason that it is consequential for the public partners in HIV initiatives to re-examine how, in the absence of school-based information about same-sex engagements, gay, bisexual and other MSM youths, particularly those without strong peer networks, access the knowledge and skills about risk behaviour necessary to navigate the world of sex. This is particularly urgent if the country is to 'reduce HIV and AIDS-related stigma and discrimination' and 'create an enabling environment for improved access to prevention knowledge, skills, treatment, care and support' (Ministry of Health 2005).

PLACING THE ISSUES OF YOUNG GAY, BISEXUAL AND OTHER MSM ISSUES IN THE EQUATION

Whitman notes that the 'human dimension of relationships and sexuality', in tandem with strategies to shape people's positive behaviour and skills early in the life cycle, could contribute to reducing infection levels in the region. She claims further that the formal education system is the primary social institution through which HIV education can be accessed by a wide cross section of students and teachers (2004). It has been reported elsewhere that education has the greatest impact on behaviour when it occurs at a young age, reflecting 'the relative effectiveness of ensuring that a child grows up to practice good health behaviors, versus efforts to achieve behavior change among adults with established risky behaviors' (World Bank 2002, 5). Thus, the school plays (and where it does not, could play) a pivotal role in creating a framework for positive actions and behaviours in students.

The promotion of risk reduction through the education system, Whitman suggests, must be premised on the provision of assistance to students to help them work to reach their full potential. Critical to this attainment is the development of knowledge and skills to make appropriate choices. She examines three initiatives that hold some promise for stemming the spread of HIV among youth. These are the Health

Promoting School (HPS) or Focusing Resources on Effective School Health (FRESH), the Health and Family Life Education (HFLE) and the Pan-Caribbean Partnership's *Regional Strategic Framework for HIV and AIDS (2002–2006)*. In these she finds options for improving the health outcomes of school populations, including teachers.

The concept of the HPS is aimed at improving the overall wellbeing of students. Institutions adopting the model extend 'teaching beyond health knowledge and skills to take account of the school social and physical environment and to develop links with the community' (Stewart-Brown 2006, 7). Premised on a theory of public health, the idea gained early acceptance at the global level through the World Health Organization, with its Global School Health Initiative. By 2000 many governments and donors started looking at it favourably. The Caribbean Network of Health Promoting Schools came into existence in 2001 (Whitman 2004).

The HFLE has a long history in the Caribbean dating back to the 1980s. Its main aim is to empower children and youth to make appropriate life choices that will guide them into adulthood. As such, it seeks to enhance the potential of young people to grow into productive and contributing adult citizens. Among other things, it seeks to promote an understanding of the principles underlying personal and social well-being, and the development of the knowledge, skills and attitudes that result in healthy social and family life (Whitman 2004). The programme includes age-appropriate instruction in specific health areas designed to promote attitudes and values alongside knowledge and skills such as 'problem-solving, decision-making, critical and creative thinking, self-awareness, the ability to empathise, cope with emotions and to refuse and resist pressure to engage in risk behaviours' (Whitman, 12).

The third initiative mentioned by Whitman is the *Regional Strategic Framework for HIV and AIDS 2002–2006*, cited earlier, designed by the Pan-Caribbean Partnership Against HIV and AIDS (PANCAP). PANCAP advocates for HIV and AIDS issues at local governmental and international levels, coordinates the regional HIV response and mobilizes resources at the country-level to address the epidemic. The *Strategic Framework* is the place where it emphasizes its priority areas. There are seven of these areas in the 2002–2006 document. These are advocacy, policy development and legislation; care, treatment and support of people living with HIV and AIDS; prevention of HIV transmission, with a focus on young people; prevention of HIV transmission among especially vulnerable groups; prevention of mother to child transmission of HIV; strengthening national and regional response capability; and resource mobilisation (CARICOM/PANCAP 2002, 14). Of special importance are priority areas three and four, since they relate to youth and especially vulnerable groups. It means that the *Strategic Framework* can serve as a platform for examining how concerns in both communities intersect.

The three initiatives highlighted by Whitman can become an articulated framework for treating with gay, bisexual and other MSM issues in the education system. It is possible to begin at the macro level of the *Regional Strategic Framework*, then cascade down to the local school system with how and why particular questions related to the gay, bisexual and other MSM community must be addressed. Perhaps because the *Strategic Framework* exists at one remove from the local context, it speaks very plainly about the challenges and risks of same-sex sexual practices in relation to HIV. In the new *Regional Strategic Framework* 2008–2012 (2008), still in draft form at the time of writing, the issues continue to be given the same attention. According to this document, the 'current stage of the AIDS epidemic in the Caribbean, suggests that the regional epidemic will be fuelled by infections within population groups that are particularly vulnerable and more at risk to infection. Therefore, there is a need to focus efforts on these vulnerable populations.' Among these groups are MSM (5).

An important aspect of the approach offered by the second *Strategic Framework* to stem the spread of HIV at the country level is the provision of a set of public goods and services. These regional public goods and services could serve as parameters within which action in education becomes possible for young gay, bisexual and other MSM. In this regard, the HFLE curriculum is an important tool in the realisation of the anticipated change. While the CARICOM model HFLE curriculum includes an important element on sex and sexuality, it is presumed that these are understood only to relate to heterosexuality. The *Strategic Framework* provides a window of opportunity for HFLE programmes to be strengthened as part of the package of regional public goods and services. Improved HFLE programmes, it notes, could work in conjunction with other vehicles towards the implementation of regional best practice in youth prevention outreach and peer education (31). Further strengthening the cause is the encouragement in the *Strategic Framework* 'of the inclusion of representatives of the Caribbean MSM … [community] at all levels of decision-making related to HIV policy and implementation' (31). The nexus between an HFLE programme that is evidence-driven rather than religion-driven and health promotion is the next critical step in such an articulated model of engagement.

CONCLUSION

The excision of homosexuality, particularly from the education system, could serve to exacerbate the vulnerability of young gay, bisexual and other MSM, many of whom appear years later in the national AIDS statistics. Indeed, the explosion of infection in the teen years of gay, bisexual and other MSM must concern all, not just non-governmental organisations such as JASL. This suggests that the framing of the HIV and AIDS epidemics over the last two decades in terms of heterosexual vulnerability must now become more nuanced, even as concerns over reinforcing the view that HIV is a 'gay disease' continue to be addressed. What, then, is obvious, is that male-to-male sex must come out of the closet, at least in the arena of HIV-prevention education. In fact, Royes (1999) proposed a decade ago that this be integrated into prevention programmes 'including media messages, street outreach, and face to face interventions,' which she noted were likely to be most effective when 'based on an assumption that male-to-male HIV and STD transmission are always possibilities and that male-to-male-to-female transmission is a logical reality in the Jamaican social and sexual setting' (1999, 9). 'This understanding is critical for two reasons.' In the first instance, it places the question of same-sex practices in discussions about HIV. Secondly, it makes the engagement with gay, bisexual and other MSM, including those hardest to reach, a matter of course in mainstream HIV outreach programmes.

Yet, transforming the Jamaican formal education landscape into one that is more supportive of and sensitive to the concerns of young gay, bisexual and other MSM presents several challenges, the most important of which is societal antipathy towards male homosexuality. This will, of course, continue to drive the country's sex education programmes for the foreseeable future. To begin to mitigate the challenge, however, it is necessary for non-governmental organisations with experience in working with MSM issues to take the lead in translating some of the good intentions stated in many national and regional policies into concrete action. It is possible, for instance, to use the new *Strategic Framework* as a base from which to design prevention programmes that transform the HFLE curriculum into a tool that empowers young gay, bisexual and other MSM to address their sexual realities. In this way NGOs could legitimately call for and/or provide the services that this group needs. This once, the transformation must start from without the education system, using existing national and regional tools.

NOTE

I would like to thank Marvin Gunter for allowing me to use his data.

REFERENCES

Barrow, C. 2007. 'Adolescent Girls, Sexual Culture, Risk and HIV in Barbados'. Retrieved March 24, 2008, from University of the West Indies, St. Augustine: http://sta.uwi.edu/conferences/salises/papers.asp

Bertrand, J. T. 2004. 'Diffusion of Innovations and HIV/AIDS'. *Journal of Health Communication*, 9: 113–21.

Blaine, B. A. 2007. 'Jamaica, beware of homosexual backlash'. *Jamaica Observer*, May 29. Retrieved March 20, 2008, from http://www.jamaicaobserver.com/columns/html/20070528T200000-0500_123615_OBS_JAMAICA__BEWARE_OF_HOMOSEXUAL_BACKLASH.asp

Boulware, J. 2000. 'Sex belongs on the beach: Textbook accepting of homosexuality is taken out of Jamaican schools'. Retrieved March 20, 2008, from Salon.com: http://

archive.salon.com/sex/world/2000/08/23/jamaica/index.html?source=search&aim=/
sex/world

Camara, B., R. Lee, J. Gatwood, H.U. Wagner, R. Cazal-Gamelsy, R. Boisson and E.
Boisson 2003. *CAREC Surveillance Report Supplement - The Caribbean HIV/AIDS Epidemic*. Port of Spain: Caribbean Epidemiology Centre.

Caribbean Vulnerable Communities. 2005. 'Vulnerable Communities'. Retrieved March
21, 2008, from Caribbean Vulnerable Communities: http://www.cvccoalition.org/
001vulcom/index.shtml

CARICOM/PANCAP. 2002. *Caribbean Regional Strategic Framework for HIV/AIDS 2002-2006*. Georgetown.

———. 2008. *Caribbean Regional Strategic Framework for HIV/AIDS 2008-2012*.
Georgetown.

Carr, R. 2003. 'On "judgements": Poverty, sexuality-based violence and social justice in
21st Century Jamaica'. *Caribbean Journal of Social Work* 2: 71–87.

———. 2002. 'Stigma, Coping and Gender: A Study of HIV+ Jamaicans'. *Race, Gender and Class. Special Issue on The Intersection of Race, Gender & Class in Social Services and Social Welfare* 9 no. 1: 122–44.

Chevannes, B. 1993. 'Sexual Behaviour of Jamaicans: A Literature Review'. *Social and Economic Studies* 42 no.1: 1–45.

Garvey, M. 2003. *Dying to Learn: Young People, HIV and the Churches*. Christian Aid/
Fabienne Fossez.

Gunter, M. 2007. 'Challenges and Opportunities for Sexual Behaviour Change
Communication amongst Young Men (15-24) who have Sex with Men in the Kingston
Metropolitan Area'. M.A. Thesis, Caribbean Institute of Media and Communication.
Kingston.

Human Rights Watch. 2004. 'Hated to Death: Homophobia, Violence and Jamaica's
HIV/AIDS Epidemic'. *Human Rights Watch* 16, no. 6 (B). New York.

Ministry of Health, Jamaica. 2008. 'National HIV Program, Jamaica Country Progress
Report To the Secretary General of the United Nations On the United Nations General
Assembly Special Session'. Kingston.

———. 2006. 'National hiv/sti control programme Facts & Figures HIV/AIDS Epidemic
Update'. Kingston.

———. 2005. 'National HIV/AIDS Policy, Jamaica'. Kingston.

Melkote, S.R, S.R. Muppidi and D. Goswami. 2000. 'Social and economic factors in an
integrated behavioural and societal approach to communication in HIV/AIDS'. *Journal of Health Communication* 5: 17–27.

Muturi, N. 2008. 'Faith-Based initiatives in Response to HIV/AIDS in Jamaica'.
International Journal of Communication 2, 108–31.

Reid, T. 2007. 'Education Ministry pulls another book - Commissioned audit finds
controversial text'. Jamaica *Gleaner*, November 18. Retrieved March 19, 2008, from:
http://jamaicagleaner.com/gleaner/20071118/lead/lead3.html

Reid, T. 2007. 'Remove it! – Ministry orders schools to stop using controversial textbook, orders full review of approved textbooks'. Jamaica *Gleaner,* November 2. Retrieved March 18, 2008, from: http://jamaicagleaner.com/gleaner/20071102/lead/lead1.html

Reid, T. 2007. 'Same-sex lessons - Ministry-recommended textbook lists homosexual unions as family option'. Jamaica *Gleaner,* October 31. Retrieved March 18, 2007, from: http://jamaicagleaner.com/gleaner/20071031/lead/lead1.html

Royes, H. 2003. *HIV/AIDS risk mapping study of men who have sex with men in Jamaica for Jamaica HIV/AIDS Prevention and Control Project (GOJ/IBRD).* Kingston, Ministry of Health.

————. 1999. *A cultural approach to HIV / AIDS prevention and care, UNESCO / UNAIDS research project. Jamaica's experience: Country report.* Kingston: UNESCO/ UNAIDS.

Stewart-Brown, S. 2006. *What is the evidence on school health promotion in improving health or preventing disease and, specifically, what is the effectiveness of the health promoting schools approach?* Copenhagen: World Health Organisation/Health Evidence Network.

USAID. 2004. *Country Profile: Jamaica HIV/AIDS.* Retrieved March 19, 2008, from USAID.

Whitman, C. 2004. Uniting Three Initiatives on Behalf of Caribbean Youth and Educators: Health and Family Life Education and the Health Promoting School in the Context of PANCAP's Strategic Framework for HIV/AIDS. *Caribbean Quarterly* 50 no. 1: 2–30.

WHO/PAHO/UNAIDS. 2006. Epidemiological Fact Sheets on HIV/AIDS and Sexually Transmitted Infections - Jamaica.

World Bank. 2002. *Education and HIV/AIDS: A window of hope.* Washington DC.

CHAPTER 14

HIV AND AIDS, VULNERABILITY AND THE GOVERNANCE AGENDA

A Critical Perspective on Barbados

PHILIP NANTON

In the context of governance and the response to the HIV epidemic, 'vulnerability' is predominantly perceived as an outcome of a failure to avoid the virus and is a term applied to individuals and groups at risk. As a term denoting a specific process of 'managing' HIV, however, it may also serve both as an instrument of hegemony when linked to governance, and as a trigger to resistance and resilience at the societal level. These alternative perspectives on 'vulnerability' arise out of the tension between the state's response to the risk intrinsic to sexual practice as requiring some form of regulation, while simultaneously struggling with the recognition that sexual practice finds expression in a variety of ways, ranging from the conventional to transgressive eroticism. My chapter examines how these tensions and blind spots are negotiated in Barbados, a place with a relatively low incidence of HIV in the wider Caribbean region, but a number of entrenched social attitudes towards sexuality.

VULNERABILITY AND HIV GOVERNANCE IN THE BARBADOS CONTEXT

It is now commonplace that the Caribbean region is experiencing an HIV epidemic that is second only in size to that affecting sub-Saharan Africa. The characteristics of the HIV epidemic in the Caribbean, including Barbados, are clearly defined. It is predominantly sexually transmitted and heterosexual, not easily detected in the early stage, and affects the most productive members of society. A central problem in responding to the HIV epidemic is how governance should manage social change to mitigate its ravages.

Barbados has experienced what has been described by UNAIDS as a more moderate HIV epidemic than other parts of the region. Between the years 2001–2006, the average number of people diagnosed with HIV each year was 184. At the end of 2006, 1,998 people diagnosed with HIV were known to be alive (Barbados Ministry of Health 2006). However, based on an estimate of undercounting, this figure is reckoned to be less than half the total number of people living with HIV in Barbados. The implication of this, as the Ministry of Health notes, 'is that the majority of PLWHA in Barbados do not know they are infected with HIV'. Two important issues in the management of the epidemic have been the context in which it is to be managed and the effectiveness of the strategy to be pursued.

Alongside its relative prosperity and stability, since the late 1990s Barbados has been experiencing a cultural crisis which has triggered the need to reassert 'moral values'. This crisis involves a host of recurring moral panics, periodically brought to public consciousness by the press and other media. They include 'ZR van culture' (privately owned, mini-van transport for the general population, identified by ZR number plates), youth sexuality, homophobia and the spread of HIV and AIDS. In 2000, an eminent newspaper columnist noted the society was facing 'a crisis of moral values that Barbados can't afford to ignore or rationalize' (Singh 2000). Since the millennium, Barbados has established two national commissions of enquiry that focus on issues of national cohesion — the National Committee of Eminent Persons to Coordinate National Reconciliation and the National Commission on Law and Order; established in 1999. In 2006, a less formal and more widely structured National Consultation to Address Societal Issues was initiated (November 27, 2003), inspired by religious leaders and NGOs. Owen Arthur, prime minister and leader of the Barbados Labour Party for three terms of office up to January 2008, repeatedly drew attention to this moral crisis. A sense of moral panic was also expressed in the form of prophetic warnings of impending calamity and destruction of the society by local religious visionaries. In 2006, these warnings increased substantially and, on September 5, Arthur chose to entertain a number of the prophets (Morris

2006). It is within this cultural context that the HIV and AIDS epidemics have continued to rise.

Barbados has implemented what has been hailed by many local and international commentators as a successful mitigation strategy in its response to the HIV epidemic. The strategy has been effective in deploying treatment to prevent mother-to-child transmission of the HIV virus and the provision of universal access to HAART treatment for people living with HIV, resulting in a reduction of AIDS related deaths. Thirdly, it is claimed that government has provided effective leadership by instituting a centralized administrative structure and multi-sector organizational change strategy.

The country's first detected case of HIV was registered in 1984. By 1997, it was second only to The Bahamas in its incidence rate of AIDS, among 14 English-speaking countries and French dependencies in the Caribbean (Barbados Ministry of Health 2000, 14). In Barbados, some 75 per cent of cases and deaths have been concentrated in the age range 20–54. In the span of 20 years, some 1,231 people have died of associated illnesses. The Barbados Ministry of Health estimated that the total number of people who had tested positive for HIV by June 2004 was 2,873 and the total number of reported cases of AIDS was 1,789. (Barbados Ministry of Health 2005). These figures, however, underestimate the extent of the spread of the virus. An upper estimate of the spread of HIV among the Barbados population is suggested by one expert as nearer 4,000 (Walrond 2005, personal communication). The pattern of distribution of AIDS cases in Barbados registers a prominent heterosexual bias at 86 per cent, with homo/bisexual AIDS cases 6 per cent and peri-natal 8 per cent (Jacobs 2004).

In Barbados, there was a reported 34 per cent reduction in the HIV-positive numbers registered between 1998 and 2001 (177–117) and over the same period a 17 per cent reduction in AIDS-related deaths. This contrasts with a regional incidence rate of AIDS among CAREC member countries which was four times as much between 1991 and 2002 (Barbados Ministry of Health 2000). Apparent success in Barbados was linked to what UNAIDS 2006 reported as a 'balanced approach' between care and treatment, involving treatment to prevent mother-to-child transmission of HIV as well as universal access to HAART treatment for people living with HIV. The outcome in 2003 was a 42 per cent reduction in AIDS mortality.

Beyond medical care and treatment interventions, much credit was given to the centralized policy pursued by the prime minister and the organizational change process that followed. In a plethora of study reports, Barbados was lauded by international agencies for taking a leading role as an advocate of this policy approach (see for example, World Bank 2001; Ameen and Lloyd n.d.; Miller 2004). The ideology of a centralized framework was further legitimized by financial support offered to Barbados by the World Bank. Thus, in 2000 Barbados obtained a US$15.5 million soft loan which has directly contributed to the availability of drugs (World Bank 2001).

This developmental perspective, encouraged by external funds and the willingness of the state's most powerful arm (the Prime Minister's Office) to take on responsibility for directing change, has widened the net of government involvement well beyond the medical field. The strategy involves the creation of a National Commission to coordinate the response to the epidemic through a 'multi sectoral' programme across the entire society — that is, public, private and NGO sectors, including exhortation of local communities and private institutions to be part of a change process, aimed at taking action to control the spread of the virus. For example, various response programmes at youth and parish levels are coordinated by the National HIV and AIDS Commission of Barbados supported by government ministries.[1]

GOVERNMENT'S PUBLIC COLLECTIVE STRATEGY RESPONSE AND ITS LIMITATIONS

In crisis management terms, a central problem in responding to the HIV and AIDS epidemics is how vertical linkages are managed on a daily basis. In 2001, the Prime Minister's Office took responsibility from the Ministry of Health for directing the national HIV-prevention strategy.

The National HIV and AIDS Commission was made the responsibility of the minister of state in the Prime Minister's Office. Its purpose is: 'To coordinate effectively the national expanded response to reduce the incidence and spread of the epidemic in Barbados.' (Interview, director June 2005.) In practice, the Commission is also responsible for inspecting annual ministerial budgets for HIV intervention programmes, developing training programmes of HIV and AIDS awareness, coordinating and liaising with civic and ministry representatives and coordinating national programmes and special HIV-awareness weeks.

Along with the centralization of this supra-ministerial body is the employment of HIV coordinators in each government ministry and department to act as committed agents of change. Informally linked to the Commission, they are responsible in line management to ministerial coordination committees. They implement mass sensitivity training programmes among civil servants, as well as a variety of public HIV information programmes. These interventions have become part of organizational orthodoxy that international agencies now recommend. Barbados is represented as the leading exponent of this strategy in the Eastern Caribbean.

Lack of civic involvement

Organizational strategies to mitigate the effect of HIV and AIDS by exerting influence through the system of government are based on the assumption that necessary change will flow smoothly from decrees issued at the centre of power for implementation at the periphery. However, it remains vague what exactly is implied by the notion of political commitment in response to HIV. 'Top-down' social prevention strategies, as employed in Barbados, appear to assume that committed leadership from the top necessarily leads to effectively implemented practice. This assumption is questionable. Headley and Siplon have recently argued in a comparison of Barbadian and Brazilian strategies that while Barbados offers universal treatment, take-up is under-utilized (one estimate for 2004 which the authors cite was that government could be under-treating by over 1,000 patients). They conclude that in Barbados: 'Though political will and a foundation of health care as a human right has brought free antiretroviral therapy to all who need it, the wider Barbadian society has failed to take responsibility and ownership of the issues of HIV and AIDS. With no input from people infected and most affected by HIV and AIDS, the universality of Barbados' programme is compromised.' (Headley and Siplon 2006, 660).

The problem of collective ownership indicated here is, however, more complex than the authors suggest. In its 2000 HIV and AIDS Action Plan, Barbados developed a 'multi-sector approach' to the crisis. The term is not clearly defined but it appears to have at least three meanings, which are elided from time to time. One meaning involves wide representation on the country's National HIV and AIDS Commission — that is, representatives on the Commission's executive drawn from media, community-based organizations (CBOs), including people living with HIV and AIDS, faith-based organizations and civic society. The second meaning suggests the involvement of all sectors of the public service to work in their own ministries and departments to respond to the issue of HIV and AIDS and the third suggests the combined working of a number of departments to solve a particular problem or aspect of a problem associated with the virus, (for example, collaborating in or jointly funding a piece of research).

The cumulative approach suggested by these three meanings is a form of 'partnership' across government ministries and between government and civic society. In each case, however, the nature of the partnership is of importance. For example, CARE Barbados, the one exclusively PLWHA organization in the island, was formed in 1993 predominantly for welfare purposes. Its members were often homeless outcasts from their families who experienced various forms of discrimination. With a small membership (30 in 2005) it has relied on the Commission (and PAHO) for financial support and advice. In practice — lacking funds and influence — the relationship is closer to patronage and dependence, useful for welfare support but a weak base from which to offer independent comment or criticism or from which to campaign for legislative change.

Distortion of goals

Another limitation of the 'top-down' strategy is that it presents a simplistic view of how power is exercised and policy implemented in large organizations. The top-down strategy ignores the implications of a range of peripheral points of power which are significant in the operation of any government service or large organization. Where these peripheral points of power have alternative priorities, or unclear goals — coordinators complain of arbitrary appointments and of being required to undertake HIV work in addition to their full complement of work — these circumstances can be sufficient to distort even the most specific requirements. Interviews conducted by the author with coordinators revealed varying rates of HIV project completion, under-spending of HIV prevention strategy budgets and rescheduling of target outputs.

THE WALROND REPORT

How might the concept of vulnerability be applied in this context of apparently effective state intervention? One way is to identify the limits to the society's capacity for resistance and resilience. My approach traces the lines of fracture that result from the conflict or tension between the society's commitment to regulation as against harm reduction. To illustrate this tension I offer the following vignette which resulted from one attempt by the Government of Barbados to institute a process of change management in response to HIV and AIDS.

In 2004, a report was commissioned as a consultation document for the Attorney General's Office aimed at bringing about legislative change, entitled *A Report on the Legal, Ethical and Socio-Economic Issues Relevant to HIV and AIDS in Barbados* and completed in June 2004, known as 'the Walrond Report'. The philosophy of the report was to be 'reasonable and empathetic to the persons affected by HIV, eschewing judgment of lifestyle and behaviour, for in most instances those persons have had little control over what the wider society finds to be immoral or criminal.' (62) Specific action that the report recommended involved rephrasing of legislation 'to begin the process of de-stigmatizing of marginalized groups such as

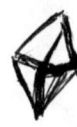
homosexuals, prostitutes and sexually active adolescents, who are at high risk for HIV infection, in order to diagnose them earlier and reduce the prevalence of HIV among them' (7).

In the context of a small conservative society the commissioning of the report by a government department was a brave and far-sighted action. Its compilation was the responsibility of a retired senior doctor with many years experience of medical practice. Begun as a confidential consultation, by the time it was completed a short version had been widely leaked. The report recommended wide-ranging legislative change to prohibit discrimination in areas of employment and service delivery in a variety of equal opportunity settings, including medical conditions. At public consultations held after the report was completed, the legislative changes that received the most public attention included the decriminalization of same-sex acts between consenting adults, the official distribution of condoms in prison, the decriminalization of prostitution, and the right to confidentiality of young people seeking medical advice from 16, the age of consent to sexual intercourse, rather than 18, the age of majority.

The report thus advocated a radical departure from existing norms. It challenged conservative opinion in the country, offered a more liberal approach to the state's regulation of sexual practices and argued for the incorporation of socially excluded groups in the interest of restricting the effects of the epidemic. The popular response to the report was hostile. Letters to newspapers and the public consultations which followed the report manifested a predominantly conservative state of opinion against the recommended changes. Other consultations with various professional and business groups were lukewarm and sometimes poorly attended. After some months, the government, caught between popular opinion in favour of the status quo and demands for liberal change, decided not to proceed with the report's recommendations.

One feature of the discussion prominent in the wake of the report was the view of homosexuality held by influential ecclesiastical leaders at the local and national level. It took the form of pronouncements made by two senior church leaders who were quick to counter any leaning towards perceived liberalism when the report was under discussion. While conservatism was

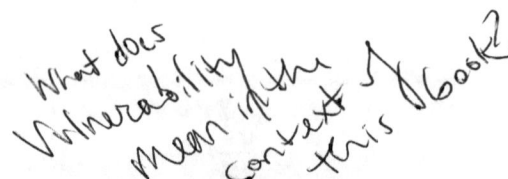

not universal, the weight of ecclesiastical opinion was with the status quo. Though one Anglican priest, a Father Carrington, was reported to observe that 'prostitution and buggery among consenting adults may be sins according to the Bible, but they should certainly not be considered as crimes (Moore 2006), this view was countered in interviews given by senior figures from two independent Pentecostal churches. The views of the leadership of these churches are important, not least because growth in their membership from small beginnings has shown a most dramatic increase in Barbados. The pattern of change in religious denominational adherence in census returns over the past 50 years indicates the consistent growth of Pentecostal denominations, from 4.8 per cent in 1960 to 18.7 per cent by 2000. (see table 14.1) This has coincided with a comparable reported decrease in church attendance (reaching 21 per cent in 2000) and a substantial decline in the once dominant Anglican denomination (from 57.6 per cent in 1960 to 28.3 per cent in 2000). Trends from the second half of the twentieth century into the twenty-first suggest that by the 2010 census, the traditionally more conservative Pentecostal adherents will have a similar proportion of adherents as the once dominant Anglican church.

The following statement by the president of the Baptist Fellowship — Pastor Vincent Wood — was therefore of some significance:

Any time a person goes against the established Laws of God, in this particular instance when God created woman for man and man for woman, when a man chooses another man as a partner the individual would have committed a crime against God. In man's sight it might not appear to be a crime, but homosexuality is an affront to God, therefore he is displeased with this behaviour. I strenuously object to Carrington's assertion that it is not a crime. It is a crime but as he rightfully said, it is also a sin. (Wood 2006).

Another church leader, a Bishop of the Bethel Pentecostal Family Church in St Lucy, expressed outspoken commitment to the idea that those who were HIV-positive were wrongdoers who had committed sin and had flouted the 'laws of nature' when he stated:

We must admit that most people who are HIV positive, they have

Table 14.1
Population by Religion: 1960, 1970, 1980, 1990 and 2000 Censuses: Barbados

	1960	%	1970	%	1980	%	1990	%	2000	%
Anglicans	133,768	57.6	124,961	53.1	96,894	39.7	81,500	33	70,705	28.3
Methodists	18,402	7.9	20,256	8.6	17,388	7.1	14,637	6	12,665	5.1
Pentecostal	11,262	4.8	14,670	6.2	18,480	7.6	31,376	12.7	46,726	18.7
Roman Catholic	6,429	2.8	9,219	3.9	10,776	4.4	10,797	4.4	10,443	4.2
Seventh Day Adventist	4,561	2.	6,174	2.6	8,511	3.5	11,134	4.5	13,726	5.5
Other	45,774	19.6	19,133	8.1	42,845	17.5	17,596	7.1	17,902	7.2
None/Not Stated	12,131	5.2	40,814	17.4	49,334	20.2	49,929	20.2	51,433	21
TOTAL	232,327	100	235,227	100	244,228	100	247,288	100	250,010	100

Sources: (i) 1960, 1970 and 1980, Table D 11, 1980 – 1981 Population Census of the Commonwealth Caribbean: Barbados Vol. 3, Preliminary Analysis of the 1980 Census, p. 35. (ii) 1990, Barbados: 1990 Population and Housing Census Vol.1, May 1, 1990 Table 02.05, Population by Sex, Age Group & Religion, pp. 144 – 145. (iii) 2000, 2000 Population and Housing Census. Vol.1, Table 02.05A, Barbados Statistical Service, Jan., 2002, pp. 34 – 37.

been caught into a trap. It is God's mercy that we have got to extend to them…But we still cannot overlook the law of nature that whenever you do wrong, the consequence you have to pay. If you stub your toe, you will bleed. (Moore 2006).

There is no space within this epistemology for the philosophical proposition of the indifference of nature.

When interviewed, Walrond recognized the extent of resistance to his report. In contrast to the widespread international agency acclaim for Barbados government policy, he observed, more soberly, that government would rather see HIV and AIDS related stigma and discrimination continue, than risk being voted against by a block of voters who oppose decriminalization of homosexuality and prostitution. Unsurprisingly, he anticipated the rejection of his report. He noted also that the rejection of condom distribution in prison where a number of HIV cases were documented 'means simply that we have moved nowhere forward in the fight against the killer disease which has infected more than 3,000 persons, nearly half of them young women.' He noted further that 'small island communities will tend to be conservative and that is why we are at greater risk'. In the context of the ecclesiastical discussion in the island he suggested, 'Any government that feels it is going to be vulnerable to the religious vote is going to shy away from this issue.' (Dear 2006)

The above case study of the report and some of the responses to it reveal that, in the context of the society's capacity for resistance and resilience, a fundamental tension in Barbados's governance response to the HIV and AIDS epidemic can be identified. This tension suggests a government caught between policy making which encourages harm reduction and policy making which favours regulation. The likelihood is that, although more lives are likely to be lost as a result of the adherence to the regulatory paradigm, regulation will dominate. Secondly, the case study highlights the problem of top-down policy making without providing scope for a sufficient groundswell of popular opinion — specifically the stimulation and recognition of sexual out-groups in the society — on which to base that policy.

The limits to vulnerability

An underlying assumption in the framing of the thesis of this collection is that advantages will flow by re-conceptualizing the analysis of HIV and AIDS in the Caribbean, from 'risk' to 'vulnerability'. Risk, with its behaviorist assumptions and its focus on incremental change, has increasingly been shown to be wanting as a dominant paradigm. A major challenge to the risk paradigm is the simple question of effectiveness, arising from its need for predictability. how do you get people to always use a condom when there is overwhelming evidence to indicate a substantial gap between knowledge and practice in this aspect of sexual behaviour? (Carter 2004) The dilemma is often complicated by the fact that lay people have substantial difficulty in explaining *why* they practise unsafe sex, often falling back on explanations such as 'it just seemed to happen' and 'the heat of the moment'.

The paradigm of risk has hitherto been an essential part of official discourse, wholeheartedly embraced by the state, the medical and caring professions. In the relatively short time of just under 30 years within which the problems of HIV and AIDS have become increasingly manifest in the Caribbean, two frameworks combining conceptual and organizational features have been used to understand their progress and to articulate a response to the spread of the virus. The first framework conceived the issue as one of health and illness of the individual; initially, the individual was the ostracized homosexual, later the focus increasingly shifted to the heterosexual working population, and especially identifiable 'risk groups', within this population. At this time — most of the 1980s and 1990s — the responsibility for a response rested, for the most part, with national ministries of health. Barbados was no exception to this early pattern in the management of the virus. An element of this reframing has sought increasingly to conceptualize the HIV epidemic as a threat to national and regional development in the Caribbean.

The second framework has shifted the focus of the problem of HIV and AIDS from an individual to a collective and national one. This developmental perspective is not necessarily in conflict with the first health ministry-based approach, as illustrated, for example, by the policy pursued in The Bahamas. However, the developmental perspective, encouraged by external funds and the willingness of the state's most powerful arm (the Prime Minister's Office) to take on the responsibility for directing change in this area, has shifted the burden of analysis well beyond the medical field into so-called 'multi-sectoral' agencies — that is, public, private, and NGO sectors, including also exhortation at the community level. This process has become for many a type of crusade. Like other crusades this one also involves a lexicon of warfare, a variety of opportunities for public dedications to the cause, as well as badges and emblems to distinguish the committed crusaders who operate at both national and local levels.

One result has been that ideologies of moralism and regulation are presented as humanitarian concerns. For example, at the national level, one manifestation of official concern is located in the ABC (abstain, be faithful or 'condomise') mantra which, when placed in the wider context of state regulation of sexuality, reveals hegemonic intentions. Those involved in the popularizing of the ABC principles invariably link them with the encouragement of voluntary counseling and testing through the ministry of health so that 'everyone' might know their HIV status. Beyond taking the appropriate blood test, those being counseled are encouraged to commit to the ABC principles. The apparent all-encompassing humanitarian concerns shown by the state are, however, circumscribed. When it comes to the selection of who the state feels it should protect from the virus and how that protection is to be provided, these concerns ring hollow, as they conveniently exclude sexual practices like buggery and homosexual out-groups. In Barbados, such practices are illegal and protection in these contexts is transformed into prosecution. As Alexander observed about The Bahamas and Trinidad and Tobago, countries with similar legislative controls, men who engage in same-sex relations and women who sell sex are 'defined as operating outside the boundaries of law and therefore poised to be disciplined and punished within it.' (Alexander 2000, 374.)

As the 'risk' framework has become increasingly recognized as a limited and tainted one, the concept of 'vulnerability' offers a potential replacement as a framework in which to locate HIV policy discourse. The concept of vulnerability in the context of HIV analysis has been presented as an outcome or a result of other practices or interventions. The 2007 UNAIDS guide to preventative practices is illustrative of this approach. *The Practical Guide for Intensifying HIV Prevention: Towards Universal Access* states that vulnerability '*results from* a range of factors that reduce the ability of individuals and communities to avoid HIV infection' (UNAIDS 2007, 4). These factors include ignorance, lack of skill, service limitations and societal norms that create or exacerbate individual and collective vulnerability. Similarly, the concept paper out of which this collection has sprung refers to vulnerability as 'a *result* of complex drivers of the epidemic'. UNAIDS has also argued that analytical provision papers need to address 'deep seated causes of vulnerability'. However, a wider framework for vulnerability can be explored.

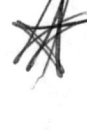

The term 'vulnerability' comes from the Latin *vulnerare*, meaning to wound. It is associated with the idea of exposure to damage, susceptibility to outside forces, lack of protection and a degree of precariousness. Inherent in vulnerability is the concept of resistance or sustainability arising from the contextual situation surrounding the hazard, as well as the concept of resilience, the capacity to adapt and respond and thus withstand the impact of a hazard. Drawing on these two elements of vulnerability, disaster management specialists utilize a systems-based framework of analysis linked to patterns of living in a society.

Specialists in disaster management define the term as combining the capacity of a society to resist a hazard with a capacity for resilience in responding to and recovering from the hazard. In disaster management terms, 'resistance' refers to the established context or patterns of governance in the society which predate the hazard but which have left an indelible mark. In the context of an analysis of sexuality, vulnerability as a lack of resistance will affect how sexual identities are formed and lived out. In the Caribbean, for example, post-colonial governments have found no reason to change colonial legislation regulating sexuality. As a result, harsh formal and informal patterns of sexual regulation continue to govern the ways in which the human condition is understood. In addition, state and church institutions reinforce simple male/female binaries, reinforce unquestioning heterosexual practices as the norm and have found a 'modus vivendi' with informal male polygyny. These conditions are so prevalent that, as recently as the1990s, critics noted how difficult it was for feminist activism to gain a foothold. Another outcome is that the start of a more public discussion on non-heterosexual orientations that has followed the HIV crisis has faced an even sterner conservatism.

Recovery or mitigation of a crisis, that is 'resilience', is claimed to be influenced by the strength or weaknesses of vertical linkages, or integration between resource holders (governments, professionals) and those lacking or having lost resources, that is, people in local communities collectively and as individuals. These relationships may operate through formal and informal networks or may be developed by local communities independently. Whether the networks are formal or informal, citizen involvement in its widest sense is considered critical to the recovery process.

It is argued that the number and range of vertical and horizontal linkages in a society determine the capacity and speed at which it is able to recover from the experience of a hazard. Researchers who have examined local recovery from natural disasters have found an important pattern to links between vertical and horizontal integration. The stronger the horizontal integration, the more effective will be the ability of vertical integration to meet local needs effectively. Neither vertical nor horizontal relationships, however, take place in a vacuum. Horizontal links from the community level to power holders can be exclusive or inclusive. Where resources are limited and there is competition for power vertical relations can be fragmented or distorted by patronage. This patronage and its effects is illustrated by the dependent relationship that has developed between the Barbados National HIV and AIDS Commission and CARE Barbados, an HIV-positive and AIDS voluntary support group.

The fact that the HIV crisis is driven by sexuality suggests specific dimensions to the hazard which requires a critique of modern sexuality and recognition of its relationship to state power. I accept Foucault's fundamental point of departure, that a critique of modern sexuality is a dispersed and de-centred field of analysis organized around multiple reference points. These de-centred points of power engage with state power, not only through conventional state structures of authority, but through language, professions and other sub-groups. This element of the discussion is also influenced by Foucault's conception of discourse, not least his recognition that the exercise of power both constrains and enables 'the will to truth', imposes boundaries on what can be known about a particular topic and shapes the style in which such claims to knowledge are articulated and subsequently communicated. Contemporary Caribbean discourse on sexuality is fragmented and can be distinguished between 'official' and 'unofficial' discourse. This distinction is important, not least because an element of the unofficial discourse involves transgressive behaviour which poses a further threat to state hegemony over sexuality. An important feature of unofficial discourse is the 'politics of desire'. Associated with notions of 'love' or pleasure, the politics of desire is characterized by instability. It is in popular consciousness a part of modern lifestyle and offers a way for its adherents to define themselves, as well as something to aspire to. Unlike the politics of risk, which stresses morality and regulation, the focus of the politics of desire incorporates pleasure-seeking and transgressive behaviour.

Some analysts argue that the politics of desire should not be represented as a simple single causative and universal element — an untainted source of sexual agency. The locations or sites of desire involve, among others, the subject, the acts, the encounter, subjectivity and passion. One site of desire, for example, is the lonely hearts and advice-seeking columns of newspapers. These are invaluable repositories of spontaneously revealed pleasure-seeking and transgressive practices.

The two frameworks of risk and desire are brought together when the search for predictability confronts aspects of sexual practice that make it enjoyable, namely elements of surprise, spontaneity, play and improvisation. These features also make it essentially unstable and thus at odds with the politics of risk's primary concern for predictability. It would appear, then, that an essential ingredient of sexual conduct and of its analysis is the recognition that it is negotiated through desire. As desire is essentially unstable and unpredictable, the challenge, then, is to analyse precisely these features in their instability. Part of that instability can involve a deconstruction of biology-based gender binaries. Judith Butler, for example, suggests that gender is more like a 'free floating artifice' and is not intrinsically linked to biology but is the performance of identity. As Catherine Waldby notes: 'Sexual practice, exactly because it involves erotic pleasure, is a potential site for...subversion or reconfiguration (of gender roles), and a correlative freeing up of their subjective implications' (271). However, in the conservative environment of Barbados, the political and administrative response to sexuality including desire (and thus eroticism) combines conservative repression with strategies of organizational fixing. These theoretical arguments and practical developments challenge the inflated claims for 'success' that inform both local and international agency perspectives on the effectiveness or otherwise of Barbados's response to the HIV epidemic. They provide a dynamic framework which can both utilize and challenge the concept of vulnerability.

In my exploration of vulnerability at the level of governance, it is apparent that it can provide a useful picture of the society's capacity to cope with and respond to the health crisis that HIV and AIDS have brought in their wake. Simultaneously, however, it is also a particularly effective tool of state and international agency hegemony for the control of sexuality in the society. In a context in which the state has claimed ownership of respectability, ultimately the systems-based framework of vulnerability accepts the hegemonic representation of the epidemic. As a result, it underplays the fragmentation and limitation of state power in negotiating legitimacy and sexual agency of those it governs.

NOTE

1. See also the independent but allied UWI HARP, UWI's HIV and AIDS Response Programme. The programme involves 'peer educators' a part of whose voluntary role is to challenge uncommitted or 'less aware' students who are considered to be potentially sexually 'at risk'. Risky behaviour may range from disloyalty to one partner, laxity in condom use or the exposure to risk by loss of inhibitions at social events involving legal or illegal substance use.

REFERENCES

Ameen A.Z. and Lloyd E. n.d. *Assessment of the National HIV/AIDS Programme of Barbados*, Caribbean Health Research Council, St. Augustine, Trinidad and Tobago.

Alexander M. Jacquie. 2000. 'Not just anybody can be a citizen: the politics of law, sexuality and post coloniality in Trinidad and Tobago and the Bahamas.' In *Cultures of Empire. A Reader. Colonizers in Britain and the Empire in the Nineteenth and Twentieth Centuries*, ed. Catherine Hall. Manchester: Manchester University Press.

Barbados Ministry of Health. 2006. Statistical Update, Bridgetown, Government Printing Office.

———. 2000. *Action Plan for a Comprehensive Programme on the Management, Prevention and Control of HIV/AIDS 2001–2006.* Bridgetown, Government Printing Office.

Butler, J. 1990. *Gender Trouble: Feminism and the Subversion of Identity.* New York: Routledge.

Carter, R. 2004. 'Report on the Secondary Schools Behavioural Survey, 2003/224, Ministry of Education Youth Affairs and Sports, Division of Youth affairs', Barbados.

Dear, K. 2006. 'AIDS Fight at Standstill', *The Nation*, June 11, 2006.

Headley, J. and P. Siplon. 2006. 'Roadblocks on the Road to Treatment: Lessons from Barbados and Brazil'. *Perspectives*, 4.4, 655–61.

Jacobs, C. 2003. Barbados: Treatment Access to Antiretroviral Therapy, Barbados, National HIV and AIDS Commission, Barbados.

Miller, B. 2004. Evaluation of the Management and Coordination of National AIDS Programmes in Countries of the OECS. Barbados, PAHO.

Moore, T. 2006. 'Priests Differ on Sin, Crime,' *The Nation*, July 24, 2006. Barbados.

Morris, R.R.. 2006. 'P.M. Flooded', *The Nation*, September 11, 2006. Barbados.

Singh, R. 2000. *Daily Nation*, January 1, 2000. Barbados.

UNAIDS. 2007. *Practical Guidelines for Intensifying HIV Prevention: Towards Universal Access.* Geneva, UNAIDS.

Waldby, C. 1995. 'Destruction: Boundary Erotics and Refigurations of the Heterosexual Male Body.' In *Sexy Bodies: The Strange Carnalities of Feminism*, eds. Elizabeth Grosz and Elspeth Probyn. New York: Routledge.

Walrond, E.R. 2004. *Report on the Legal, Ethical and Socio-Economic Issues Relevant to HIV/AIDS in Barbados: A Consultation for the Attorney-General's Office.* Bridgetown: Government Printing Office.

World Bank. 2001. Barbados HIV/AIDS Prevention and Control Project, Technical Annex, Barbados.

CHAPTER 15

HIV AND AIDS IN THE CARIBBEAN – AN ASSESSMENT OF THE RISK ENVIRONMENT

The Case of Trinidad and Tobago

ROGER MCLEAN, KARL THEODORE,
CAROLINE ALLEN, MARTIN FRANKLIN,
CHRISTINE LAPTISTE

BACKGROUND AND INTRODUCTION

The current HIV and AIDS crises continue to present unique challenges to policymakers, international experts, aid-donors and caregivers, alike, because of their reach and impact on families, communities and entire societies. The changes spawned have reconfigured long-standing social and economic structures and now threaten the very social fabric of countries.

For the countries of the English-speaking Caribbean, early advances made in the field of health led to the reduction and, in some cases, the eradication of key infectious diseases thereby significantly enhancing the quality of life. The spread of HIV and AIDS now threatens to erode these gains and, ultimately, short-circuit the development processes in many countries. The epidemics continue to be rooted predominantly among the young and productive cohorts of the population. In acknowledging this fact the paper focuses on some of the causal factors that make this group vulnerable to the disease. Central to the discussion on vulnerability, specifically as it pertains to HIV and AIDS, is the issue of the risk environment and those factors that influence this environment.

The chapter will, therefore, begins by examining a conceptual framework for assessing the vulnerability of persons infected and affected by, and at risk of HIV and AIDS in Trinidad and Tobago. This entails an assessment of the risk environment itself, looking specifically at key socio-cultural and economic drivers. The overall objective is to gain a better understanding of the dynamics driving the epidemics so as to identify ex-ante patterns about future trends.

METHODOLOGY

The chapter draws from both primary and secondary data sources. The latter involves the use of local and international documents and reports that capture the nature and trends of the HIV and AIDS epidemics. These include country reports of the National AIDS Coordinating Committee (NACC) of Trinidad and Tobago and the National Surveillance Unit of Trinidad and Tobago. With respect to the primary data collection process of the main tool is a quality of life survey which was conducted among a cross-section of the community of people living with HIV and AIDS (PLWHIV). This exercise was led by the Caribbean Health Research Council (CHRC) and done in collaboration with the Health Economics Unit of the University of the West Indies, St. Augustine campus. The quality of life survey was conducted on behalf of the Caribbean Regional Network for People Living with HIV and AIDS (CRN+). Primary data were also compiled through a number of techniques, including key informant interviews and focus group discussions with stakeholders in Trinidad and Tobago.

A BRIEF EPIDEMIOLOGICAL REVIEW

The Caribbean's epidemics vary considerably in extent and intensity with HIV prevalence ranging from three per cent in The Bahamas and Haiti and two per cent in Trinidad and Tobago, to one per cent and less in some of the islands of the Eastern Caribbean (CAREC, 2004). Trinidad and Tobago stands among those countries with the highest rates in the English-speaking Caribbean with 29,000 persons infected. The epidemic is also estimated to have claimed between 4,500 and 5,000 lives during the first 19 years of its existence (CAREC 2004, 170).

The first AIDS cases in Trinidad and Tobago were reported among homosexual men in 1983. From then to the end of the third quarter of

2007, a cumulative total of 18,378 HIV-positive cases, 5,835 AIDS cases and 3,604 deaths due to AIDS were reported to the National Surveillance Unit of the Ministry of Health (Ministry of Health 2007). The epidemic continues to be concentrated in the age group 15 to 49 years. Females also continue to be the group most at risk accounting for 45 per cent of new infections, and 70 per cent of new infections among 15–24 year olds. UNAIDS estimated the HIV prevalence rate in adult population of Trinidad and Tobago at approximately 3.2 per cent and the PLWHIV population is estimated at approximately 29,000 (Ministry of Health 2007).

The highest reports of AIDS deaths occurred between the years 1996 and 1998, numbering 256 and 254, respectively. There has since been a decrease, both in the number of reported AIDS and HIV-positive cases as well as in AIDS morbidity and mortality. From 1996 to 2004 there was a 50 per cent decrease in reported deaths due to AIDS and from 2001 to 2004 there was a 44 per cent decrease in reported AIDS cases. In fact, in 2001 there were 440 reported AIDS cases, with 418 and 246 being reported in 2003 and 2004, respectively (Ministry of Health 2004).

This trend points in large part to the significant inroads being made in the areas of treatment, care and support. More importantly, it also points to the significant number of persons living with HIV and AIDS and raises questions as to the quality of life that is being experienced by this growing pool. Addressing the issue of vulnerability, therefore, requires a look at the situation of those infected and living with the HIV disease. Before doing so, however, we will explore further the concepts of vulnerability and risk behaviour, and the linkages between them, so as to provide the contextual framework for the assessment of risk behaviour among this group.

A SOCIAL COHESION FRAMEWORK FOR ASSESSING VULNERABILITY AND THE RISK ENVIRONMENT

A risk environment is one in which the chances of disease transmission change as a result of socio-cultural, behavioural and economic factors

(Whiteside and Sunter 2000). This environment is, therefore, key in the determination of both the rate at which an epidemic is propagated and the extent of its impact at the micro and macro levels. Linked closely to this is the issue of *vvulnerability,* which measures the resilience against a shock that may result in a decline in wellbeing (World Bank 2001, 139). When applied to society at large, vulnerability describes those features that make it more or less likely that increased mortality and morbidity will adversely affect the society, or segments of it. Ultimately, it determines the extent of the 'impact' of these features (Whiteside and Sunter 2000).

There are certain social and economic characteristics which determine the nature and extent of an epidemic, whether concentrated or generalised, and therefore influence the degree of vulnerability of the society to the epidemic. These determinants are in turn closely tied to the characteristics which make the society more likely to suffer adverse consequences resulting from increased illness and death; its vulnerability. These characteristics are what Keating and Mustard (1993) refer to as their social and physical environment, which they identify as the key determinant of the health and well-being of populations. Citing the example of the tubercle bacillus virus they note that infected individuals in poorer social environments appear to be most vulnerable to expression of the disease. It is this social environment that determines what constitutes the risk environment, and in turn the 'riskiness' of the environment in which the individual lives and works.

The environment, therefore, plays a critical role in determining the coping potential of individuals and the minimizing of their risk of contracting diseases or any other social ill, as it impacts on, and determines the degree of vulnerability. The expression of any disease is, therefore, influenced by how well the individual copes with the challenges of living (Keating and Mustard 1993).

The issue of the environment is, therefore, critical to determining the extent to which perceived vulnerability will translate into preventative behaviour. The framework being discussed here postulates that an important determinant of the risk environment is the level of social cohesion that exists within the group, nation or region in question. Social cohesion is central in the determination of vulnerability as it represents the degree to which members of the community experience a sense of belonging and being cared for. Critical components of this definition are variables such as access to education, health care and social protection (IADB 2006). In addressing the issue of social cohesion in Latin America and the Caribbean the IABD (2006) identified two broad categories; the first represents the degree of socio-economic differentiation while the second category captures the level of social capital in the country.

Socio-economic differentiation speaks of distributional opportunities and includes such measures as poverty incidence (relative and absolute poverty), the Gini coefficient which captures the extent to which income is equitably distributed, the size of middle class and equality under the law (IADB 2006).

Social capital is defined as the structure of relations between and among actors in society, the focus being not on the actors themselves but on the nature of the interrelationships among them. Social capital exists in the relations among persons (de Vylder 1995). It is embodied in the skill and knowledge of an individual and captured through such measures as trust in public institutions, involvement in organizations and interpersonal trust (IADB 2006). Social capital therefore provides an environment for greater interaction and coordination among members thereby reducing opportunistic behaviour among members in a community (de Vylder 1995).

The role of social capital in achieving the goal of economic development has also been acknowledged by Sir Arthur Lewis. Acknowledging the critical role of human behaviour in determining development, Lewis linked this not to culture, but to social capital (Meier 2002). Lewis divided social capital into civil social capital and government social capital. Civil social capital relates to individual values, attitudes, norms and behaviours, while government social capital relates to rules, procedures and organizations as embedded in institutions (Meier 2002).

Social cohesion, by virtue of its facilitating role in innovation, strong institutions and building consensus, impacts significantly on the quality and sustainability of growth with social capital playing a vital role (IADB

2006). Low levels of social cohesion among individuals can distort the appraisal of costs and benefits associated with different types of behaviour, which can result in harmful choices being made by those individuals. This observation is of importance and most relevant particularly to those groups most at risk. Low levels of social capital and socio-economic differentiation are here linked to poor judgement and risky behaviour, in such a society people lose hope and are less likely to see a future in which they can invest present sacrifices. Social cohesion is therefore central in the determination of vulnerability as a negative correlation exists between the two. That is, high levels of social cohesion are likely to be reflected in low levels of vulnerability in the population and vice versa.

Gerrard et al. (1996) in their work on vulnerability and sexual behaviour explored the linkages and relationships between risk behaviour, whether manifested in terms of increased or decreased risk taking activity, and perceived vulnerability, the latter being informed by experiences in the past. Based on the recognition that risky behaviour can impact vulnerability, their work focused on a number of theories on health-protective, risk avoidance or preventative behaviour, which result from a perception of the vulnerability that is associated with a negative event. Central to these theories is what is referred to as the motivational hypothesis, which states that perceived vulnerability is a major motivational force behind preventative behaviour (Gerrard et al. 1996).

However, a number of factors and situations challenge the effectiveness of this hypothesis. These include instances of extremely menacing diseases for which there is no cure or where precautionary measures are either unavailable or perceived to be difficult to implement or sustain. In the case of HIV we are faced with a disease that has reversed gains in life expectancy and improvements in child mortality transforming the demographic profile in many countries. With between 30.6 and 36.1 million persons estimated to be living with the virus and over 6,800 persons estimated to become infected with the virus daily, the HIV and AIDS epidemics have been identified as the worst plagues in history and the most serious of infectious disease challenges to public health (UNAIDS 2007).

Additionally, the literature has shown that there are other factors that also pose challenges to the motivational hypothesis as it relates to HIV and AIDS. Two of these are mentioned here; one being an environment that is characterized by unacceptably high levels of stigma and discrimination towards PLHIV. In such an environment, those infected, as well as affected, are less likely to acknowledge their status and openly commit to preventative behaviours that may require divulging their status.

The other factor is the gender dynamic associated with the epidemic, where precautionary sexual behaviour will require a significant degree of negotiation between sexual partners and confronting deeply engrained beliefs and habits that can put woman at greater risk (Gerrard et al. 1996). This factor has, in large part, been responsible for what has been acknowledged as the 'feminization' of the epidemic over the last two decades. As Plummer (2007) points out, risk and vulnerability are socially embedded partly because of gender roles.

SURVEY BACKGROUND AND METHODOLOGY

We have thus far provided a review of the conceptual framework from which we will evaluate the links between HIV risk and vulnerability and specifically the impact of perceived vulnerability to the epidemic, as a major motivational force, on preventative behaviour. We have also identified some of the unique challenges posed by HIV and AIDS pandemic to this hypothesis. In an attempt to assess the validity of this hypothesis in the Trinidad and Tobago context, we turn to the findings of the survey on the quality of life among members of support groups for persons living with HIV and AIDS (PLHIV). Specifically, we will look at a series of socio-economic and quality of life variables within a framework of social cohesion, which can provide some insights into the degree of perceived vulnerability felt by the group. These variables will then be evaluated against the degree of risky behaviour displayed by the group which, for the purposes of this study, will be evidenced by the use or non-use of condoms at last sexual encounter.

The empirical data were drawn from a study that was coordinated and implemented by the Caribbean Health Research Council (CHRC) on the quality of life of PLHIV. The study investigated health-seeking and risk behaviours among this group across three Caribbean territories, Antigua and Barbuda, Grenada and Trinidad and Tobago. For the purposes of this chapter we will focus on the results from Trinidad and Tobago.

The respondents for this cross sectional study were drawn from non-governmental organizations (NGOs) with PLHIV membership that were affiliated to the Caribbean Regional Network of Persons Living with HIV (CRN+). Data were captured by means of a structured questionnaire with all interviews being conducted by members of the NGO support groups for PLHIV. Interviewers were involved in an extensive training session on the nature and objective of the study as well as on the administering of the instrument prior to commencement of fieldwork. A total of 321 respondents form the basis of the analysis that follows.

ANALYSIS OF SURVEY FINDINGS

Socio-economic profile

Of the total respondents, 59 per cent were female with the remaining 41 per cent being male. Just under one half of persons infected (48.6 per cent) were employed, with more male respondents being employed than their female counterparts (51.2 per cent vs. 46.3 per cent) as shown in table 15.1 below.

Table 15.1
Employment status by sex of respondent

Employment Status	Sex			Total
	Male	Female	Not stated	
Employed	51.2%	46.3%	100.0%	48.6%
Unemployed	48.8%	53.7%	.0%	51.4%
Total	100.0%	100.0%	100.0%	100.0%
Base	129	190	2	321

Additionally, as it relates to their income and living expenses, over one half of the respondents indicated that they had just enough money to live on, with sacrifices being made, while 28 per cent indicated that they did not have enough money to live on. This implies that over 78 per cent of the persons supported by these NGOs were unable to live comfortably. Linked to employment status, it was also discovered that female respondents were more likely to be living below an acceptable level than the males (86 per cent vs. 69 per cent) as shown in table 15.2.

The data indicate a significantly low degree of socio-economic differentiation among the respondents. This is evidenced by a high unemployment rate of 51.4 per cent alongside a statistic that indicates that 78 per cent of respondents are struggling financially to make ends

Table 15.2
Income level of family by sex of respondent

Income Level	Sex			Total
	Male	Female	Not stated	
Family does not have enough money to live	24.0%	30.5%	.0%	27.7%
Family has just enough money to live, but with sacrifices	45.0%	55.8%	.0%	51.1%
Family has sufficient money to live without making sacrifice	11.6%	2.6%	.0%	6.2%
Family has enough not to go without anything important	7.8%	2.6%	.0%	4.7%
Not stated	3.9%	1.1%	0%	2.2%
Prefer not to answer	6.2%	6.3%	100.0%	6.9%
Response Not Given	1.6%	1.1%	0.0%	1.2%
Total	100.0%	100.0%	100.0%	100.0%
Base	129	190	2	321

meet. In addition, the low social cohesiveness here is experienced more by females 86 per cent of whom were living below acceptable levels.

QUALITY OF LIFE PROFILE

Over 28 per cent of the respondents rated their overall quality of life as neither good nor poor, while 21.8 per cent rated the overall quality of life as poor or worse. A review of this variable on the basis of sex of respondents revealed that among the PLHIV, interviewed males rated their quality of lives higher than the female respondents. This is reflected in the significantly higher percentage of women who rated their quality of life as neither good nor poor and higher percentages among the men who rated their quality of life as good or very good. With an overall 50 per cent perceiving their lives as neither good nor poor and poor or worse, the social cohesion indicators are very low. See table 15.3 below.

As it relates to their quality of health, 24 per cent of the respondents indicated that they were not satisfied, while an additional 43.6 per cent

Table 15.3
Quality of life by sex of respondent

| Quality of Life | Sex | | | Total |
	Male	Female	Not stated	
Very poor	7.8%	4.2%	.0%	5.6%
Poor	16.3%	16.3%	.0%	16.2%
Neither good nor poor	21.7%	33.2%	.0%	28.3%
Good	40.3%	35.3%	50.0%	37.4%
Very good	10.9%	7.4%	.0%	8.7%
Don't know	.0%	2.1%	50.0%	1.6%
Not stated	.0%	.5%	.0%	.3%
Prefer not to answer	2.3%	.5%	.0%	1.2%
No Response Given	.8%	.5%	.0%	.6%
Base	129	190	2	321
Total	100.0%	100.0%	100.0%	100.0%

Table 15.4
Satisfied with health by sex of respondent

Satisfaction	Sex			Total
	Male	Female	Not stated	
Very dissatisfied	6.2%	2.6%	.0%	4.0%
Dissatisfied	23.3%	18.4%	.0%	20.2%
Neither satisfied nor dissatisfied	14.0%	22.1%	50.0%	19.0%
Satisfied	38.0%	47.9%	.0%	43.6%
Very satisfied	14.7%	7.9%	.0%	10.6%
Don't know	.0%	.0%	50.0%	.3%
Not stated	.0%	.5%	.0%	.3%
Prefer not to answer	3.1%	.0%	.0%	1.2%
No Response Given	.8%	.5%	.0%	.6%
Base	129	190	2	321
Total	100.0%	100.0%	100.0%	100.0%

were neither satisfied nor dissatisfied. Female respondents appeared to be less dissatisfied with their quality of health than their male counterparts (21 per cent vs. 29.5 per cent).

With respect to experiences as a result of their HIV status, just over 36 per cent of the respondents indicated that they were exposed to either physical or verbal abuse. While a significant 86 percent made new friends, 72 per cent experienced rejection by family, including a brother, sister or spouse. Additionally, more than 12 per cent of the group lost their job. The fact that almost one in four respondents indicated dissatisfaction with their health status, and over one-third encountering physical or verbal abuse, points to relatively low levels of the social capital component of social cohesion.

When it comes to specific emotions felt as a person living with HIV, 71 per cent identified with the community of PLHIV and indicated that they viewed HIV as another chronic disease. However, a significant

Table 15.5
Feelings about living with HIV disease

	Think About HIV and AIDS When I am Feeling Unwell	Sense of Connectedness with Other People With HIV and AIDS	Being HIV+ is an Important Part of My Sense of Self/Identity	HIV Infection is Just Like Any Other Chronic Manageable Condition	Being HIV+ is a Form of Disability	I Cry or Feel Like Crying Most of the Times	I Don't Enjoy Things the Way I Used To	Changes in My Body Due to HIV Made Me Feel Unattractive	I Never Think about HIV
	%	%	%	%	%	%	%	%	%
Strongly Agree	5.3%	29.9%	21.2%	21.8%	10.0%	11.8%	16.2%	7.2%	4.4%
Agree	22.4%	40.8%	41.4%	49.2%	23.7%	22.4%	37.7%	21.5%	11.8%
Neither Agree nor Disagree	4.0%	4.0%	6.9%	2.8%	5.0%	8.4%	6.2%	3.7%	4.7%
Disagree	46.4%	13.7%	17.8%	13.4%	45.2%	38.0%	28.0%	46.1%	52.3%
Strongly Disagree	19.0%	1.9%	7.8%	7.2%	12.1%	13.1%	8.1%	15.3%	24.6%
Don't know	.6%	6.9%	2.8%	4.0%	2.2%	.9%	.3%	2.5%	.3%
Not stated	.6%	.3%	.6%			2.2%	.3%	.6%	
Prefer not to answer	1.2%	2.2%	1.2%	.9%	1.2%	1.9%	2.2%	2.5%	1.2%
No Response Given	.3%	.3%	.3%	.6%	.6%	1.2%	.9%	.6%	.6%
Total	100.0%	100.0%	100.0%	100.0%	100.0%	100.0%	100.0%	100.0%	100.0%

proportion (33.7 per cent) of the respondents referred to HIV as a disability while some expressed feelings of sadness (34.2 per cent) and unattractiveness (28.7 per cent).

Profile of risk sexual behaviour among persons living with HIV

In evaluating risk behaviour among the group of persons living with HIV, the use of a condom at last sexual experience was assessed. While well over 53 per cent of the respondents indicated that they did use a condom at their last sexual encounter, it is worth noting that a significant 40 per cent of this group did not use a condom at their last sexual act. Female respondents were less likely to have used a condom (44.9 per cent) than males (33.6 per cent) at their last sexual contact.

The level of education plays an important role in determining the degree of risk behaviour displayed by the PLHIV population. A clear pattern emerges in table 15.7, with the more educated displaying a greater likelihood of using a condom at their last sexual encounter with condom use increasing from just under 50 per cent of the respondents who reached the primary school level to over 83 per cent for those who had reached as high as university level education.

Table 15.6
Used condom at last sex by sex of respondent

Used Condom Last Time Had Sex	Sex			Total
	Male	Female	Not stated	
Yes	57.0%	51.4%	50.0%	53.7%
No	33.6%	44.9%	50.0%	40.3%
Don't know	2.3%	.5%	.0%	1.3%
Not stated	2.3%	.5%	.0%	1.3%
Prefer not to answer	4.7%	2.7%	.0%	3.5%
Total	100.0%	100.0%	100.0%	100.0%
Base	128	185	2	315

Table 15.7
Used condom at last sex by highest level of education

Used Condom Last Time Had Sex	Highest Level of Education						
	Never went to school	Primary	Secondary	Technical/ Vocational	University	Don't know & Other Responses	Total
Yes	.0%	49.5%	49.3%	68.6%	83.3%	0.0%	53.7%
No	100.0%	44.0%	43.3%	29.4%	16.7%	66.6%	40.3%
Don't know	.0%	4.4%	.0%	.0%	.0%	.0%	1.3%
Total	100.0%	100.0%	100.0%	100.0%	100.0%	100.0%	100.0%
Base	2	91	150	51	181	3	315

Condom use at last sexual encounter was generally found to be positively correlated with the socio-economic status of the respondents in the study. Higher reported usage was found among those in the higher income classification, among those who were employed and among those who reported a higher quality of life as shown in table 15.8.

Since social cohesiveness encompasses both educational and income distribution components, the indications from the data are startling and point to the need for structured educational and economic independence programmes for the vulnerable in the society.

The HIV status of current partner was also identified as influential in determining condom use at last sexual encounter. Based on table 15.9, 76.2 per cent of the respondents whose partners were known to be HIV-negative, used a condom at their last encounter, while a far less 58 per cent engaged in protected sex if their partners were known to be also HIV-positive. A positive correlation was also noted between condom use and those respondents who identified with the community of persons living with HIV and AIDS. Stated condom use was also notably higher among those persons living with the disease and who felt and saw HIV as a disability.

Table 15.8
Use of condom at last sex by income level of family

Used Condom Last Time Had Sex	Income Level of Family							Total
	Family does not have enough money to live	Family has just enough money to live, but with sacrifices	Family has sufficient money to live without making sacrifice	Family has enough not to go without anything important	Not stated	Prefer not to answer	Response Not Given	
Yes	40.4%	58.4%	75.0%	93.3%	50.0%	28.6%	33.3%	53.7%
No	55.1%	39.8%	20.0%	6.7%	16.7%	28.6%	66.7%	40.3%
Don't know	2.2%	.6%	.0%	.0%	.0%	4.8%	.0%	1.3%
Not stated	2.2%	.0%	5.0%	.0%	16.7%	.0%	.0%	1.3%
Prefer not to answer	.0%	1.2%	.0%	.0%	16.7%	38.1%	.0%	3.5%
Total	100.0%	100.0%	100.0%	100.0%	100.0%	100.0%	100.0%	100.0%
Base	89	161	20	15	6	21	3	315

Discussion

Several factors in the risk environment heavily influence the extent to which perceived vulnerability can be translated into precautionary sexual behaviour. To validate and further investigate this relationship we drew data from the findings of the Quality of Life survey among PLHIV who are members of NGO support groups. Using condom use at last sexual encounter as the risk indicator, Chi Square tests revealed that among the factors displaying the highest level of significance, were those that determine socio-economic status, in particular the variables that captured income, employment and educational status of the group. From the tables, a clear pattern emerged with respondents in the lower income and educational status less likely to engage in precautionary sexual practices.

As it relates to other 'influencing factors', the HIV status of the respondent's partner also stood out as key in informing precautionary behaviour, the extent to which this translated to a change in behaviour is again influenced by the socio economic status of the PLHIV.

Table 15.9
Used condom at last sex by knowledge of current partner's HIV status

Used Condom Last Time Had Sex	Know Current Partner's HIV Status										Total
	Yes, HIV positive	Yes, HIV negative	Yes, but will not tell interviewer	No, I have not asked	No, s/he has not had a test	No, s/he has not told me	Don't know	Not stated	Prefer not to answer	No Response Given	
Yes	58.0%	76.2%	25.0%	53.3%	28.6%	75.0%	38.5%	42.9%	31.6%	45.5%	53.7%
No	42.0%	23.8%	50.0%	40.0%	71.4%	25.0%	61.5%	42.9%	15.8%	47.7%	40.3%
Don't know	.0%	.0%	.0%	.0%	.0%	.0%	.0%	14.3%	.0%	3.4%	1.3%
Not stated	.0%	.0%	.0%	6.7%	.0%	.0%	.0%	.0%	.0%	3.4%	1.3%
Prefer not to answer	.0%	.0%	25.0%	.0%	.0%	.0%	.0%	.0%	52.6%	.0%	3.5%
Total	100.0%	100.0%	100.0%	100.0%	100.0%	100.0%	100.0%	100.0%	100.0%	100.0%	100.0%
Base	88	63	4	15	14	4	13	7	19	88	315

While a number of quality of life markers was evaluated and shown to be significant, no clear pattern emerged as to their impact on condom use at last sexual encounter. The link between condom use and sex of respondent was also significant at the 10 per cent level, identifying it as well as a variable also worthy of assessing. Here a clear pattern has emerged which highlights a level of 'unevenness' across gender lines and across the key socio-economic indicators. This is reflected in a higher level of dissatisfaction in the quality of life expressed by women in the survey and ultimately resulting in a clear difference in adoption of precautionary sexual behaviour across gender lines.

These findings underscore a degree of inequity among a group that benefits from being in an environment that provides information and support to ensure its members can live safely with HIV. The unequal access to employment and other related opportunities and its impact on the degree of social cohesion within this group can, if not addressed, accelerate the feminization of the epidemic resulting in the possible risk of new and deadlier strains of the virus being exposed. This points to an urgent need for policy to address the social and economic needs of this group in general and specifically the gender imbalance as it relates to these indicators.

REFERENCES

Barnett, Tony and Alan Whiteside. 2000. *Guidelines for Studies of the Social and Economic Impact of HIV/AIDS*. Geneva: UNAIDS.

———. 2002. *AIDS in the Twenty-First Century: Disease and Globalization*. Basingstoke: Palgrave Macmillan.

———. 2006. *AIDS in the Twenty-First Century – Disease and Globalization*. Palgrave Macmillan, New York.

CAREC. 2004. *Status and Trends: Analysis of the Caribbean HIV-AIDS Epidemic 1982-2002*. Port of Spain: CAREC/ PAHO/ WHO.

Calvo, Cesar and Stafan Dercon. 2005. 'Measuring Individual Vulnerability'. University of Oxford, Department of Economics Discussion Paper Series. Number 229, March 2005.

Camara, Bilali, Sheldon Nicholls et al. 2001. *Modelling and Projecting the Macroeconomic Impact of HIV/AIDS in the Caribbean: The Experience of Trinidad and Tobago and Jamaica*. Port of Spain: CAREC/PAHO/WHO.

Dinkelman, Taryn, James Levinsohn and Rolang Mejelantle. 2006. 'When knowledge in not enough: HIV/AIDS information and risky behavoiur in Botswana'. National Bureau of Economic Research Working Paper Series. Working Paper 12418. http://www.nber.org/papers/w12418. Massachusetts Avenue. Cambridge, MA 02138. July 2006.

Dutta, Gautam. 2001. 'Inequality and Health'. *Two Eyes* 3, Spring. http:/home.earthlink.net/~twoeyesmagazine/issue3/health.htm

Gerrard, Meg, Frederick X. Gibbons and Brad J Bushman. 1996. 'Relation Between Perceived Vulnerability to HIV and Precautionary Sexual Behaviour'. *Psychological Bulletin* 119, no. 3: 390–409.

Hall David R. 2002. 'Risk Society and The Second Demographic Transition'. *Canadian Studies in Population* 29, no.2: 173–93.

Health Economics Unit. 2001. 'Situational and Response Analysis of HIV-AIDS in Trinidad'. University of the West Indies, St Augustine, Trinidad and Tobago, August.

Inter-American Development Bank. 2006. 'Social Cohesion in Latin America and the Caribbean'. *Analysis, Action, and Coordination*. Washington: IADB.

Keating, D and J. Fraser Mustard. 1993. *The National Forum and Family Security: Social Economic Factors and Human Development*. Toronto, Ontario: Canadian Institute for Advanced Research.

Meier, Gerald M. 2002. 'Sir Arthur Lewis and Development Economics: Fifty Years On'. In The Eastern Caribbean Central Bank (eds) *Economic Theory and Development Options for the Caribbean. The Arthur Lewis Memorial Lectures 1996-2005*. Kingston: Ian Randle Publishers.

Ministry of Health, the Republic of Trinidad and Tobago. 1992. *KAP Survey Report: Trinidad and Tobago*. Port of Spain: Ministry of Health.

Ministry of Health, the Republic of Trinidad and Tobago, National Surveillance Unit. 2004. 'HIV/AIDS Morbidity and Mortality Report'. Quarterly Report, Ministry of Health, Port of Spain.

———. 2007. 'HIV/AIDS Morbidity and Mortality Report.' Quarterly Report, Ministry of Health, Port of Spain.

Mustard, J Fraser. 1999. 'Health, health care and social cohesion'. In *Health Reform: Public Success, Private Failure,* eds Danial Drache and Perry Sullivan. UK: Routledge.

Padmore, J. and A. Jones. 2004. 'The Social Work Implications of HIV-AIDS: National Human Development Report'. Research Paper (unpublished).

Plummer, David. 2007. 'How risk and vulnerability become socially embedded: Insights into the silent gap between awareness and safety in HIV/AIDS'. UWI, mimeo.

Ratna, Jalpa and Susan B Rifkin. 2005. 'Equity, Empowerment and CHOICE: From Theory to Practice in Public Health'. Presentation made at Forum 9, Mumbai, India, September 12–16 2005. http:/globalforumhealth.org/finesupld/forum9/CD%20furum%209/papers/Rifkin%205.pdf

Republic of Trinidad and Tobago. 2007. Five-Year National HIV-AIDS Strategic Plan – – January 2003-December 2005.

Sharpe, Jacqueline and Joan Bishop. 1993. *Situation Analysis of Children in Especially Difficult Circumstances in Trinidad and Tobago*. St. Michael, Barbados: UNICEF.

Theodore, Karl. 2000. 'HIV-AIDS in the Caribbean: Economic Issues-Impact and Investment Response'. Discussion Paper Number 1, Health Economics Unit, UWI.

UNAIDS. 2007. *Report on the Global AIDS Epidemic*. UNAIDS.

———. 2006. *United National General Assembly. Republic of Trinidad and Tobago HIV/ AIDS - Country Report January 2003–December 2005*. United Nations General Assembly Special Session on HIV/AIDS.

Vylder de , S. 1995. 'Sustainable Human Development and Macroeconomics: Strategic Links and Implications'. A UNDP Discussion Paper. UNDP. Washington.

Whiteside, Alan and Clem Sunter. 2000. *AIDS: The Challenge for South Africa*. Johannesburg, South Africa: Human and Rousseau.

Wilkinson, R.G. 1999. 'Income Inequity, Social Cohesion and Health: Clarifying the Theory. A Reply to Muntaner and Lynch'. *International Journal of Health Services* 29, no. 3: 525–43.

World Bank, The. 2001. *World Development Report 2002/2001. Attacking Poverty*, New York: Oxford University Press.

Contributors

Caroline Allen is health research scientist at the Caribbean Health Research Council (CHRC) in Trinidad and Tobago. She is a social scientist who has published widely on HIV and AIDS in the Caribbean and East Africa.

Rose-Marie Antoine is professor of Labour Law and Offshore Financial Law, Faculty of Law, University of the West Indies, Barbados. She publishes mainly in the area of labour law, including discrimination in employment, offshore financial law and laws and legal systems.

Christine Barrow is professorial fellow, Sir Arthur Lewis Institute of Social and Economic Studies (SALISES), University of the West Indies, Barbados, and campus chair, UWI HARP, University of the West Indies, Barbados. Her research focuses on social development in the Caribbean with emphasis on family, gender, child rights, HIV and vulnerability.

Marjan de Bruin is Director and Senior Lecturer at the Caribbean Institute of Media and Communication (CARIMAC) and Deputy Chair of UWI HARP, both located at the University of the West Indies, Mona, Jamaica. Her research areas are: communication for social and behaviour change, and media violence and its effects on children. She leads the working group Communication and HIV of the International Association of Media and Communication Research (IAMCR).

Robert Carr is Senior Lecturer and Coordinator Graduate Programme Unit, Caribbean Institute of Media and Communication (CARIMAC), University of the West Indies, Jamaica, and Executive Director, Caribbean Vulnerable Communities Coalition (CVC). His work focuses on human rights for women and other marginalized groups in the Caribbean context, as well as globally.

Marcus Day is Director, Caribbean Drug and Alcohol Research Institute, Saint Lucia. Caribbean Harm Reduction Coalition. He researches and writes on issues surrounding access and utilization of primary health care (including HIV care and treatment) of indigent crack cocaine users in the Caribbean.

Martin Franklin is a Lecturer in the Department of Economics, University of the West Indies, St. Augustine, Trinidad and Tobago. He has undertaken research in HIV and AIDS in Trinidad and Tobago, and other related topics including aging, poverty reduction, remittances and development.

Andil Gosine is Assistant Professor, Department of Sociology, York University, Toronto. His research considers the collaborated production of sexuality with 'race', gender and class in various contexts, including international development and environmentalism.

Kamala Kempadoo is Director, Graduate Programme in Social and Political Thought, and Associate Professor, Division of Social Sciences, York University, Toronto. Her research emphasizes sexual labour and sexual-economic relations, gender and race in global development, and transnational feminism.

Christine Laptiste is Lecturer in the Department of Economics and a Senior Researcher at the Health Economics Unit, University of the West Indies, St. Augustine, Trinidad and Tobago. Her research interest is in Health Economics with an emphasis on the costing of health services, equity and poverty.

R. Anthony Lewis is a Lecturer in French and Communications at the University of Technology, Jamaica where he also heads the Foreign Languages Division. He studies and writes on language ideology, creolisation and translation as well as HIV and vulnerability. He is one of the directors of the Caribbean Vulnerable Communities Coalition (CVC).

Roger McLean is Lecturer, Department of Economics, University of the West Indies, St. Augustine Campus, Trinidad and Tobago and Health Economist attached to the Health Economics Unit (HEU) at that campus. He has conducted research in the area of development economics, specifically health economics.

David A.B. Murray is Associate Professor of Anthropology at York University, Toronto. His research focuses on the politics of sexual identities and the state, currently on homophobia and changing sexual moralities in Barbados.

Philip Nanton is an occasional Lecturer in Cultural Studies at University of the West Indies, Cave Hill and formerly Project Officer, UWIHARP, University of the West Indies, Barbados. He has written widely on Caribbean Social Policy and Culture.

David Plummer is the former Commonwealth/UNESCO Caribbean Professor in Education (HIV Health Promotion). He is based at the School of Education, the University of the West Indies, Trinidad and Tobago. His research is in gender, sexual health, marginalization and health, and stigma and discrimination. He is a member of the UNAIDS Global Reference Group on HIV Prevention and has worked in HIV in Australia, the Asia-Pacific Region and the Caribbean.

Tracy Robinson is a Senior Lecturer in the Faculty of Law, University of the West Indies, Barbados where she researches and teaches in the areas of family law, constitutional law, Commonwealth Caribbean human rights law, and gender and the law.

Karl Theodore is the Coordinator of the Health Economics Unit (HEU) at the University of the West Indies and Professor of Economics in the Department of Economics on the St. Augustine campus. Under his leadership the HEU has conducted research on estimating the economic impact of HIV and AIDS, and the cost of responding to the epidemics at the individual, sector and country level for a number of Caribbean territories.

Robin Vincent is Senior Adviser, HIV and AIDS programme at Panos London. His current work focuses on the communication dynamics of HIV and other social movements, complex systems theory and social change, and facilitating learning forums on good practice and innovation in HIV communication.

Gloria Wekker is Professor of Gender and Ethnicity, Department of Gender Studies, Faculty of the Arts, and Director of Expertise Center GEM (Gender, Ethnicity and Multiculturality) in Higher Education, Utrecht University, The Netherlands. Her research engages with constructions of Afro-Surinamese and black diasporic female sexual subjectivity; and with gendered and ethnicized knowledge systems in the Dutch academy and multicultural society.

INDEX

ABC approach: to HIV prevention, xix, 289–290

Accommodation: HIV and the principle of, 53–54

Adolescent boys: AIDS among Jamaican, 265–267; and peer pressure, 247–249

Adolescent girls: AIDS among Jamaican, 265–267; vulnerability of, xxvii, 215–234; sexuality of, 223–231

Africa: response to AIDS, 168–169; and CFSC, 170

African diaspora: sexuality in the, 198–200

Afro-Surinamese women: sexual culture of, 192–211

AIDS: in Barbados, 278, 279–280; communication strategies and theories to prevent, 136–148, 153–173, 216–218; difference between HIV and,72–75; drug use and, 24, 28–31; feminization of, 216; global response to, xix, 95–97, 167–169, 171–172; and governance, 277–293; MSM and, 98–99, 104–106; social dimensions of, 154–161, 164–167

AIDS Alliance International Report: *Between Men*, 107; in Barbados, 117–127

AIDS and the Ecology of Poverty: Eileen Stillwagon on, 164–165

Alexander, M. Jacqui: critique of the T&T Sexual Offences Act, 3; on heteropatriarchy, 98

Allen, Caroline, 314

Alleyne, Sir George: preface by, xi–xiii

American Anthropological Association (AAA): and sexuality research, 195

Anal sex: Caribbean law and, 14–15, 123–125; rape and, 16

Anti-discrimination legislation: PLWHIV and, 51–58, 60–62. *See also* Unfair dismissal legislation

Antigua and Barbuda: Offences Against the Person Act 1840, 6

Antoine, Rosemarie, 314

Aputku: in Afro-Surinamese culture, 198

Arthur, Prime Minister Owen: and Barbados's cultural crisis, 278–279

Autonomy: and sexuality, 3

Bahamas, The: child prostitution in, 47-48; cocaine and HIV infection in, 29-30, 130

Bahamas Sexual Offences and Domestic Violence Act 1991, The, 3–4, 13–14, 16

Barbados: governance of HIV and AIDS, 277–293; HIV education in, 280–283; HIV rates in, 278, 279–280; MSM in, 125–127, 128; National HIV and AIDS Commission, 117, 281, 282, 291; National Strategic Plan and HIV, 141–142, 143–144; vulnerability of adolescent girls in, xxvii, 215–234

Barbados Family Law Act: marriage and, 10; Industrial Relations Code of Practice, 49; Sexual Offences Act 1992, 13, 14

Barbados Plan of Action: and drug use in the Caribbean, 25

Barrow, Christine, 314

Bashment: femininity and adolescent girls, 221–223, 231–233

Behaviour change communication (BCCC): and HIV, 139–141, 143–145

Behaviour Surveillance Survey (BSS): in Jamaica 199/2000, 132–133

Belize: buggery in, 12

Belize Criminal Code 2001: sexual offences and the, 17

Benoit: on homosexuality, 108

Bermuda: homophobia in, 101

Best, Robert: on sex workers, 84–85

Between Men, 107

Biomedical approach: in HIV prevention, xx; in sexuality, 182–184

de Bruin, Marjan, 314

Buggery: Caribbean law and, 6, 12–17, 99, 120

CARE Barbados: and PLWHA, 282, 291

Caribbean: and drug control, 33, 34; drug use in the, 24–27, 28–31; governance and social exclusion, 77–89, 277–293; HIV infection in the, 27–28, 72–74, 130–149, 260–262, 296–297; homophobia in the, 99–103, 119–120; KAP gap in the xxviii, 72–74, 132–134, 182–183, 218–219, 239–243; response to HIV prevention, xvii–xxii, xxi, xxii, xxviii, 97–98; response to MSM, 1004–106; rights and freedoms in the, 76–78; sexual abuse of girls in the, 217; sexual offences legislation, 3–21; sexuality studies, 179–188; vulnerabilities, 74–76

Caribbean Epidemiology Centre: report on HIV, 122–123

Caribbean Health Research Council (CRHC), 296

Caribbean Network of Health Promoting Schools, 271

Caribbean Regional Network for PLWHIV and AIDS, 296

Caribbean Regional Strategic Framework: and HIV and AIDS, 142, 266–267

Caribbean Vulnerable Communities Coalition (CVC), 267

CARICOM: and the free movement of labour, 63–64; and gender equality, 8–9

Carr, Robert, 314

Centres for Disease Control (CDC): and HIV prevention, 73

Chalk v USDC: and PLWHIV, 45–46

Chevannes, Barry: HIV research, 134

Child prostitution: in The Bahamas, 47–48

Chin, Lascelles: on regularizing sex work, 86–87

Church: and sexuality, 78–79, 101–103; and the Walrond Report, 285–286. *See also* Religion

Class: HIV and, 47–48

Cocaine: and HIV infection, 28–32; trafficking, 25–27, 28

Cohabitation Relationships Act: T&T, 10–11

Common-law unions: law and, 8, 12

Communication: and community, 80–87; defining, xxiv–xxv, 140, 142–145; gender and, 159–161; and HIV prevention, xxv–xxvi, 130–148, 216–218; theories on HIV prevention, 147–148

Communications for Social Change (CFSC), 155–157, 169–171

Communications Framework for HIV and AIDS, 137–138, 155–157

Compulsory testing: and HIV, 66–67

Concubinage: law and, 8

Condom use: adolescent girls and, 228–231; and HIV prevention, xvii, xix, 72; issues influencing, 135–136; in Jamaica, 132; in the OECS, 133; among PLWHIV in T&T, 308

Conjugality: definition of, 10–11, 12

Constitution: and protection of PLWHIV, 58–60

Creole elite: and state power, 77–79

Criminal Code of Barbados, 120, 127–128

Criminal Code 2004: Saint Lucia, 14–15

Cuba: HIV rates in, 130; treatment of PLWHIV in, xviii

D v UK, 65

Day, Marcus, 315

Department for International Development (DFID): and HIV communication strategies, 139

Discrimination: combating, 157–162; homosexuality and, 121–123; against PLWHIV, 50–60

Dismissal: PLWHIV and unfair, 60–62

Domestic Violence Act 1999: T&T, 11

Domestic violence laws: Caribbean, 8

Dominica Sexual Offences Act 1998: rape and the, 9

Dominican Republic: HIV rates in, 130;

Drug control conventions: international, 32–35

Drug users: human rights and, xxii, 23–31

Economic power: and risk, 250–252

Education: MSM and HIV prevention, 259–274; and risk

behaviour among PLWHIV in T&T, 307–308

Employment: and anti-discrimination legislation, 51; PLWHIV and, 39–52

Employment Act 2001: The Bahamas, 49

Employment contracts: PLWHIV and, 62–63

Empowerment: of adolescent girls, 231–234

Enslaved See Slavery

Environment: vulnerability and, 299–301

Equal Opportunities Act 2000: T&T, 17

Equality: of treatment and the law, 45–46

Equality of Opportunity and Treatment in Employment and Occupation Act 2000: Saint Lucia, 51

Erotic autonomy: and gender equality, 16; and human rights, 3–6; 98

Ethiopia: CFSC and HIV and AIDS in, 156

Europe: and drug control, 33

European Convention on Human Rights, 65

Family law: marriage and, 10; reform, 4, 11, 12, 19

Family patterns: during slavery, 201–203, 205–206

Fear and myths: surrounding HIV, 52–53

Femininity: normative, 220–223, 231–233

Feminist movement: Caribbean, 18

Fidelity: adolescent girls and, 227–228

Focussing Resources on Effective School Health (FRESH): and risk education, 270–271

Franklin, Martin, 315

Free movement of workers: and HIV, 63–64

FreeForum, 106

Freedom: in Caribbean context, 76–78

Gay: identity, 111–112, 125–127

Gay cruises: Caribbean reaction to, 101–103

Gender: defining, 17–19; and economies of risk, 250–253; and Human rights, xxiii, 44–45; roles and risk, 243–249; and sexuality, xix–xx, 181–182, 204–206

Gender discrimination: ILO and, 54–55

Gender inequity: and HIV, 153, 159–161; law and, xxiii, 8–9,

18; and poverty, 47–48; and vulnerability of adolescent girl in Barbados, 215–234

Gender neutral: rape laws, 9, 14

Girard and the St Lucia Teachers Union v. A.G., 44, 59

Girls: influences on sexual behaviour of, 134–135

Gleaner: Debate on regularization of sex work, 86–87

Global School Health Initiative, 271

Gosine, Andile, 315

Governance: and HIV and AIDS, 277–293; social exclusion and models of Caribbean, 77–89

Gross indecency: and law, 6, 14, 15

Guyana: HIV rates in, 130; law and sexual behaviour in, 6; Prevention of Discrimination Act 1997, 51; SASOD in, 101

Haiti: HIV rates in, 130

Health: social patterns and public, 163–164

Health and Family Life Education: and HIV and AIDS education, 264–265, 271, 272–273

Health Economics Unit, UWI, 296

Health Promoting School (HPS): and risk education, 270–271

Health systems. *See* Public health

Heteronationalism: defining, 98, 111

Heteropatriarchy: defining, 98

Heterosexual population: and HIV, 260, 251

HIV: in Barbados, 117–127, 216–218; in the Caribbean, 27–28, 72–74, 130–149; communication strategies and theories, 136–141, 146, 153–172; and crack cocaine, 27–28, 29–31; difference between AIDS and, 72–75; and gender, 153, 159–161; and governance, 277–293; in Jamaica, 260–275; and MSM, 97–112; and risk, 38; social dimensions of, 154–161, 164–167; and sexual orientation, 57–58; at the workplace, 39–40

HIV policy: heteronormative framework of, 119

HIV prevention: ABC approach to, xix, 289–290; communication and, 136–148; and condom use, xvii, xix, 72; education and MSM, 259–275; and gender inequality, 215–233; and sexual behaviour, 131–134

HIV transmission: in the Caribbean, 130–131, 182–183, 185, 260–262; interpreting, xvii, 122–123

Hoffman v SA Airways, 53

Ho Lung, Father Richard: and the regularization of sex work, 87, 88

Home Economics: C-SEC and Beyond – Management, 262–262

Homophobia: in the Caribbean, 99–103, 119–120

Homosexuality: in Barbados, 119–127; Caribbean law and the, 4–5, 6, 121–123; in Jamaica, 259-275; lack of education on, 268–270

Homosexual sex: criminalization of, 12, 14, 123–124

Human rights: erotic autonomy and, 3–6; gender and, xxiii; HIV and, 40–47; homosexuals and, 125–127; state and, 89; war on drugs and lack of, 32–33

'I Am a Gold Coin', 196–197, 205

Identity: Afro-Surinamese culture and, 197–198; sexuality and, 3

Industrial Relations Code of Practice: Barbados, 49

International Centre for Research on Women (ICRW): initiatives to combat stigma and discrimination, 158

International Covenant on Civil and Political Rights (ICCPR), 34

International health organisations: and AIDS, 117–118, 139–141, 260

International Labour Organisation (ILO): and gender discrimination, 54–55; human rights at the workplace, 40–41;

Jamaica: HIV in, 260–275; homophobia in, 98–99, 259; KAPB study (2004), 132; MSM in, 259–274; National Strategic Plan, 141–142, 143, 144; policy on HIV and AIDS, 264–256

Jamaica AIDS Support for Life (JASL): and risk education, 267, 268, 269, 273–274

Joint United Nations Programme on HIV/AIDS, 72–73

Judicial review: and protection of PLWHIV, 59–60

KAP Gap: HIV and the, xxviii, 72–74, 132–134, 182–183, 218–219, 239–243

Kempadoo, Kamala, 315

Labour Code of Saint Lucia: and HIV, 49

laptiste, 315

Law: and drug abusers, xxiii; employment and anti-

discrimination,51–58; gender equality and, xxiii, 8–9, 18; and HIV,39–50; and rights of PLWHIV, 40-47; and sexuality, 3–6, 13–21, 120, 290–291

Lewis, Anthony R., 315

Long, Scott: on homophobia in Jamaica, 100

Love: and adolescent sexuality, 223–224

Males: HIV infection among Jamaican. 265–267

Male gender: and peer pressure, 247–254; and risk, 243–246

Marginalized groups: HIV and, 73–90. See also Social exclusion

Marital rape: definition of, 9–10

Marriage: in Afro-Surinamese culture, 206–209; and law and, 7–8; during slavery, 201–209

Masculinity; and peer pressure, 247–254; and risk, 243–246

Mati work: sexual culture of, 193

McLean, Roger, 316

Media: and community, 81–87; homophobia in the, 119–120

Men who have sex with men (MSM): in Barbados, 125–126, 127; HIV prevention and, xxv, 259–273; vulnerability of, xxviii, 97–98, 259–274, 259–260, 267–270, 273–274

Messam, Van: on homophobia in Jamaica, 100, 102

Migration: and PLWHIV, 63–66

Ministry of Education and Youth (Jamaica): and alternative family units, 262–265

Ministry of Health (Jamaica): data on HIV and AIDS rates, 259–261

Morality: human rights and, 43–45; regulating, xxiv, 289

Mother to child transmission (MTC): HIV and, 130; rates in Barbados, 216

Mothers: and daughters' sexuality, 221

Mottley, Mia: on HIV and discrimination in Barbados, 121–123, 126

'MSM No Political Agenda', 106–112

Multiple partnerships: adolescent girls and, 227–228; and HIV, 136

Munoz-Laboy: research on MSM, 110

Murray, David, 316

Myths: surrounding HIV, 52–53

Nanton, Phillip, 316

Nation, The: on legalizing sex work, 82–85

National AIDS Coordinating Committee of T&T, 296

National Commission on Law and Order (Barbados), 278

National Committee of Eminent Persons to Coordinate National Reconciliation (Barbados), 278

National Consultation to Address Societal Issues (Barbados), 278

National HIV and AIDS Commission (NHAC): Barbados, 118, 120, 122, 127, 281

National HIV and AIDS Policy (Jamaica): and same sex relationships, 253–264

National Strategic Plan: Barbados, 141–142, 143; and HIV prevention, xvi–xxii; Jamaica's, 141, 143; T&T, 141–142, 143

National Surveillance Unit of T&T, 296

Nationalist movements: and colonial governance systems, 77–79

New Steps in Religious Education for the Caribbean Book 3: and same-sex relationships, 263

Nicaragua: CFSC in, 156, 171

Nicaragua Round Table Conference (2001): on communication strategies for HIV prevention, 138

Normative femininity: and
    adolescent girls in Barbados,
    220–223, 231–233

Offences Against the Person Act
    1840: Antigua and Barbuda, 6
Organisation of Eastern Caribbean
    States (OECS): condom use in
    the, 133
Ottowa Charter for Health: and
    public health, 166–167

Pan Caribbean Partnership Against
    HIV (PANCAP): regional
    strategic framework, 147
Panos Institute: on HIV
    communication strategies, 138
Peer pressure: adolescent males and,
    247–254
People living with HIV
    (PLWHIV): Caribbean law and,
    15–17; and compulsory testing,
    66–67; and discrimination, 50–
    60, 158–159; and drug abuse,
    23–31; human rights and, xxiii,
    40–47; judicial review and
    protection of, 59–60; treatment
    of, xviii–xix; vulnerability of,
    40–47, 295–311
Power: gender relations and, xvii,
    xix–xx
Post-colonial studies: Subaltern
    group, 77–80

Plummer, David, 316
Policy framework: and HIV and
    AIDS governance, 277–293;
    HIV prevention, xxviii, 141–
    148
Poverty: HIV infection and, 47–48
Practical Guide for intensifying HIV
    prevention: Towards Universal
    Access: UNAIDS, 73, 290
Preparing for the Vibes in the World
    of Sexuality: and anal sex, 263
President's Emergency Plan for
    HIV and AIDS Relief
    (PEPFAR): US, 167
Prevention education: and HIV,
    xix; moral agenda of, xxv–xxvi
Prevention of Discrimination Act
    1997 (Guyana), 51
Princess Apiaba: in Afro-
    Surinamese oral history, 207
Privacy: and compulsory HIV
    testing, 66–67; PLWHIV and
    the right to, 46
Prostitution: The Bahamas and
    child, 47–48. See also Sex work
Public education. See Prevention
    education.
Public health: and HIV prevention,
    xvi, xviii, 107–109, 117–119,
    128; social patterns and, 163–
    167
Puntos de Encuentro: and CFSC,
    171

Quality of life profile: of PLWHIV in T&T, 304–307

R v The London Borough of Hackney, 65

Rajkumar et al v Commissioner of Police, 60

Rape: and Caribbean law, 16; and the Dominica Sexual Offences Act 1998, 9

Reggae music: violence against homosexuals in, 99–100, 101

Regional Action Plan:

Regional Strategic Framework (RSF): HIV prevention and the, xxii–xxiv, 271–273

Relationships: and sexual stigma, 55–56

Religion. *See* Church

Report on the Legal, Ethical and Socio-Economic Issues Relevant to HIV and AIDS in Barbados, A, 283–287

Reproductive sex: social attitudes towards, 7

Research: HIV and Caribbean KAPB, 132, 218–219, 239–243; on MSM, 109–112; on males and risk, 243–254; on the risk environment in T&T, 295–311;on sources of HIV education, 267–270

Risk: behavior, xxi, 38, 288, 307–308; defining, xvi–xvii ; economies of, 251–253; education, 270–273; same-sex relationships and, 267–270; socially embedded, 243–254;

Robinson, Tracy, 316

Rockefeller Foundation: and HIV communication framework, 137–138

Rubin, Gayle: on sexuality studies, 196

Saint Lucia: Criminal Code 2004, 14–15; Equality of Opportunity and Treatment in Employment and Occupation Act 2000, 51; homophobia in, 108

Same-Sex couples: Ministry of Education and Youth and, 262–265

Self-concept: in Afro-Surinamese culture, 197

Serious indecency: Caribbean law and, 15

Sex: definition of, 14, 17

Sex work: in the Caribbean, 79; Caribbean law and, 5

Sex workers: vulnerability of, 73–75

Sexto Sentido: and CFSC, 156

Sexual behaviour: of Afro-Surinamese women, 192–211;

changing, 137–138, 143–145;
of adolescent girls, 134–135,
215–234; and HIV prevention,
xvii–xvii; risk and, xxi–xxii,
125–127, 131–134, 300–301;
of PLWHIV in T&T, 307–309
Sexual culture: of Afro-Surinamese
women, 192–211
Sexual initiation: adolescent girls
and age of, 225–227
Sexual offences legislation:
Caribbean, 3–19
Sexual orientation: discrimination
and, 57–58
Sexual praxis,180–182, 185
Sexual relationships: and stigma,
55–56
Sexual stigma: and relationships,
55–56
Sexuality: of African-Surinamese
women, xxvii, 192–211; in
biomedical approaches, 182–
184; and law, 3–6, 13–21,
120,187; and the Church, 78–
70; and HIV prevention, xvi:
and the state, 117; during
slavery, 199–203; studies on
Caribbean, 179–188, 192-211;
in West African culture, 199,
203–206
Silence: HIV and the culture of,
46–47

Slavery: sexuality under, 199–203,
205–206, 208
Social capital: definition of, 299,
300
Social change communication: and
HIV and AIDS, 155–157
Social change: and HIV rates in
Barbados, 278
Social cohesion: vulnerability and,
299–3300
Social dimensions: of HIV and
AIDS, 154–161; of
vulnerability, 298–300
Social exclusion: vulnerability and,
87–90. See also Marginalized
groups
Social life: complexity theory on,
161–164
Society Against Sexual Orientation
Discrimination (SASOD): in
Guyana, 101
Socio-economic profile: of
PLWHIV in T&T, 302–304
Sodomy. See Buggery
Spivak, Gayatri: subaltern studies,
76–87
St Maarten: and homosexualiy,
102
State: and human rights, 98–99;
and sexuality, 117
Stigma: combating, 157–161;
HIV and, 252

Stillwagon, Eileen: *AIDS and the Ecology of Poverty* by, 164–165

Suriname: sexual culture of Creole women in, 192-211

Surrat v AG of Trinidad and Tobago, 57–58

Subaltern Studies: on the marginalized, 76–87

Suriname: colonial, 200–203

Surinamese women: sexuality of working-class African-, xxvii

Tambiah, Yasmin: and homosexual sex, 15–16; study of the T&T Sexual Offences Act, 3–6

Teenagers at risk. 216–234

Theodore, Karl, 316

Tolerance: and human rights, 78–79

Trinidad and Tobago (T&T): cocaine and HIV infection in, 29; Domestic Violence Act 1999, 11; equality legislation in, 57–58; HIV and AIDS in, 296–298; homophobia in, 101; MSM in, 106; National Strategic Plan, 141–142, 143; research on the risk environment in, 295–311; Sexual Offences Act 1986, 3–5, 12; and sexual violence, 16

UNAIDS: and HIV communication strategies, 139–141, 145–146, 155–157, 290

UNAIDS Policy Position Paper: Intensifying HIV Prevention, 73

UNICEF: and CFSC, 156

United Nations: and drug control, 32–33, 34; and national responses to MSM, 104

United States of America (USA): and AIDS, 170; and drug control, 33; and PLWHIV, xviii; PEPFAR, 167–168

Uganda: respons to AIDS, 169

University of the West Indies (UWI): HIV study, 56

'Unnatural crime': definition of, 6, 12–17

Unfair dismissal legislation: PLWHIV and, 60–62

US Centre for Disease Control (CDC): and high-risk groups, xviii–xix

US National Drug Threat Assessment, 33

Vincent, Robin, 317

Violence: against homosexuals, 99–103; against women and law, 8–9, 217

Visiting relationships: law and, 12

Vulnerability: of adolescent girls, 228–234; defining, 116–117, 290–291, 298–300; of drug users, 23–24; of girls, 134–135; and HIV, 153–154, 277–293; of marginalized groups, 73–90; of MSM, 104–112, 259–274; of PLWHIV, 40–47, 295–311; social exclusion and, 87–90; socially embedded, 243–254; understanding, xvi–xvii, xxi, xxiii; of women, 54–56. *See also* Risk

Wade v Roches, 59
Walrond, Professor E.R.: on discrimination and homosexuality, 121–123, 126
Walrond Report: on HIV and AIDS in Barbados, 283–287
'We All Have Aids' Campaign, 95
Wekker, Gloria, 317
West African culture: sexuality in, 198, 203–209
Western culture: sexuality in, 196, 201–203, 205
Whitman, C: on risk education, 269–272
Winti: in Afro-Surinamese culture, 197
Women: and AIDS, 215–234, 265–267; moral regulation of, 98–99; and sex, 18; and sex work, 81–87; sexual culture of Afro-Surinamese, 192–211; violence against, 8–9; and vulnerability to HIV, 54–56
Women who have sex with Women (WSW): sexual orientation and, 104–105, 198–199
Workers: and HIV, 39–64; HIV and free movement of, 63–64
World Bank: on HIV communication strategies, 139–141
World Cup Cricket (WCC): The *Nation* on sex work and, 82–85
World Health Organisation (WHO): and public health, 166–167

Young and Meyer: research on MSM, 110–112

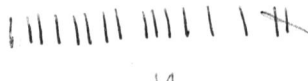

14

CPSIA information can be obtained at www.ICGtesting.com
Printed in the USA
BVOW04s1248210115

384325BV00008B/28/P

9 789766 373955